"And Neither Have I Wings to Fly"

Labelled and Locked Up in Canada's Oldest Institution

Thelma Wheatley

INANNA PUBLICATIONS AND EDUCATION INC.
TORONTO, CANADA

Canada Council for the Arts Conseil des Arts du Canada

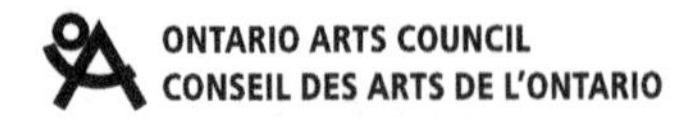

We gratefully acknowledge the support of the Canada Council for the Arts and the Ontario Arts Council for our publishing program.

We are also grateful for the support received from an Anonymous Fund at The Calgary Foundation.

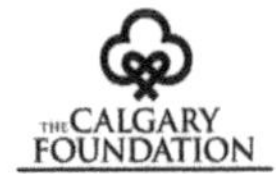

Cover design: Val Fullard
Interior design: Luciana Ricciutelli

Library and Archives Canada Cataloguing in Publication

Wheatley, Thelma, 1941-
And neither have I wings to fly : labelled and locked up in Canada's oldest institution / Thelma Wheatley.

Includes bibliographical references.
Issued also in electronic format.
ISBN 978-1-926708-58-4

1. People with mental disabilities—Ontario—Orillia—Biography. 2. People with mental disabilities—Abuse of—Ontario—Orillia—History. 3. People with mental disabilities—Institutional care—Ontario—Orillia—History. 4. Huronia Regional Centre—History. 5. Eugenics—Canada—History—20th century. 6. Involuntary sterilization—Ontario—Orillia—History. I. Title.

HV3008.C32O75 2013 362.3'80971317 C2012-904532-4

Printed and bound in Canada

Inanna Publications and Education Inc.
210 Founders College, York University
4700 Keele Street
Toronto, Ontario, Canada M3J 1P3
Telephone: (416) 736-5356 Fax (416) 736-5765
Email: inanna.publications@inanna.ca
Website: www.inanna.ca

For "Daisy,"
and all who have passed this way.

TABLE OF CONTENTS

AUTHOR'S NOTE

The terms used throughout this book that refer to developmentally and intellectually challenged persons are those that were used from the early 1900s up to the 1970s, and do not reflect the author's own usage or attitude.

Classification Terms, 1900s:

Term	I.Q.
Idiot	below 20 or 25
Imbecile	20-25
Moron/ Half-Moron	50-70 or 75
Dull Normal	80-90

(Average I.Q. on Stanford-Binet Scale: 100)

The labels "feeble-minded" and "mentally defective" were general terms that had different meanings in various countries in the early twentieth century. Canadians and British tended to use these words to denote those with a higher level of intelligence, I.Q. in the 70 range on the Binet Scales of Intelligence, or a mental age of twelve years. Americans used these words to denote all mental defectives generally. "Retarded" was another general term in use. People in the institution were invariably referred to as inmates, patients, and residents.

Pseudonyms have been used for "Daisy" and members of her family, nursing staff and attendants at Orillia, Salvation Army workers at "The Nest," and social workers, excepting Vera Moberley of the Children's Aid Society, to protect their identity. Patient file numbers for this book have been recoded in accordance with the *Freedom of Information and Protection of Privacy Act* of theprovince of Ontario.

Mentally defective children should be separated from the normal at an early age ... and what better place to send them than the asylum in Orillia?

—Dr. Helen MacMurchy, Inspector of the Feeble-Minded in Ontario, 1906-1919.

PROLOGUE

"YOU KNOWS WHAT TO WRITE, Thelma, you knows legal." That is what Daisy Potts said to me in 2006, the day she sought me out. She was in her early sixties at the time. Daisy gripped my arm. "You c'n get my file from Orillia, please and thank you and kindly." She said she had been in Cottage O.

At once Cottage O came to mind from my research: a dull, red brick, three-storey building with rows of windows, next to Entrance B. In its time, it had held thousands of girls, the long wards locked at night. Daisy Potts had been institutionalized in Orillia as a child, and now that institution was slated to be permanently closed by the government of Ontario in 2009. Daisy wanted my help to get her records, before it was too late. She had never been allowed to see them and she wanted finally to know what was in them.

The institution — which most people simply called "Orillia" — had originally been called the Asylum for Idiots and Feebleminded (a former branch of the Provincial Lunatic Asylum in Toronto), the oldest in Canada for "mentally retarded" people, dating back to 1876. Heralded as innovative and humane, a "fine place" for idiots and epileptics, the asylum had provided custodial care and protection for the thirty or so inmates at its opening. Before that time, "mental defectives," as they were often called, whose families could no longer care for them, often ended up in the county lunatic asylum, or worse, the work house or local gaol, or were left roaming the countryside at will. The new asylum was meant to mitigate such horrors, and provide not just custodial care but vocational training for the more "educable" ones, with the intent of eventually returning them to their families.

By the early 1900s, however, attitudes toward mental defectives had begun to change as the effects of the Industrial Revolution took its toll on the cities: slums, unemployment, crime, and disease gave rise to fears of a new underclass. Orillia became a big custodial institution, a useful place to put the unwanted in society, the so-called "feeble-minded," that included a mix of indigents invariably found on its wards: paupers, incurables, alcoholics, syphilitics, the old and infirm, and unmarried girls and their babies who had nowhere else to go.

Renamed "Ontario Hospital School" (OHS) in 1936, it had a population of nearly 3,000 when Daisy was housed there in the 1950s. A grim sort of place for a child, I always thought on my visits, with its vast grounds, over two hundred acres, and towering Administration Building much praised for its fine front. There were double-glassed doors at the top of a flight of steps through which all the new admissions passed.

It was hard to imagine Daisy in such a place.

"But Daisy, you're not retarded!" At once I regretted the word, so outmoded, anachronistic in definition. A look of bewilderment crossed her face.

"Yeah, well, that's what Children's Aid in T'ronto said too, Thelma. They promised I wouldn't be with the retarded ones; I'd be kept sep'rate on the ward."

I was silent. This sounded much like the placating of parents so familiar to me as a former teacher. There was obviously much here left unsaid, perhaps lost to the understanding of a small child, even duplicitous.

"First I was taken away, 'cause I was the oldest. Then Lizzie and my baby brother, Pips. But Children's Aid kept them together in a foster home in Richmond Hill an' I never really saw much of them again."

Daisy sounded aggrieved. It was what she most wanted to know: why had she been the only one singled out for Orillia, and why had her mother signed her over? Why hadn't she been placed with the Wilsons, too? The records would explain, the records would tell, said Daisy.

She wanted to know about her mother especially — a no-good, low-down sort according to Daisy. All she'd wanted was a good time while their dad was out working all hours, Daisy added. "One cock wasn' big enough for 'er." She wanted her mother's records from Orillia as well; she knew she had also been there as a patient, along with other members of her family.

Daisy wanted the truth. She wanted to know whether they had written about the rapes and the tortures that took place on the wards.

I glanced sharply at Daisy — mother and daughter both in Orillia. However, she seemed unaware of the implication: two generations possibly deemed "feeble-minded."

I had known Daisy since the late 1990s, though only casually, through the Women's Auxiliary Club run by the local church to which I belonged for a while. I sometimes gave Daisy rides home in the rain, or helped her with her shopping, or took her to the food bank. I had become fond of her. She was a responsible mother of two and a grandmother. Though uneducated — I was not sure how well she could read; I often helped her find her place in the song book at the club — she had supported herself all her life cleaning offices with her husband, Joe, managing the family income, and attending church, something she seemed proud of. Unlike her mother who was a Catholic, she once confided, Daisy was Anglican. "My dad said is better to be a Protesterant, Thelma, you get a better edjucation," she explained.

Now, somehow, the focus of our friendship had shifted in some implicit way, disturbing when she confided to me after a meeting that she was an "institutional girl," as she put it. "I tell you 'cause I trust you, Thelma, you're a mother of a handicap." She meant my adult autistic son whom she had met on occasion at special club festivities.

I sensed the secret Daisy had obviously kept for years — "Only Joe knows, Thelma" — from neighbours, and especially from the ladies at the Women's Auxiliary Club whose acceptance she especially desired and valued. ("That woman's not sixteen ounces to the pound," Moira Witherspoon, the club's social and flowers convener, had once said somewhat cuttingly of Daisy when Daisy mixed up the opening songs. Daisy had sung all the louder, in confusion.)

Dear Daisy, with her worn cardigan, flip-flop sandals, and grey woolly hair. She was given to crossing herself effusively during the singing of "O Canada" at meetings; perhaps she thought she was in church. A lovable character, with undeniable quirks and oddities, not so unlike the rest of us as I liked to say at the club.

"Thelma, you understands, you has a retarded boy what you kept," Daisy was doing her best to persuade me.

It occurred to me that Daisy and I were linked by similar motives, the same need to know about Orillia, about placing children there against their will. I was the mother of a child who could well have ended up in the institution, but had not. We had been urged to place him in a regional centre when he was age four. "He'll never amount to anything." I burned with indignation at the callous doctor. It was perhaps what had driven me subsequently to investigate Orillia over the years, something I realized Daisy intuitively understood. I was a mother who had said "no" to putting her child away, and her mother had said, "yes." "And that was the difference," said Daisy tersely. But was it that simple?

Of course I agreed to help Daisy. It was a moment in time, if we but knew, that we were about to embark unwittingly on a voyage that would take us ultimately to the very heart of Orillia.

But for now, a signed, witnessed letter and a copy of Daisy's Health Card for identification purposes, to be sent to the Records Office, which was still in operation at the institution, sufficed. From my years of research into the Orillia institution, I was well acquainted with the intricacies of the *Freedom of Information and Protection of Privacy Act* of Ontario and the process of accessing records. It was not as complicated as Daisy seemed to think. In the case of older files, such as her mother's, which went back to the 1930s, the Archives of Ontario provided access.

But I wondered if Daisy understood the implications, the danger, of opening up old records, since what might be revealed she might not necessarily wish to know. "Are you sure you want this, Daisy?" Even more important, would her mother?

Daisy was certain her mother would sign. "Course, she only uses an 'X', Thelma; she had no edjucation," she added nervously. "Me an' Lizzie told her to go back to school an' learn but she wouldn't. Says she's too old and stupid."

I was surprised. I had not realized that Daisy was still in touch with her mother, or that she had a sister living here in Toronto. The way Daisy had spoken of them on other occasions, they had seemed estranged, as so many former patients of Orillia often were from their families.

"Oh, well, yeah, they're here in T'ronto. My mother's jus' down the road, at Gerrard an' Sumach Streets, Regent Park, same old place. She calls all the time bugging me she's lonely and stuff, but I don't reply, I don't really *know* her. Or my sister. On account of bein' in Orillia so long."

Last time she had heard from Lizzie she was living in a room off Sackville Street.

We went down steep broken steps below street level to a basement flat; sodden leaves caught against the gritty window. Lizzie was now on a street off River Street, by the railway lines and the canal. The street was old, lined with brick row houses, some with rotting garbage behind them, and unpainted doors. This was a rental area like much of Toronto's lower Cabbagetown, though some of the houses had recently been renovated by professionals, who brought a more tony air to the neighbourhood. There was a hum from the Don Valley Parkway below.

"Well, come on in. Watch the steps, the rail don't work."

It had seemed opportune to call on Lizzie on the way to visit Mrs. Lumsden (Daisy's mother), though Daisy had not seen her sister in years, not since a party for one of Lizzie's children back in the 1980s. Lizzie might have some information or insight to offer on their childhood. Daisy hoped she could provide some of the answers Daisy sought in the records, as if Lizzie could maybe validate her existence in Orillia.

But Lizzie sat stiff, tight-lipped. She did not want "nothing to do with Orillia" or her mother, she said. Daisy had brought cigarettes and chocolates. Lizzie, at once, snatched up the Players and lit up.

Dim light filtered at a slant from the street above into the tiny living room, quite different from Daisy's big, cosy, old apartment crammed with chesterfields and arm-chairs, ornaments and photos, knick-knacks everywhere. By contrast, Lizzie's was almost ascetic, with bare white walls, plain wood floor.

"I mean, I never even remembered I even *had* a sister until 1966, when I was seventeen," she said. "Then staff at Lorimer Lodge told me Daisy been released from the institution and I was to meet her."

At that time, Lorimer Lodge had been a half-way house on St. George Street aimed at helping mentally-retarded women learn how to adapt to community living after being released into the neighbourhood, something that Lizzie herself may not have known. It was where she, too, had lived for a time, after she left the foster home. That Lizzie may have also been deemed "retarded" was the kind of information that could be revealed in the records; did Daisy understand that? That she could be privy to so much more, not only about her mother, but also about Lizzie and any number of other members of her own family. I tensed. "She was no fucking mother to me." Lizzie took a long drag on her cigarette; did not care if her mother lived or died. "She was *incompetent,*" she said, bitterly.

And where had that come from? Perhaps Lizzie, as a child, and a ward of the Children's Aid Society (CAS), blinking behind her glasses, had caught the professional lingo of the adults talking over her head in the Wilsons' living room, as the social worker checked up on Lizzie and her brother, Pips, arranging the next visit of their biological parents, Ella and Ernest Lumsden?

Daisy sat very still, staring at Lizzie.

"Mrs. Wilson was my mother. She was the best anyone could have! I can't say enough for 'er, nor Pips."

Yes, one could well see the neat suburban bungalow in Richmond Hill with its manicured lawns and basketball net in the driveway, the nice local school Lizzie and her brother Pips no doubt had attended, perhaps placed in a Special Class that maybe Lizzie had not been aware of (the records would tell). Then her parents, the Lumsdens, would arrive.

"They come up every two weeks on the bus. Soon as I got old enough I told them to fuck off, I didn't want them in my life. First thing I done when I was free was change my name. I didn't even want their fucking name, Eliza Lumsden."

Yet, Lizzie had returned to Cabbagetown in Toronto on her release from the half-way house at first chance, I noted, to the very neighbourhood of her parents and grandparents with its old streets and taverns. Her first room had been but blocks from her parents on Sumach Street.

"Oh-h, I saw her once, in the Winchester, years ago..."

Lizzie seemed bemused. It was as if this was what we had really come to hear: to hear Lizzie tell us what the records could not reveal.

"She was drinking with some men at the bar and I thought: 'I know that woman, it was my mother.' And sure enough she comes over and says: 'Are you Lizzie?' I says, 'Yes, and I know who you are.' And I says, 'Don't I have a sister somewhere?'"

(So she did care then; Daisy sat up straighter.)

"And she said, 'Oh, Daisy's dead.' She wanted me to join her for a beer, and I told her, 'You stay at your end of the room and I'll stay in mine.'"

Lizzie's mouth set in a thin tight line. She was unlike Daisy, tall and thin with long platinum blond dyed hair. She had been divorced a long time now from Arnold, "the bastard." "Went to jail over 'im," she said dryly.

"*Jail!*" Daisy leaned forward excitedly.

"Did two months in Women's Detention, Owen Sound, Assault an' Battery," Lizzie drawled. "Worth every single day. My only regret is I didn' finish him off with a hatchet."

Daisy squeaked. "You know, our mother was in jail once. For prostituting herself."

Lizzie's cheeks turned dark pink. "That's not true!" She glanced quickly at me in confusion.

"Is so. My dad told me. I went to him and said, 'Dad, you gotta tell me the truth, was my mother ever in jail? And he said, 'How did you find out?' angry-like. And I said Lizzie told me. And he said, 'Your sister was right, she was arrested an' put in detention in the Don Jail."

"I never said any such thing!" Lizzie flushed and glanced at me, embarrassed.

Daisy held her tongue, but as soon as Lizzie went out to the kitchenette for the sandwiches, Daisy whispered, "Did you see that, Thelma? Can't face it."

It was hard to read Lizzie. Was she of "normal" intelligence? Could she read and write? Though perhaps this was irrelevant. She had survived thus far in life, she said wryly, married and divorced with four children, and three grandchildren.

She screwed up her thin, fair face. Despite her tough words, one could sense all was not well. Though Lizzie seemed to have been raised in a kind foster home with a loving foster mother, Daisy seemed the more secure, despite the experience of Orillia and a difficult childhood. She was affluent, even, by comparison, in her own small way. Daisy and Joe Potts' apartment on Rose Avenue near Wellesley and south of Bloor Street, once trendy in the 1960s, must have been a come-up in the world for Daisy, certainly superior to life in a rooming house.

I struggled with the seeming paradox — Daisy with a husband of forty years, a home and social circle, despite being what she called "a institution girl." I saw now how important the Women's Auxiliary Club was for her socially, and worried how opening up the records of her institutionalization might affect her view of herself and her social standing if these records included the results of any I.Q. tests that might have indicated she was indeed "retarded."

"I c'n always get money," said Lizzie quickly. "I'm moving out soon." She took another drag at her cigarette, glancing sideways at Daisy who still sat excitedly on the sofa next to her.

Daisy had been particularly thrilled to see Lizzie again. "After all, she's my *sister!*"

"You're like *her,*" said Lizzie, slowly. "Like mother."

"No! No, am not!" Daisy's lip trembled. "I'm like my dad."

"N-no. Me and Pips is like him, strawberry blond," persisted Lizzie, her glasses glinting. "I had red hair to my waist as a kid," she turned to me.

"I'm like my dad!" Daisy was tearful.

"No, you're not."

"I'll tell you something about Lizzie," Daisy confided angrily, as we drove away. "She's a lesbian."

"A lesbian?"

"Yep. And you won't believe how I knows, Thelma. I was just out of Orillia and back in T'ronto. It was 1966. I was twenny and didn't know nothing. And she calls and says for me to come on over and meet her friends, get to know each other, go for a drink, and I thinks yes, this is my only sister."

They went to an old pub on Queen Street, a bit of a dive. "She left me at the bar by myself, said she had to go to the loo, and time went by. I was thinking what's going on?" After a while Daisy went to the washroom to find out. "There was Lizzie with some woman sucking her tits, on top of the toilit, a whole bunch of them sucking each other I won't tell you where, Thelma. But then I thought, I don't know what happen to her over the years but she's my sister, and it don't harm me so I forgive her."

The last thing Lizzie had called out from the doorway was: "Don't you dare give that woman my phone number!"

Daisy was anxious about seeing her mother again. "She got a boyfriend, Ron, living with her," she warned. "Pretends it's her brother. It's disgusting, him sixty and her eighty and all."

Ella Lumsden was not what I imagined. She turned out to be a tall, powerful, big-boned woman, with insane-looking eyes due to a stigmatization, a piercing squint like Lizzie's. Dyed blond hair, long aristocratic nose, round face like Daisy's. Her legs were sheathed in nylons and she wore a twin-set and tartan skirt, the stylish clothes of another era likely bought from the second-hand shop on Queen. She usually wore sweatpants, whispered Daisy. She had dressed up for us.

It was a desperate sort of place, Regent Park. Low-rental housing from the fifties built in blocks, with numbers inset in the red brick walls: Building 49, Building 26, Building 37 (not unlike Orillia). There had been another murder there that week.

The apartment in Building 247 was stifling hot, the windows tightly locked. The apartment's contents included a sofa, an armchair, a huge console TV with a talk-show on, a sideboard, and a table.

"Nothing has changed," marvelled Daisy softly. Her mother sat on the sofa with her boyfriend, who grinned.

The dusty sideboard is crammed with mementos: photographs of Daisy and Joe on their wedding day; Lizzie aged eighteen, blond hair backcombed in a sixties bouffant. Lizzie, age four, squinting in the sun in a dirty dress. What had happened to Pips? Who knew? On the wall hung a faded picture of the Sacred Heart of Jesus, and another of the Solidarity of the Blessed Virgin.

"I think Pips is dead!" said Ella suddenly

"Dead?" blinked Daisy.

Ella Lumsden straightens up suddenly on the sofa next to Ron. Ella then seemed to forget Pips as quickly as she remembered him. She smiled coyly, "This is Ron, my half-brother."

Daisy scowled.

"He helps with the rent," smiled Ella. We kept up the pretence. Ron, smaller than Ella, kept grinning, toothless.

Her "fancy man," hissed Daisy. "How can she sit there with him under her and dad's wedding photo?"

I was secretly admiring of eighty-year-old Ella, intrigued by the charade she demanded. Twice a day Ron gives Ella her medication, we learned. A cleaning woman comes in each week to tidy the apartment, and a nurse from the Victorian Order gives her a bath, all paid for by Social Services. She has a small disability pension. Ron has her Health Card, for safe-keeping, he hinted.

"Look, Ma," Daisy cut in. "We wants you to sign a letter to get your records from Orillia, to find out what happen."

"What happen?" Ella looked up, suspicious.

"*You* know," said Daisy fiercely. This was a new Daisy I was seeing, stronger, even aggressive.

But Ella did not want to talk about Orillia, the old Hospital for the Feeble-Minded. She wanted to talk about Lizzie. Lizzie and Daisy. They were in a bar, the Isabella on Sherbourne Street, decades ago. She looked dreamy, her eyes clouded.

"Daisy sat nicely with you," she said distantly, as if Daisy was not there. "But Lizzie. You take her for a drink and she'd go to some man across the room and start talking, making up to him like. I calls to her, 'Do you *know* that man, Lizzie?'" Ella leaned toward me on the sofa, indignant at the memory now. "'No,' says Lizzie, all saucy-like, 'that's why I'm talking to him!' That was Lizzie. But not Daisy. Daisy would stay with you nice and quiet. I think she's dead now, Lizzie, dead an' gorn."

"Never mind Lizzie," Daisy said, her voice firm.

And, of course, there was another story here, beneath the story, the words rambling on as Daisy whispered to me, Ella slumped and stared at a repeat of *The Oprah Winfrey Show*. "It still makes me so mad thinking of it, my dad out on night-shift working all hours and her in the pubs."

Daisy pushed the letter into her mother's hands. "You remember Orillia."

"Hey, she gotta 'ave her medicashun," Ron fluttered. He pattered to the kitchen, then brought back a glass of water and some little orange pills.

"Shutup, lover-boy." I had never known Daisy to talk like this. "You go photocopy the Health Card down at the office."

Ella Lumsden came alive: *Orillia*. Her eyes flashed, her lips curled in a sneer. For a moment she remembered. What did she remember? What of the girl Ella Hewitt, before she married Ernest Lumsden? Young Ella Hewitt's memory of the 1930s, and the institution she had known as the Hospital for the Feeble-Minded, was the memory we needed.

"All they did was drug you!" she hissed. "Drugs, drugs, drugs. And them nurses bossing you around morning to night, do this, do that!"

We waited for more, but nothing came. She sank back on the sofa. That was it; yet it said so much.

"Look, Ma, just put an 'X' by the dot," said Daisy impatiently, her round face flushed.

Ella nodded; this woman who wished her children dead. Her bony fingers gripped the pen. Slowly, painfully, she drew the 'X,' perhaps the only letter of the alphabet she knew, a large unwieldy scrawl like that of a child. It was the 'X' that would release the past.

Daisy and her mother were, I realized, a living testament to Orillia.

I warned Daisy about the possible consequences of opening up records marked "Confidential," records that had never been meant for her eyes: *Daisy Lumsden, Case #65043*. "Are you sure you want this, Daisy?"

But Daisy was adamant. She wanted to know what they had *written* about her.

PART ONE
DAISY'S STORY

ONTARIO HOSPITAL SCHOOL

ORILLIA, 1951-1966

I promise to pray, to read my Bible, and to abstain from all intoxicating drink and tobacco.

—Daisy Lumsden, age eleven, Junior Soldier's Pledge, Danforth Corps, Toronto, December 1, 1957

1.

MRS. LUMSDEN WAS THE PROBLEM, always would be, of course, being the mother. One could understand how Miss Prewse at the Toronto Children's Aid Society saw it, for there seemed little doubt from the outset on that day in 1951 that Ella Lumsden was a sex delinquent (possibly even dangerous).

It was Mr. Lumsden, Ernest Lumsden — or "Ernie" — the children's father, a short, slight man, "obviously retarded," wrote Miss Prewse, who had brought in the children that February morning: a little girl he called Daisy, about four-and-a-half; her sister Lizzie, age three, both clinging to his legs; and a baby, Pips, in his arms. He said he wanted to give them up; he was worried about the "babby." The children were dirty and unkempt, tear-stained. The baby was listless, possibly undernourished.

Extraordinary. Apparently he had found his way by memory across the city from Cabbagetown, first to the old Infants Home on Charles Street East, then to their new offices on Isabella Street. He had gotten off the streetcar at Yonge Street and walked through biting wind and cold with the children. Mrs. Lumsden, it seemed, was holed up in a room somewhere down on Jarvis with a man; or more than one, Mr. Lumsden had hinted.

Miss Prewse tightened, at once on the alert.

Mr. Lumsden claimed that his wife had fits. Miss Prewse duly recorded: "Wife has fits periodically, and Mr. Lumsden frequently arrives home to find her in a coma, the furniture smashed and her clothes torn off..."

He had known at once something was wrong as he had turned the doorknob and noticed the darkness. It was a Friday. He had learned the calendar in Auxiliary Class for the feeble-minded as a boy and he knew Sunday started the week. The children were huddled sobbing in the centre of the room in the dark, frightened and hungry. They had not had their tea, and the babby was in Daisy's lap with a dirty, empty bottle in his mouth. Ella was sprawled on her back naked on the living-room floor, her tits hanging sideways like balloons, her legs sprawled.

At once he covered her bush of hair there with his coat. Everything was smashed: the lamps, the pictures, the delicate Virgin Mary from the Catholic Women's League. One chair had four broken legs.

Daisy ran to him sobbing, "Dada, oh, Dada!"

"Well, what have I got for my little girls?" He pretended not to see, then pulled out some biscuits he had taken when the boss wasn't looking. He worked daytime at Christie's Biscuits on Lakeshore.

Lizzie snatched the biscuit out of his hand and Daisy let her. "Now let's share nicely," he chided.

Then he lifted Ella up and half carried, half dragged her (for she was heavier and taller than himself) into the room off the kitchen that was their bedroom, and clumsily dropped her on the bed. He saw at once how it had been. Her brassiere tossed. Her skirt ripped fiercely. The sheets were crumpled. Then there was the telltale smell. He knew how his wife shook during orgasm, often tearing the sheet in her frenzy, falling to the floor in her pleasure as she was straddled, before passing out.

He hurried back to the children who were crying again. The baby lay still, his dirty bottle fallen off his chest, the thin milk congealed. He washed that first in the sink, then took some milk from the milk bottle on the shelf. The littlest daughter, Lizzie, stood stiff and unblinking as he put the kettle on to boil; for her, he would mix hot water with dried milk the way they had shown at the Mother and Baby clinic up on Parliament Street. Soon he put on baked beans and some chopped wieners for their tea, cut the last bit of bread and mixed up some orange juice from a dark little bottle from the clinic. He remembered what they told him: "Give them a teaspoon mixed with water every day." He then noticed that she had let the fire die out in the grate.

The tiny row house had three rooms: kitchen, parlour and a small bedroom. But they had more than most folks, he knew because he worked regular. They had a nice used sofa from the Society of St. Vincent de Paul store, as well as an armchair, a deal table and hard chairs from the Women's Auxiliary Club. The wallpaper peeled in tatters, cockroaches got at the linoleum floor and bugs crawled up the wall, but no matter.

"What happen to your ma?" he asked, though he had already guessed.

At his words Daisy burst into sobs and shook. She had shit and wet herself again. Lizzie's thin tight face was pinched, her long hair straggled with grime, her knickers also soaked with piss. He held the baby close and pushed the bottle in his mouth, but the baby, Pips, would not take it; there were deep circles under his eyes. Ernie sighed. Ella had been shown at the clinic up on Parliament Street how to breastfeed him, but she gave up after a few weeks, said she could not stand that milk dribbling all over. He just wanted to fuckin' suck suck all day.

He found dry underwear, though not clean, and changed the girls, then went back to the bedroom while they ate, leaving the baby in a small box by the stove. He pushed his wife's breasts into her brassiere and pulled on another skirt to cover the long heavy legs he knew so well, and then a sweater. He could not manage the girdle or the suspenders. His fingers couldn't work the claw-like metal grips. He smelled her smell and felt suddenly dizzy with desire. And anger at the man.

He heard the tenants next door on the other side of the wall. They were yelling, children screaming. Babies were crying. There were thuds. Ernest knew the old man's fists were on poor Mrs. Eagleston. She cried hoarsely.

"Let's go see Ganny," he said. He had a decision to make: which Ganny? Ganny Hewitt or Ganny Lumsden? He had to be at the docks for his second job, the night shift down at the wharf on Cherry Street loading vans. He was known as a steady worker who never asked for no raise. He did not want to lose his job.

His parents, the Lumsdens, lived furthest away on River Street. He would have to carry the kids past the icy bridge at Queen Street, about a twenty-minute walk he knew by his big watch. Ella's mother, Florrie Hewitt, lived closer down on Sumach Street. Florrie was a nervous woman, fearful of her husband Henry, as was Ernie. Their house was tiny, and there was no bedding for the little girls, let alone a baby. Ernie was afraid of his father-in-law; he knew how much he beat Florrie. Much depended on his drinking, and how much he'd had. He was older now, over sixty.

Daisy began to cry as soon as he got the jackets and boots. "Wanna Dada."

"S'okay, Do-do, Dada sees you t'morrow morning, have a nice time at Ganny's."

Lizzie stood frowning. Who was Ganny? She was only three and did not have glasses yet, so her father was a blur. She was to have her too-big second-hand coat (passed down from Daisy) put on her and a woolly hat and newspaper wrapped round her feet with string to keep out the wind.

He held Daisy close to him. She was to hang on to his pocket. The baby was wrapped under one arm, and Lizzie was in the other, and in this formation they plodded slowly down Berkeley Street to Shuter Street, past the old Wesleyan Methodist Church on the corner. It was snowing lightly in the crisp afternoon. The streetcars rumbled and clanged their bells. Vendors sold vegetables near the sidewalks. Fumes, grey and acrid, drifted from the factories. A wind rose over the bridge at Queen Street, the Don River far below a long stretch of ice and dark grey. Somewhere down there beyond the girders and Eastern Avenue, Ernie knew lay the dockland where he sojourned nightly amongst the ghostly ships and cargo.

Soon they had reached Lower Sumach Street, a rundown place, the houses in long drab rows. Garbage bins were outside and trash was blown around. Papers and beer bottles were strewn along the gutter; refuse clogged the pavement.

The city was supposed to be building a housing complex some day soon for the poor, to be called Regent Park.

"What the bleedin' hell has the devil brought in now?" grunted Henry Hewitt whom they all feared. You never knew what he would do with his fist. He was a thin hard-bodied man with a lean face and light blue eyes.

"Ella's not well, Dad ... had the fits agin"

"Out bloody whoring again, you mean."

Florrie Hewitt gasped trembling, full of fear of her husband, but fluttering softly with delight as she took the baby. "Oh, 'Enry, jus' look at him, the dearie," she cried.

She was a tiny, toothless woman with washed-out, greying hair. Ernie knew she was also half-deaf from the many beatings she had received from her husband. A worn frazzled woman of fifty-nine, she'd had at least twelve children, plus one that had died, one that had been adopted, and two "miscarriages," which Ernie had heard about over the years. ("They was abortions," Daisy once told me in conversation.)

Ella's brothers and sisters had long left home, so there was room of sorts in the house (although the upstairs was rented to a family from Russia). But it was poor; all they had was an old chesterfield from the Salvation Army store, a weathered chair, a small table, and a bed in the other room. There was a coal fire going in the pot-bellied stove and the little girls suddenly ran to it for the warmth, their arms round each other. Ganny brought them biscuits and a cup of milk.

"If they could jus' stay the night or so 'til Monday." Ernie raised his voice so his mother-in-law could hear. "I got my jobs."

"What's he bloody shouting at?" bawled Mr. Hewitt.

Ernie had slurry speech himself. He knew why too; his own father had beat him as a child. Arthur Lumsden had worked at the Woodbine racetrack picking up the garbage and there had not been much love there, not like Ernie's own love for his kiddies, Daisy and Lizzie, but especially the babby, Pips. Daisy ran back to his legs and pushed her face against his crotch. But Lizzie moved cautiously toward her Ganny, not sure who she was, but sure she was somebody who could give her something more.

"Let's see the little devils, then," Henry Hewitt said gruffly, pulling up the girls. "Well, she's a little looker," he said of Lizzie. "Boys'll be on 'er later; but this older one's spit of Ella, poor bugger. Hope she don't grow up like 'er. Bloody whore needs a good hammering."

Ella woke with a headache. The house was still. Then excitement flooded back. He had left dollars, lots of them. She was not sure how much or how to count, but she had done extra on him. She could smell his tobacco and oil. She pulled on stockings and clipped the tops into her suspenders. She put on lipstick and some scent her friend Maggie on Bleeker Street had given her. Then she went out through the back door and down the snowy path. She would find Maggie at the green door of the pub a few streets away.

She could not read, but she knew the shop windows, the corner grocery, the taverns with their billboards advertising beer and Black Cats. It was getting dark. Friday nights were band nights and dancing at the Isabella Hotel or Canada House Tavern on Sherbourne where there were fights when the Irish boys came. ("Oh, she used to go to the pubs all the time," said Daisy. "The Winchester Arms, the Carlton down on College there — oh, that was a bad place!") The rooms thick with cigarette smoke, Player's Lights and Cats, the thrum of bands.

This particular night, Ella went to the Isabella Hotel, its front door a dark green. The Isabella Hotel had two bands, one up in the turret and one downstairs in the basement. Shoes clicked loudly on the linoleum. The walls, dark and sweaty, were stained with beer and tobacco. There was a long banquette to sit on, and on the glass-topped tables the spilled beer was shiny under the lights. Men and women got up to rumba on the tiny dance floor at a dizzying pace.

"Where's th' kids then?" asked Maggie.

Ella was confused. The kids? "Oh, Ernie got 'em. I want some fun before I knock off. I ain't ending up like my mother with ten kids 'n' nothin' to show for it."

A swarthy man smelling of drink squeezed her arm and his hand slid down her thigh. "How about a beer, lovie?"

Ella knew what he wanted, what men wanted, and laughed loudly, her mouth opening wide. He was looking at her tits, they all did. She had big ones, and they liked that. Men at dark tables smoked in the back bar, but they would sidle over; a little wank out the back passage? And later perhaps, yes, down Jarvis Street to the big house with veiled windows and a cardboard sign in the front glass door that she knew said: "Room for rent by the week, by the day, by the hour. Two dollars a night." She had learned that from Maggie.

Ernie paused and felt a whirl of snow and icy breath from the lake upon his face. He had to cross back under vast iron girders on the construction sites under the highway up from the docks. His shift over, he walked the lonely roads, and a thick smoky haze fell in long blue spirals over the warehouses. It was two in the morning and he hurried up Cherry Street past Gooderham and Worts and across to Eastern Avenue and Parliament Street, thinking of Ella where he had left her. Desire for his wife filled him, for her large open mouth, and loose, big breasts.

She was gone. He knew it right away. He slumped on the mattress in the dark, felt her absence, and began to sob. But now he knew what he had to do, for he loved the babby.

2.

IT WAS OBVIOUSLY AN EMERGENCY. Miss Prewse, in keeping with her training, went into action: the baby was assigned to the Infant's Home on Grosvenor Street, at least until the mother could be found, and the girls were to be admitted to the old Receiving Center at 15 Huntley Street on a temporary basis. The Infants' Home, founded in 1875 by J. J. Kelso, and the Children's Aid Society of Toronto were, in 1951, still in the process of amalgamating and of moving into the new centre on Isabella Street. The Infants' Home helped out in emergencies, if there was space.

Ernie nodded, relieved. "I jush can't do two jobs an' look after the kids," he mumbled. "I took time off already grinding sugar at Chrissie's B'scuits." He meant Christie's Biscuits factory on Lakeshore Road West, well known by its sweet aromas wafting through the area.

The older girl, Daisy, clung to her father's legs, sobbing. The littlest one, a pretty child with long fair hair, pursed her lips.

"Now then, you'll be all right. You'll be seeing Daddy again some time soon." Miss Prewse paused; she knew from experience it was best not to make too many promises. "You'll have children to play with and you'll be with each other," Miss Prewse urged brightly.

Every effort would be made to keep the sisters together, she assured Mr. Lumsden. A volunteer was already at hand with fresh diapers, clothing for the baby, and baby formula. Miss Prewse noted the yellow-brown seepage through the children's pants. This family would have to be followed up on.

It had become increasingly evident, from interviews over the next few months, that Mrs. Lumsden might be mentally retarded. Ella had eventually surfaced in a certain rooming house on lower Sherbourne Street, found by police officers dressed in a half-buttoned scarlet blouse and slit skirt, declaring she was not bloody well going back home.

According to her father, Henry Hewitt, in his mid-fifties, of Sumach Street, Toronto, Ella had been put in the institution in Orillia as a girl, as had two older brothers before her. This, of course, put an entirely different face on the situation. Mr. Hewitt himself was from England and had reached Junior 111 education in a board school, equivalent to grade three in Ontario, and could therefore be regarded as reasonably reliable. He was an acetylene welder by trade but "drank."

Miss Prewse put a call through to the Catholic Children's Aid Society on Bond Street requesting any information regarding Ella Lumsden, "*née* Hewitt," circa 1930s. Ella Hewitt had been registered as a Roman Catholic like her mother, explained Mr. Hewitt. The two CAS societies were used to cooperating in the sharing of client information, a quiet exchange of information among professionals that could provide immediate knowledge of clients' backgrounds and histories otherwise time-taking to retrieve.

At the same time, Miss Prewse decided to check their own CAS of Toronto archives for the Lumsden family history, for Ernest Lumsden had intimated in his interview, somewhat innocently, that he'd had a sister, Effie, and a brother in Orillia.

Both families retarded. Miss Prewse recoiled. The Hewitts and the Lumsdens seemed to have had at least twenty-one defective children between them, a generation back. They had lived, she noted, in the same neighbourhood together, no doubt intermarrying. Miss Prewse realized she was privy to certain intimacies in the files marked "Confidential," but she had to consider what kind of support for the children these obviously mentally deficient relatives could provide, if any.

Effie Lumsden's records (Case #5721), from the Orillia Asylum for Idiots, subsequently showed she had been deemed an "Imbecile," as was reportedly her brother, Albert. On the Admission Forms and Family History Form 120, a psychiatrist had noted of the Lumsdens: "All the children are backward." Even poor Mr. Lumsden, whom Miss Prewse was beginning to recognize as a decent sort, reliable and caring of his children, had been cited as "mentally deficient." The mother, Violet Lumsden, another "Imbecile" (I.Q. 42 on the Stanford-Binet Intelligence Scale), was illiterate, "terrified of her husband," and stuttered, as did Ernest and all the siblings.

The Hewitt file was even more perturbing. Miss Prewse turned once again to the Family History Form 120. It seemed Mrs. Lumsden had not only torn her clothes to shreds as a child, but had been given to throwing them in the flames. A psychiatrist at the Toronto Psychiatric Hospital clinic had written in 1932 that "this girl is fascinated with fire."

Miss Prewse pursed her lips. With such early dangerous proclivities, should Mrs. Lumsden be allowed her children back? She read on.

Mr. Hewitt, Mrs. Lumsden's father, had "brutalized his wife Florrie and children on three occasions." It did not elucidate. She thought of Florrie Hewitt in the interview a few weeks earlier, a thin drawn woman looking older than her years. Her face had screwed up with anxiety, when Mr. Hewitt said their daughter Ella had always been after cock.

Miss Prewse closed the file for now. It might be well to have the stenographer type up a discreet letter to Dr. Stanley R. Montgomery, Medical Superintendent of the Ontario Hospital School in Orillia, concerning Mrs. Lumsden (*née* Ella Hewitt).

The letter was still in Daisy's file, dated 1951, stamped: CHILDREN'S AID SOCIETY OF TORONTO, a minor but important document that was to change the course of Ella's children's lives forever, part of a network of confidential information exchanged between institutions, and unknown to the Lumsdens themselves, for whom it was not meant.

CHILDREN'S AID SOCIETY OF TORONTO
Telephone Midway 0921 ... 32 Isabella Street
TORONTO 5, CANADA

April 20, 1951
Private and Confidential
(Please reply attention: J. Prewse)

Dr. Stanley R. Montgomery,
Superintendent,
Ontario Hospital School, Orillia.

Re: ELLA LUMSDEN, née HEWITT

Dear Dr. Montgomery:

We understand that Mrs. Ella Lumsden, née Hewitt, was admitted for Training to the Ontario Hospital School, Orillia, in 1937. Mr. and Mrs. Lumsden have recently separated and at Mr. Lumsden's request we admitted their three children.

We are concerned as to whether Mrs. Lumsden is capable of caring for the children should they be returned to her. Therefore, we would appreciate any information you could give us regarding her capacities and capabilities which would enable us to determine the plans that should be made for the children.

Mr. Lumsden reports that his wife has fits periodically and that frequently he has arrived home to find her in a coma, the furniture smashed and her clothes torn off. We have been unable to determine the nature of these fits or whether there is any history of epilepsy. Consequently, any help you could give us in this respect would be of great assistance.

Yours very truly,
CHILDREN'S AID SOCIETY OF TORONTO
D. Eisenfeld, M.D., Specialist in Psychiatry

The reply was immediate, arriving within the week, and marked "Private and Confidential." It bore the black circular stamp from the Orillia mailroom.

"School, Orillia"
Attention: Ms. Prewse
Re: ELLA LUMSDEN, née HEWITT

The above-mentioned was admitted to the Ontario Hospital School, Orillia, on August 10, 1937, and was diagnosed as a Mental Defective of Imbecile Intelligence, with an Intelligence Quotient of 40. There is definite evidence of mental deficiency in the family, two older brothers having at one time been patients at the Ontario Hospital School, Orillia.

Due to the patient's degree of mental deficiency, it is very unlikely that she is capable of giving her children adequate care and attention.

Yours very truly,
H. F. Frank, M.D.
Assistant Superintendent.

An addendum noted: "No fits or epilepsy were observed in this patient while at this hospital."

3.

MISS PREWSE EYED THE LUMSDENS cautiously. They were sitting across from her desk, looking somewhat bewildered; Mrs. Lumsden, in particular, seemed not to understand. Though she had been taken to visit the children several times over the past months, she did not seem to have any idea where they were or why. Miss Prewse thought to herself, how could she?

"Where's the chil'ren?" Mrs. Lumsden cried wildly again, looking around the office, the large desk with its sheaves of papers and files, important papers full of words about them she couldn't read, suddenly anxious: "Where's Pips?" she fretted. "Where's the babby?"

Whereupon Ernest Lumsden's eyes filled with tears, and he began to sob that the "babby didn' know 'im no more."

Miss Prewse was momentarily discomfited by Mrs. Lumsden's unexpected evident pain and her plea to take home Daisy's little doll, given to the little girls at the shelter, to wash — Mrs. Lumsden who had not a bar of soap in the house. She knew it was essential to remain calm and objective for, of course, there was no possibility that the children could be returned to them under the circumstances. But Miss Prewse felt regret, too, for Mr. Lumsden had turned out to be a decent man, even if deemed "backward." He never missed a visit to the children, and was a reliable wage earner: a call to Christie's Biscuits had confirmed that he was a respected worker grinding sugar in the cake-making department.

"I'm sorry, Mr. and Mrs. Lumsden." Miss Prewse spoke slowly, carefully, explaining again that for now the three children would remain in the foster home in Richmond Hill, a suburb north of Toronto, where they had been for the past months. The littlest girl, Lizzie, was just starting to call Mrs. Wilson "Mommy," a detail Miss Prewse did not divulge.

The children had not done well there at first, and there had been serious problems in particular with Daisy, much wetting and soiling and vomiting. She also masturbated and ground her teeth at night. The vomiting was a particular problem, according to the worker's report in the records, occurring in relation to any upset concerning her father whom she loved, particularly after his visits, when it was leave-taking time.

She had been "completely unable to build up a relationship with her foster mother," continued the report, but carried over from her relationship with her father a "freedom" to relate to her foster father, Mr. Wilson, the only one she had endeared herself to. This had caused a strain between Mrs. Wilson and her husband because of her sense of rejection, and her husband's physical closeness in his relations with Daisy. Because of this, explained Miss Prewse, they had decided to remove Daisy in June 1951 and place her in the Toronto Children's Aid shelter on St. Charles Street, so she could be nearer her father.

Of course, not all this was necessarily explained to the Lumsdens, it was just in the records that Miss Prewse was privy to. She put it in simple terms for them: Daisy would remain that summer in the Children's Aid shelter until a place became available at Earlscourt Children's Home in the Dufferin-St. Clair area. Lizzie and Pips would remain with the Wilsons.

"But where's Pips?" persisted Mrs. Lumsden, in that heavy nasal voice of hers, bewildered again. "Where's the chil'ren, are they coming back?" She jerked her head around, looking for them. Mr. Lumsden looked worried.

Once again Miss Prewse remained collected, patient. The Lumsdens might have to sign forms and appear in court, for these children would have to be made temporary wards of the CAS of Toronto, and later on, permanent wards, in keeping with the *Child Welfare Act* that only allowed temporary wardship for two years. (Her mother, Daisy noted to me, would have had to sign with an "X".)

"You'll still have visiting rights, of course, Mr. and Mrs. Lumsden."

The Lumsdens had recently separated. Mrs. Lumsden was living in a room on River Street while Mr. Lumsden had moved into one on Bleeker Street, their previous rooms having already been rented to new tenants.

The CAS of Toronto would, of course, do all it could to help them in their marital difficulties by providing counselling and practical help, assured Miss Prewse smoothly. The CAS of Toronto had a history going back to 1895 of working with families in their own homes to avoid separating children from their parents. J. J. Kelso himself, the founder of the movement in the nineteenth century, had stressed in the Annual Report of CAS in 1894, that if a family "failed ... the authorities should firmly and unhesitatingly remove the child and place him or her in wholesome and kindly surroundings, the entire purpose being the protection of the child."

"You may see the children regularly."

But what did "regularly" mean to someone who could not count? Mrs. Lumsden let out a wail and pulled at her hair.

Miss Prewse stiffened, but she was prepared for anything. What had to be kept firmly in mind was that Ella Lumsden was a classified "Imbecile," with a mental age of five. Moreover, the reason for her committal to Orillia at age twelve had been: "Parents fear she will become a sexual delinquent."

4.

IT WAS THAT MRS. LUMSDEN AT THE DOOR AGAIN, husband in tow, demanding to see "'er daughta." Miss Prewse was not with her.

"What is it, Mrs. Lumsden?" called out Captain Rawlings. "What are you doing here, banging on the door like that?"

"Wants ter see Daisy."

Mr. Lumsden shuffled about, looking lost.

"You have to have an appointment through your Children's Aid worker. You can't just turn up at The Nest like this, it disturbs the whole house."

Daisy flew past her mother into her father's arms. "Dada! Dada! Oh, I knew you come!"

In her office on Isabella Street, Miss Prewse checked the files. It was 1958. The time had come to make a decision concerning the three Lumsden children, now permanent wards of the CAS of Toronto, particularly Daisy who was almost twelve and who was slated for Orillia. Over the years, the girl had settled in quite nicely at The Nest, the Salvation Army Home for Girls on Broadview Avenue, at the corner of Pottery Road, where she had been sent in 1954. It accommodated up to thirty-five young girls, age seven to eleven, as Captain Rawlings, the Matron, had explained.

Captain Rawlings, or "Cap" as she liked to be affectionately called by the girls, remembered the very opening of the Salvation Army Home in 1941, attended by Lady Eaton herself, a generous benefactress. There was a photograph of Captain Rawlings in *War Cry* at the time, surrounded by a circle of healthy, smiling girls, and the caption: "Home for Wee Maids at Newly Opened Home ... 21-room mansion for little girls in Toronto." It had twenty-two acres of land that included a beautiful old coach house, once used for servants, and now a playroom. The back overlooked the Don Valley, with a vista of the city's skyscrapers through the trees.

The beautiful old mansion cited attractive bedrooms containing up to three or four girls. The former gracious front room downstairs now sported seven or eight beds, with a small adjoining room for night staff. There was a scullery, a main kitchen, a Matron's office, and a gracious staircase. The emphasis was on instilling good Christian values in the girls who were often from broken homes, and were emotionally disturbed; some were there temporarily due to financial stress in the home, or were awaiting adoption. The Nest provided the same care and training, stressed Captain Rawlings, that they would receive in a good middle-class home, and an education at the local school that would help them find jobs later on at age sixteen.

The Salvation Army did not, however, serve the mentally retarded, but in 1954 an exception had been made for Daisy for she did not *look* retarded, as Captain Rawlings had noted. Miss Foster, Placement Officer for CAS of Toronto at the time, had explained to Captain Rawlings that Orillia had been thought of. Meanwhile, Daisy would hopefully fit in unnoticed. Of course, as time went by, Captain Rawlings had been concerned that her girls, all normal, some quite bright, would become aware of Daisy's retardation or that Daisy might herself.

Daisy shared a bedroom with Jessie, Isabelle, and Patsy; it was painted white and pink and had picture on the walls of a young Jesus nestling little lambs in his arms. She had her own bed with matching coverlet, a small white bedside table for her personal things, a hairslide, a plastic comb, and a Bible card. Too, she shared a large closet where her Sunday clothes hung.

Finances had been settled: her board was $40 per month, and she received 75 cents "spending money," all paid for by cheque by the Children's Aid Society.

Daisy had blossomed, noted Miss Prewse on a recent visit. She was now, at age eleven and a half, turning out to be quite a pretty child. All the bedwetting, vomiting, headbanging, and certain other unpleasant behaviours had stopped. A charming pencil portrait of her sketched by one of the lieutenants, dated 1956, showed curved cheekbones and full lips, deep-set eyes and straight nose, and soft brown hair. Wonders what correct nutrition, sleep, discipline and affection, as well as daily prayers and Bible readings did for a child, Miss Prewse thought. The girls polished their shoes every Saturday night in readiness for church Sunday morning.

Daisy Lumsden was a lucky girl. She now lived in a neighbourhood that was affluent compared with that of her family. East York was a lower middle-class area, originally populated by British immigrants buying their first homes. Residents lived on quiet streets in small two-bedroom brick bungalows in neat rows with flowery gardens and hedges. There were small parks on the corner for their children to play in nicely.

This was a far cry from the Lumsdens' grimy apartment on squalid Sumach Street in Regent Park, a public housing area on the east side of the city that was once the original old Cabbagetown before the government had razed it to the ground and built public housing: grim utilitarian housing blocks shadowed by frowzy trees, their back alleys strewn with broken glass, scrap iron, beer bottles and other unmentionable refuse, all coated with city soot. Crime and prostitution was rampant.

And yet. Nearing Christmas at The Nest when Isabelle and Patsy and others were excitedly preparing little gifts wrapped in cheerful red paper covered in pictures of holly and reindeer to place under the tree in the playroom downstairs, Daisy had written an anxious note to her parents. It was printed in the round childlike letters she had learned at school:

> *To Dear Mother and father —*
> *I witer I could go home for aver*
> *because I crie ever night and I miss*
> *momy and Daddy and my sister and*
> *my brother,*
> *from Daisy*

There had followed a pyramid of kisses and zeroes no doubt learned at school, and then a "P.S." *Now I say Gooay-by and I will see you.*

She handed the note to the Captain. "Please and thank you, will you send it to my parents, Cap."

Captain Rawlings read it through quickly in the privacy of her office, as she did all the girls' mail. She hesitated. Mrs. Ella Lumsden and her garish red-lipsticked mouth came to mind, and the slovenly rooms the Lumsdens inhabited that she knew only too well. She also knew that Mrs. Lumsden spent nights out with "other men." She quietly slipped the note into Daisy's file, where it lay for decades, untouched.

Daisy waited out the days that holiday in 1958. Snow fell over the swings and slide in the garden. Great light white swept over the city, its churches and Army citadels, filling the Don Valley below, blotting out the landscape. She pressed her face secretively against the playroom window. Dada would come. Mommy would ring the front bell (she sensed rather than knew by now that Dada and Mommy could not write letters). "But they comin' you'll see," she confided to Patsy.

But no reply to her letter. Slowly, as Christmas came and went, and she received the same parcel of coloured pictures of Jesus and his disciples, and a stocking stuffed with toys to be shared nicely with all, and candies and an apple, and had praised baby Jesus in his crib at the Riverdale Corps Citadel on Broadview Avenue, something quietly and imperceptibly closed over her heart: parents did not necessarily come for their children. "*Jesus loves me this I know, because the Bible tells me so*," Daisy sang along with the girls in the Citadel.

The days went quickly by. The young and pretty Lieutenant Lovering often put her arms around her at bedtime prayers in the dorm and comforted her. The girls sat together in their dressing gowns with glasses of warm milk and sang the final evening hymn, Lieutenant Lovering's favourite from her childhood: "*Now the day is over, night is drawing nigh, shadows of the evening steal across the sky.*" Daisy sang too, but sadly, though she loved Lieutenant Lovering with all her heart.

So that when her mother and finally father appeared, bewilderingly, after such a long time, accompanied by the social worker, Daisy went loyally but cautiously with them for the day, holding her father's hand tightly.

5.

CAPTAIN RAWLINGS GLANCED at her fellow Army comrades. First Lieutenant Lovering and Second Lieutenant Newsome, and Miss Prewse, from the CAS and Infants' Homes of Toronto (amalgamated in 1955), had gathered in her office behind the sitting room for the conference on Daisy Lumsden. All agreed that Daisy was a sweet-natured, affectionate child who always tried to be good. (Daisy wept on reading this. "Yes, I was a good little girl.") Miss Prewse marvelled at how wonderfully Daisy had come along. "Easy to manage if surrounded by affection," proffered young Lieutenant Lovering. The bedwetting, head-banging and vomiting exhibited on admission had almost entirely ceased. "Daisy was a disturbed little girl when she first arrived in The Nest in 1954," intake officer Lieutenant Newsome noted.

Of ongoing concern were Ernest Lumsden's weekly visits. It was observed by both lieutenants that Daisy "lived for her father." She watched for him at the windows and talked of him constantly. After each visit she often had "upsets," and resumed her vomiting. However, it was noted that she ate greedily when out with her father. She also ate greedily afterwards at The Nest and did not chew her food well. It was questionable, therefore, observed Captain Rawlings, whether the "upsets" could be labelled as only "emotional."

The new CAS of Toronto case worker, Miss Tidwell, had queried Daisy's attachment, and was in favour of cutting back visits from Mr. Lumsden, something, she confided to the Captain and the lieutenants, that would prepare Daisy realistically for the day when she would be in Orillia and no longer in touch with him. There had, in fact, been a recent incident in which Daisy had checked for letters from her father by the hour and waited at the door for him to come only to discover that Miss Tidwell had thought it appropriate to cancel the visit for Daisy's own good, and Daisy had sobbed.

At this point, Miss Prewse reviewed Daisy's history: that Miss Foster, Placement Supervisor of Children's Aid and Infants Homes had requested a placement for Daisy in the Salvation Army Home for Girls in 1954. Daisy, a temporary ward then, had been unable to adjust to the foster home in Richmond Hill. It was thought that Daisy would ultimately be placed in the Orillia Hospital School, as well as her sister Lizzie, though this of course was not divulged to the Lumsdens. Lizzie, however, had subsequently been allowed to stay at the foster home permanently with her brother Pips as she was doing so well there. In March of 1954, Daisy (despite several undesirable traits) had been admitted to The Nest though Captain Rawlings had reiterated that being responsible for mentally retarded girls was not a prime function of the Home. It was then that the Captain had learned that Daisy and her siblings had been made permanent wards. A psychological examination done by the CAS in 1951, when Daisy was five and was in the process of being sent to the Wilson's foster home in Richmond Hill, had given Daisy an I.Q. of 66. In 1954, when she was seven and a half and had been transferred to The Nest, the resident psychometrist assessed her I.Q. at 62, which meant she was functioning at the mid-moron level and warranted placement in Orillia.

The agency went ahead with its application to the hospital. However in 1955, when Daisy was nine years old, it was acknowledged that admission to an overcrowded Orillia was somewhat remote given her age, and that she was best off for the time being in The Nest, where, since she was Protestant according to her father, Mr. Lumsden, she could attend the Opportunity Class in William Burgess Public School nearby.

The topic now switched to the issue at hand: Ernest Lumsden's visits. Once again, all agreed that Ernest Lumsden, despite his mental retardation, was a conscientious father, doing his best under the circumstances, unlike Ella Lumsden. Here Miss Prewse had noted in the records that, "Mrs. Lumsden was just released from the Don Jail for soliciting." It seemed she had been apprehended by police officers in a bawdy house, something Mrs. Lumsden denied, claiming she had been "duckled" by some drunk. By contrast, Mr. Lumsden had faithfully visited Daisy every week up to the summer, when he and Mrs. Lumsden had got back together again; after that, his visits had become less dependable. Mr. Lumsden had also been taking Daisy to visit her sister and brother in Richmond Hill without the worker's knowledge or permission, and this had upset the Wilsons.

Captain Rawlings wondered whether Daisy's retardation was not becoming more evident, though still not as yet detected by the other children. Here Miss Prewse felt the application to Orillia should be pushed forward, and agreed with Miss Tidwell that the Lumsdens' visits be curtailed to once every two weeks, in preparation for Daisy's separation from her father.

Daisy had admittedly become bewildered, and asked daily after her father, said Lieutenant Lovering. She pointed out gently that surely one had to take into consideration that Daisy had been in four schools, two Toronto CAS shelters, including a stint from 1952 to 1954 at Earlscourt Children's Home before coming to The Nest. Yet Lieutenant Lovering had been amazed at how quickly Daisy had learned the words of "The Young Soldier": "He went about / He was so kind / To cure poor people who were blind..." And Daisy had recently taken the Junior Soldier's Pledge at the Danforth Corps in front of Brigadier Stanfield. Daisy had promised to forsake her sins, trust in Jesus Christ, and be a faithful soldier who always helps others. Most importantly, she had promised to pray, read her Bible, and abstain from all intoxicating drink and tobacco.

There was a favourable rustle of concern.

It was decided that since Orillia was still a way off — at least a year, until she reached age twelve or so (the age of menarche), the usual age for admission for a girl like Daisy — her father's visits should resume back to once a week since this meant so much to Daisy. Lieutenant Lovering noted that Daisy had a strong sense of family. In fact, Mr. and Mrs. Lumsden were pressuring for the children to be returned home and were "very anxious for their return."

Miss Prewse was in a quandary. The Children's Aid Society of Toronto was dedicated to restoring family relations and returning children as soon as possible to their natural families. There was the issue of Mrs. Lumsden's "operation." She claimed she was feeling much better after she had gotten her "hystrect'my." She seemed to understand the significance of what had been done: "No more babbies." Now she wanted her children back, so there seemed little excuse or reason not to comply, her stint in jail notwithstanding.

Miss Prewse added cautiously that there was no doubt that Mrs. Lumsden loved her children. The Lumsdens were at present living upstairs in a house on Shuter Street with Mrs. Lumsden's parents. It seemed that

Henry Hewitt, Ella's father and Daisy's grandfather, was in support of the children returning, and vowed to help his daughter. He knew from his son-in-law, Ernest, that Daisy was the most retarded of the three grandchildren, according to the I.Q. tests. And yet, according to CAS of Toronto records, Mr. Hewitt had once tried to swallow a bottle of Lysol and throw himself off the roof of a house. Miss Tidwell, the CAS's visiting case worker, had noted that Mrs. Lumsden's housekeeping had "improved."

It was decided, therefore, that the children would be returned to their parents on a trial basis over that summer, in 1958, when school would not be interrupted, beginning with Daisy. Captain Rawlings' private opinion was that Mrs. Lumsden affected an interest in the children only in order to get her husband back, and needed watching.

It was hopeless, of course. Ella Lumsden, though she had tried her best, was incapable of looking after three lively young children, concluded Miss Tidwell. Children had to be fed three times a day, every day, not just when you felt like getting around to it. They had to be bathed and changed. The laundry had to be done in order for them to have clean clothes. The shopping had to be done in order to provide them with food. But all Ella Lumsden wanted to do was to go out and enjoy herself. She could barely look after herself. Miss Tidwell reported that, "Mrs. Lumsden was just unable to cope with three young, unsettled children," adding somewhat obliquely, "the parents have lived and worked in downtown Toronto."

But Daisy's memory was different. "Oh, it was fun!" to be back as a family with Mommy, Dada, and Lizzie, who was now nine and had lovely long red hair and pretty horn-rimmed glasses, and little Pips, who was about seven. She didn't care about the dirt and grime, or the back alleys with their broken bottles and rubbers and mangy cats, or the old mottled building on Sumach Street, or the cramped rooms they shared with Granpa and Ganny Hewitt. Ganny was deaf, and you had to shout into her left ear, but she always had treats for them in her fridge.

"Lizzie an' me used to sneak out early morning before peoples was up an' go round the doors stealing the cream off the milk bottles. Ooh, it was good! Til we was found out and oh boy there was hell to play."

Dada took them to Riverdale Zoo up the road. There was a stone necropolis and wrought iron gates among trees; they'd played on the grass in the dappled sun. And Uncle Robbie — "He was nice" — sneaked

Chiclets out of the factory for them. He always had some in his pockets for his little nieces and nephew, Ella's kiddies. He was a big man with big shoulders, thick curly brown hair, and a loud laugh. He threw Pips into the air like a kid himself. They were a "fam'ly," Daisy felt, satisfied. Uncle Robbie, Uncle Edgar, and Auntie Agnes made much of the children upstairs on Sumach Street, especially of Lizzie who was slender, fair, and blue-eyed with hair to her waist, who insisted at mealtimes on a knife and fork. "Eats like a real little lady!" Uncle Robbie had said admiringly.

Every night Lizzie brushed her golden-red hair a hundred times in front of an adoring Daisy, though Daisy noticed she couldn't count beyond twenty correctly. "Fifteen, sixteen, eighteen, twenny, sixty… "

"Tha's not right, Lizzie, is twenny-ONE, twenny-TWO," cried Daisy.

Lizzie put down her brush.

"You're like *her,*" she flashed triumphantly. "You're not my sister, I don't really know you."

Daisy's eyes filled with tears.

At once Lizzie pounced. "Me and Pips is like Dada. That's why we're together."

"No! No!"

Lizzie gave a short laugh. When the time came to return to school in September and the case workers picked them up, Daisy sobbed inconsolably at the loss of Lizzie. But Lizzie turned at the door of the Hewitt apartment and said archly to a bewildered Ella that she was glad to be going back, back to her "real mother" in Richmond Hill. Pips was happy everywhere with everyone. He had been made much of by the family, and petted by Granpa and Ganny, but he was also loved by Mrs. Wilson in Richmond Hill.

The following year, in April 1959, six months before Daisy turned thirteen, Mr. Stanstead, the psychologist at Toronto Psychiatric Hospital Outpatient Clinic recorded the then twelve-year-old Daisy Lumsden's I.Q. as 53, and that was being generous, he said. She had been given every benefit of the doubt.

Captain Rawlings paused. The fact was, at nearly thirteen, Daisy had the highest education of any member of her family other than her grandfather, Henry Hewitt, who had managed to reach Junior 111 in England. Daisy had done surprisingly well in the Opportunity Class at the local William Burgess Public School on Torrens Avenue, a solid, massive turn-of-the-century building with wide stone stairs and fan-shaped windows. It had a special class for "backward" children who were "behind," run by Miss Webb, a dear old teacher with a row of little white curls across her forehead that Daisy loved. The day at William Burgess began with the standing to attention for the national anthem, "God Save the Queen," a recitation of the "Lord's Prayer," and a Bible reading by Miss Webb, often from the Psalms of David: "Blessed is the man that walketh not in the counsel of the ungodly..." all highly approved of by the Captain. The school's Religious Instruction and Moral Training followed the Public School guidelines that every teacher was to "inculcate by precept and example respect for religion and the principles of Christian morality and the highest regard for truth, justice, loyalty, love of country, humanity, benevolence, sobriety, industry, frugality, purity, temperance and all other virtues." Captain Rawlings could not have formulated it better herself. The Nest was an open secret among the William Burgess students, and they were on their honour not to mention to the children at The Nest that they were separated from their families to avoid stigmatizing them.

Daisy had learned cursive handwriting, could read various morals and exhortations in the *Young Soldier*: "The greatest iceberg once was just a tiny flake of snow." Her school report card showed she had a B in Comprehension; a C in Spelling ("Keep trying, Daisy," Miss Webb had written); and a B in Arithmetic ("Accuracy improving," Miss Webb had written). "Good guidance at home in The Nest is helping," Miss Webb had added. At the Danforth Corps, Daisy had also shown improvement in reading and comprehension, reaching Level Blue in Bible Class, noted Captain Rawlings approvingly.

Her last report card, signed by the Captain herself—"*Mildred Rawlings, Captain*" — had given Daisy a B in Effort and a D in Reading. "Passed to Grade Two in Arithmetic. New Reader is *Come Along*, at the Grade Two level. Very good indeed for her ability," Miss Webb had written.

But Daisy could not stay at the William Burgess School. It was now 1959 and she was over twelve years of age. Her time was virtually up at The Nest as the Salvation Army mandate did not allow for girls over age twelve, and preparations would soon have to be made for Daisy's admission to Orillia. Miss Tidwell, Daisy's new social worker at CAS of Toronto, had hinted to Daisy about the possibility of being sent to a new school over the coming year, meaning Orillia. It had been awkward since Daisy had taken that to mean a new senior school in the neighbourhood and she constantly talked about it excitedly. Behind closed doors there had been sharp anxious whisperings between Captain Rawlings and Miss Tidwell. It seemed unfair, Miss Tidwell had admitted in a low voice, to lead Daisy on. But one could not possibly tell her the truth yet for she would be sure to tell her mother. When broached with the subject of Orillia, Mr. and Mrs. Lumsden had been upset. Mrs. Lumsden admitted to having been a patient there herself, and that it was a place for violent and mentally sick people and that the children in Orillia were neglected. Mr. Lumsden had nodded anxiously. Daisy was a sweet girl, eager to please and she did not belong there. She could tie her shoes, make her bed, and even read and write. The Lumsdens wanted her to go to the vocational school on Boyden Avenue, which once had links to the Haven, the refuge for feeble-minded girls run by the Salvation Army before it became Lorimer Lodge on St George Street. She could live at home with them as they had an extra bedroom.

One could not possibly send Daisy back to her retarded relatives. There had, apparently, been a grandmother on the mother's side, an idiot, incarcerated in Rainhill Asylum, England, an infamous place for paupers. Captain Rawlings had long since digested the contents of Daisy's family records forwarded by the Toronto CAS. The entire family was of low repute. The CAS had, perforce, kept arrangements for Daisy's admission a secret until the last moment, when only Daisy and Mr. Lumsden would be notified as he'd always been cooperative with the caseworkers.

Captain Rawlings' lips tightened. Working for Jesus was not for the lily-livered, Jesus was no milksop, and doing this work meant making hard, tough decisions. She, who had once had occasion to visit Orillia as a young lieutenant, nevertheless, thought of the long hard dormitory that lay in store for Daisy as she signed the release form.

As a lieutenant and then Captain of many years with the Salvation Army, Mildred Rawlings was more than familiar with family strife, break-ups, rape, murder, incest, and general mayhem. One but thought of General William Booth, the Army's founder, and his cry: "Around me were wretchedness, misery, blasphemy, and poverty, poverty, poverty." The Captain loved to recite one of his favourite poems at the Citadel:

> While children suffer and cry for bread,
> I'll fight till they're warmed and clothed and fed;
> While stricken women in sorrow weep,

While lost girls wander in anguish deep...

and so on, until the last moving lines:

While one dark soul is without the light,
To the very end I'll fight — I'll fight!

General Booth had once visited the Holy Land itself and hoisted the Army flag on Mount Calvary. Falling to his knees, he had prayed under the Tree of Agony in the Garden of Gethsemane.

That August night in 1959, after the social worker's visit from CAS to arrange for Daisy's admission to Orillia, Daisy wept softly under the blankets, after saying her prayers, not wanting the other girls to know her shame of being the only to be one sent away. She had not even Lieutenant Lovering's arms to comfort her, to sing and pray together, "*Now the day is over...*" She was away on her summer holidays.

The last thing Constance Lovering, now a Junior Captain, had done before setting off for the Haliburton Highlands at the beginning of August 1959, had been to write to Miss Fickles at Children's Aid Society of Toronto, 33 Charles Street West, concerning Daisy's final release. "Enclosed is a form which was sent to us in connection with transfers to Orillia. Perhaps you would be good enough to complete this with reference to Daisy Lumsden. Sincerely, Junior Captain Constance Lovering"

Unlike Captain Rawlings, Constance Lovering had little knowledge of the institution in Orillia; she had never been there. She only knew that Army Chaplain Officer Dinsmore took the Sunday morning services up there for the Protestants.

6.

THERE WERE THREE LONG ROWS OF IRON BEDS with grimy coverlets. Daisy tried not to cry, to be strong and brave for Jesus, as Captain at The Nest had urged. In the centre of the ward were two nursing stations, said the aide, who was dressed in blue with a blue-and-white headband, which was how you knew she was an aide. Aides wore blue, nurses wore white, assistants wore green stripes. Opposite the stations were the four Punishment Rooms, two on each side, so the nurse on duty could keep watch. "You don't want to end up in there," warned Nurse Chalmers, supervisor for Ward O-3, from her station in the Cottage.

Inside the guard, or punishment, room was a narrow bed and a window. Daisy told me that she and the girls would often sneak in and look out of the window. The dorm had long drab walls with shards of plaster peeling from the ceilings. The ward was separated into one area for those who were unclean and incontinent — Daisy would not be with them as an ex-Army girl — and those who were clean in their habits. The drugs were kept next to the Nursing Office where Daisy had no business ever to be.

"This is your bed. Use only this," said the young nursing aide, not unkindly. "Do not switch beds, and always answer your name at Roll Call." Her name was Miss Abbeyfield, but Nurse Chalmers had called out "Abbey" to her. "The other girls will be up soon."

The bed was like the others, crammed inches away from the ones on each side. It was an iron bed with oval iron bars at the head. It had one grey blanket and a hard pillow. There was a strong odour of urine, poop, stale blood, and dust that Daisy was not used to after her fresh room at The Nest, where Captain had insisted on the windows being kept open one inch whatever the weather for "fresh air."

"Where's my, my bedside table?" Daisy asked timidly, putting down her small cotton overnight bag between the beds. She couldn't see any down the long dorm.

"Ugh. Hey, Vera, this one wants a bedside table!"

"Where she think she is, Château Laurier?"

"Use under the mattress, for your lipstick," whispered a thin young girl later, who had something wrong with her lips. Daisy didn't want to look at her. She did not want this terrible, ugly girl called Alice — there was something very wrong with her — for a "buddy." She did not want to be in this terrible ward with all these girls and young women who had come shambling and stomping into the dorm, hundreds of them it seemed. They were loud, ugly, misshapen girls, frightening really. They grabbed at their tooth-brushes and surged to a doorway at one of the dorm where there was a bathroom. Too, they were pulling down their knickers already, pushing for the toilets — there was no door to the toilets, Daisy was alarmed to see. She was shocked to understand that you had to pee in front of everybody, at a row of open cubicles, the nurses and aides watching, opposite a row of filthy sinks. And once the door was locked at the end of the room at night, you couldn't get up and pee again until the morning, even if you wanted to badly. You had to keep the pee in.

She felt sobs coming; she wanted to go home, back to The Nest and First Lieutenant Lovering, she whimpered to Abbey, who, with her round kindly face and rosy cheeks, surely must be kind.

"You're in Ward O-3, Daisy, in Cottage O, and this is where you'll stay."

Ward Admission Record, Ontario Hospital School
(Department of Health – Hospitals Division)

Daisy Lumsden:
Ambulatory female. Admitted 3:00 p.m. August 23, 1959.
Height: 64 inches. Weight: 80 lbs.
Condition of person (indicate cleanliness, vermin etc.): Clean, no vermin.
Condition of hair: Brown, free from vermin.
Admission care given: Routine tub bath.
Articles on Patient: None.
Attitude of Patient on Admission: (cooperative, resistive, disturbed, excited, violent, threatening, etc.): Cooperative, but can be explosive.
Signed: Beatrice Gormers, Reg. Nurse.
(Supervisor in charge, Infirmary.)

Dr. William Serson had been the medical doctor on duty that August day in the new Infirmary where Daisy, a first admission under the guardianship of the Children's Aid Society of Toronto, had been held with other girls in the isolation ward until the assessments were done. The old Infirmary where Daisy's mother, Ella, and other Hewitt relatives, as well as her father's sister, Effie, had been kept, stood further down a steep slope on the institution grounds, unbeknownst to Daisy. It was occupied now by the overflow of patients from other Cottages, for the population of the hospital had reached almost 3,000 by 1959.

Dr. Serson had sifted quickly but decisively through Daisy Lumsden's documents, including the two Physicians' Certificates of Incompetence as per section 12 of the *Mental Hospitals Act* that had been forwarded from the Toronto Psychiatric Hospital: "...the certificate or certificates, when accompanied by the forms mentioned in subsection 1 of section 20, shall be sufficient authority to any person to convey the patient to the institution ... and to the authorities thereof to detain him therein..."

"Another member of this family for you, and who knows how many more there are in the hospital," the psychiatrist, Dr. Edmunds, at the Toronto Psychiatric Hospital had written dryly in the accompanying note. The Lumsdens and the Hewitts had produced, apparently, at least twenty-one retarded children between them, which meant that Daisy was the third generation designated as retarded.

Three generations mentally retarded! Both sides of the family affected, though "the parents were not blood relations," the psychologist, Mr. Stanstead, at TPH had commented under "Family History." Mr. Gooding, the psychologist at Orillia, had been most interested in the genetic aspect of the case, and drawn up a family tree of the Lumsdens and Hewitts going back to the patient's great-grandmother, who had been an inmate at Rainhill Asylum in Liverpool, England. This "tree" was still in Daisy's file.

There was no end to the degeneracy of this family. The Lumsdens were all backward or mentally deficient. On the maternal side, the patient's mother, Ella Lumsden, *née* Hewitt, an "Imbecile" and potential arsonist in childhood, had been a patient in the Hospital for the Feeble-Minded in 1937, along with her brothers and an illegitimate nephew. Her older sister, Henrietta (a patient at the Cobourg Asylum) had had an illegitimate son at age sixteen named Cuthbert who was placed at the Orillia Hospital for the Feeble-Minded by the Toronto Children's Aid Society at age six. An incorrigible child by all reports; he had bit the teacher in the Backward Class and called her a "sod." Cuthbert Hewitt was still in Orillia, in his twenties now, a patient in Cottage B (for low-grade males), something that Daisy Lumsden need not know, of course. Dr. Brillinger, colleague and fellow physician, agreed.

As to the rest of the Hewitts, the Toronto Social Service Index (TSSI) on Adelaide Street had put out a call for information on the younger boys Oswald and Wilfred, now men in their late thirties, who had attended Jarvis Vocational School and done fairly well there in the Backward Vocational classes; TSSI wanted to follow through on them for the records.

Mr. Gooding, the psychometrist, had assessed Daisy 's I.Q. at 54 — mid- or half-moron level — even though at one point the psychologist at CAS had given Daisy a score of 66 when she was nearly five, and Mr. Stanstead, at Toronto Psychiatric Hospital, had given Daisy a score of 62 on the Stanford-Binet Intelligence Scales when Daisy was seven and a half. Mr. Gooding seemed not to notice the discrepancy in results, the dramatic drop in Daisy's performance, or make allowance for a child in shock over the journey from Toronto, over the affront of an intimate physical examination, or over finding herself cast into a new life in the middle of nowhere.

She had been too frightened she would fall off the narrow examining table to cry out as she lay with her feet in the stirrups, legs apart. "This won't take a minute."

"They brought you into a room in isolation in th' Infirm'ry with other girls. Oh, there was about seven of us," Daisy recalled. "Then they told you to undress for th' physical. You had to line up in a straight line and step forward when your name was called. Girls and boys separate. They put their hands and fingers all over you, in your ears, in your mouth, up your vagina, everywhere, you lay on your back upon a table. You had to open your mouth wide and say, 'Ahh.' And be weighed on a scale and measured. Their hands was all over your breasts squeezing — mine was small, I was just a kid of twelve nearly thirteen," she said. "What right did they have ter do that? I was just a kid."

"Physical completed: 11:45 am," the report stated. She had been given the usual mandatory tub bath, her hair shorn. Short stumpy tufts now stuck out from her head down to her ears. She was ugly now, she knew.

She remembered crying after her hair was shorn, to stop nits and lice, they had said. "I want to go home, I want to go back to my Mommy and Dada," she had wept. And they'd laughed and said, 'Your parents are no good. You've been taken away from them and that's why you're here.' An' I cried all the harder."

She had been "withdrawn and dull," Mr. Gooding had noted during the psychological examination: "A defective-looking girl. Conversation limited due to intellectual defect."

Yet the physical examination had also shown a strong, healthy girl, noted Dr. Serson as he went over the results from Mr. Gooding. ("Head size normal: circumference 53cms"). Inoculations were in place; the Wassermann test was completed ("Negative"); her genitourinary system NAD ("No Apparent Disease"). Number concepts good. She could spell simple words like "cat" and "dog." Overall, a sweet and obedient girl, he noted (this was important). Some masturbation.

Dr. Serson hesitated on the final pronouncement. First Admissions into Orillia that year, 1959, had been in the ten to fourteen age range, all "moron" level: twenty-four males and only twelve females; thirty-six in total.

There was a shortage of menial help on Ward O-3 in Cottage O for the female patients. He wrote down briskly: "Classification, Half-Moron. Placement: Ward O-3, Cottage O."

Without hesitation, he assigned Daisy to morning academics in the Orillia school in Group 20, moron group, and Ward Work in the afternoon, adding: "Custodial" ("*for life*").

7.

THE NEST WAS A DREAM, and Lizzie and Pips — a more grown-up Lizzie than the one she had seen that summer at the foster home in Richmond Hill — phantoms. Captain Rawlings had agreed with the CAS of Toronto's caseworker, Miss Prewse, that Daisy could spend her last month with her siblings before going to Orillia. Lizzie had not seemed to remember her, nor Pips, now age nine.

"It were lovely in th' foster home in July when I was there with my sister an' brother before I come to Orillia, but I was scared at first. I pretended I didn' know my name when my sister asked me. I wasn' sure it *was* my sister, but I thought it might be. Then I never wanted to leave an' come to Orillia, I wanted to stay forever with Lizzie."

Eleven-year-old Lizzie was taller, imperious in her new green horn-rimmed glasses. "Are they really my brother and sister?" Daisy had wondered as they played house together and poured tea in Lizzie's tiny plastic tea set in the Wilsons' den. She was no longer sure, yet she felt she knew Lizzie. Mrs. Wilson said she could ask the caseworker if she was allowed to be told. Miss Prewse had said it was all right for Daisy to know, and for Lizzie to be told who Daisy really was, too. "Oh I cried an' cried when they took me away in the van, I wasn' to see them again. Why couldn' I of stayed there?"

"She was the most retarded of the three children," Dr. Serson had recorded in Daisy's Admission Records, noting that the CAS social worker, Miss Prewse, had observed: "Does not miss her mother and father but likes to be with her sister and brother."

The third floor of Cottage O was what was real now. Cottage O was on the south side of the big administrative building, said an aide when Daisy asked, "Where is I?" Daisy tried to grasp south and north, but she could not. She felt only the oppression of a huge, red brick building surrounding her; a building that she could not yet understand contained administrative offices, and Cottages with Wards that held the younger children. Somewhere, at the back, were the schoolrooms.

"You'll get used to it," said a kindly nurse's aide, dressed in blue. The new patient looked promising; she was ambulatory, and could talk and toilet herself.

Her mother and Aunt Effie had been in Cottage O before her, long ago, her mother had told her that before Daisy left, and Uncle Robbie and Uncle Edgar had been in Cottage D, but Daisy tried not to think about that, of their presence in this place, their shame, and hers.

Daisy learned to follow the other girls down the back stairs to breakfast, holding on to the iron railing, feet clattering down to level O-2, which meant the second floor. There was Ward O-1 and Ward O-2 below her ward, which was occupied by younger girls. The dining room was on the second floor, and was shared with the O-2 girls. Ward O-1 had its own dining room for the littler girls. Daisy at once wanted to be with the younger girls as they reminded her of Lizzie. But the rules were that you followed the monitor assigned to your group, in Daisy's case, a tall, important girl called Stacey, who stood at the head of the table, the morning sun filtering through the dingy windows. You stood to attention while Stacey said "Grace," before tackling your bowl of porridge, your bread and butter, and your tea.

"Have your periods started yet?" Supervisor Nurse Chalmers came up to Daisy in dorm, clipboard in hand. Daisy shook her head. Lieutenant Lovering had told her and the other girls in the Rosebud Room at The Nest all about God's special love for girls and Daisy's special duty to stay good and clean once she menstruated.

If blood came between her legs at night in Ward O she was to go straight to the nursing station and tell, said Nurse Chalmers. If it came on in the daytime she was to tell the teacher or an aide (they were the ones in the blue uniform, Daisy tried to keep this in mind). It seemed the blood could come at any time, now that she was nearly thirteen.

"You had to put up your hand at Roll Call if you was menserating. They wrote down when you started and ended, how many days you bled and how many pads you used. If you missed two months you were marched down to the Infirmary," Daisy said to me.

"You didn't have Kotex available in a cupboard in the dorm?" I asked.

"Nope, you had to ask. It was locked up and they had the key." In a large institution with thousands of girls in its care, thousands of Kotex pads had to be ordered and accounted for.

Daisy was hurried back upstairs to the dorm with hundreds of girls, and it was confusing. Some groups were to go to the school and the rest, the "ward workers," began putting on canvas aprons and over-dresses for Ward Work. Daisy was in the morning "school" group, said Nurse Chalmers. She was to put on a navy serge tunic and white blouse tossed to her from a large cupboard at one end of the ward which contained "school clothes," explained Alice, kindly Alice with the terrible lips Daisy was, by now, getting used to. That was what was so awful: that soon she would not notice at all, she thought, frightened. Alice would look normal to her. She had to wear heavy black shoes too big for her — she had not known her shoe size, so she just accepted what was given to her by the aide, along with a long black knee-socks. "Hurry," the aide had hissed.

The schoolroom was behind the locked door that led to the central corridor. The corridor was a shock, filled with lines of noisy boys from Cottage A. Daisy looked at them, startled. Some were mongoloids; she saw their eyes and tongues just like Alice's, and she was frightened again. What were they doing here? "Children's Aid had promise me I wouldn' be with them ones," Daisy said. But here she was, plodding heavily with them. One of them smiled and waved at her. She nodded cautiously; he had a happy face. The Captain at The Nest had not spoken of what Jesus thought of these ones but that He did suffer all. More lines were coming outside because of the lovely weather, from other Cottages, led by attendants. A bell rang.

Daisy was in Group 20. She found herself in a large airy room with big windows. She sat at a wooden desk next to Alice. All the girls were dressed the same in tunics and blouses, their short hair cut above the neck, and held off the face in the front with a clip if necessary. No adornment was allowed: no earrings, no necklaces, no bangles, no hair ribbons, and certainly no lipstick. Girls at the front; boys at the back. They stared at the teacher, Mrs. Mead, a stout woman: "Use your *teeth* and your *tongue* and your *lips*." She grimaced, baring her teeth.

Mrs. Meade held up two dolls, to demonstrate the words "In" and "Out" as she pretended to push them in and out of a pretend house. A few aides and attendants stood to the side; they supervised, whispered

Alice. "I want you to put your tongue *behind* your teeth now and say after me 'in' and 'out!'..."

After recess, she followed the attendant leading the line back upstairs to the dorm through the doors that locked behind you. "KEEP LOCKED AT ALL TIMES," she read. The keys hung around a nurse's waist, clinking. "RING BUZZER FOR ENTRY," said another sign. Daisy was to change quickly and not waste time. She had to get out of her tunic and blouse, which were thrown into the cupboard — one of the ward workers was to hang them up on hooks — and join the other girls in the Training Programme for Ward Work. Today, she would help to feed the severely retarded ones on the other end of Ward O-3.

"Try not to let them touch you," Nurse Chalmers advised Abbey, the new, young nurse's aide assigned to O-3. "They do like to cling." Personally, Nurse Chalmers doused her outer garments thoroughly afterwards with disinfectant. Some you threw away *at once*.

There was a small group of mothers in the ward that Fall afternoon, volunteers from the town. They were known as "The Mothers Volunteer Group" and they came in once a month bringing books and toys for the patients, and helped with the children downstairs. Today they were helping the staff with the patients who were always kept separate, the low-functioning girls and teenagers behind the screen at the end of the Ward O-3. Daisy took up a mop and bucket and filled it at a filthy tap; soiled nappies lay in the gutter filled with poop and slime. She tried not to look as she bent over the tiles to wash away what was all over it; other girls were scrubbing the bathroom area, holding their aprons over their noses when the nurse in charge was not looking.

But the most horrible were the ones in the center of the floor, their legs apart or tied up in knotted sheets; such knots at the back that Daisy had trouble figuring them out. The girls sat rocking and spitting, grunting and howling; some peed themselves, while others grovelled for food. Some of the staff laughed, and said to the two mothers who were standing there holding the pathetic cookies that they had baked back at their church, "Huh, watch them go for it!" The aides threw pieces of cookies and candy into the centre of the floor. The girls at once squealed and grunted, grabbing at the food, "like animals," said the aide, "aren't they, Vera?"

Only Abbey seemed uncomfortable with the scene and wanted the patients to be fed at a table, but it was dangerous to allow cutlery for these girls, the other aide warned her and the mothers, they would chop each other up with the knives, or eat the napkins, or plunge forks into each other's eyes. "You had to watch," she hastened to add.

One girl, about fifteen Daisy guessed, lunged at the aide in an effort to grab more candy. "What the — hey, Abbey, get her!" cried Vera, but Abbey was too late. An aide grabbed the girl by the shoulders and the two scuffled. Then the girl bit the aide, snarling like an animal. Daisy gripped her mop. What was happening? The aide, who still had the girl by her shoulders, suddenly bashed her head against the wall, back and forth, yelling, "You little fucker!" Abbey pressed the bell on the wall for Nurse Chalmers, dazed and shocked.

Mrs. Blaine, the leader of the Mothers Volunteer Group, gasped. She knew better than to intervene or complain to the supervisor, of course, otherwise visiting privileges of the Mothers Volunteer Group would be cancelled.

Even more horrible, the dentist, Dr. Moyne came in, breezily calling for the first young woman to be put in the chair. But it was not any dentist's chair that Mrs. Blaine had ever seen; it was an old wheelchair with a wooden foot-step. The first girl was strapped in — a loose, fleshy, helpless sort of girl with a lolling mouth — and she had little idea of what was to happen to her. No anaesthetic was used that Mrs. Blaine could make out, just a quick screwing motion inside the girl's gagging mouth, and a groan.

When the straps were loosened, the girl came staggering across to a horrified Mrs. Baine holding her jaw. "Catch 'er, Mrs. Blaine," but Mrs. Blaine could not bring herself to even touch this bloodied human flesh gagging at her feet. Daisy, the shorn patient on Ward O-3 whom Mrs. Blaine recognized at once as a new girl, poured some water over the girl's face and said the most remarkable thing: "That's what Jesus would a done, Miss."

Mrs. Blaine knew, of course, that there were always a certain number of normal girls on the wards used by the aides to do the lowly work, such as scrubbing and cleaning up the refuse and human offal to relieve the stench, while the aides took a bit of a break. Such girls, Mrs. Blaine had been given to understand, would work their way up and eventually become "Monitors." Monitors got special privileges, such as the honour of being allowed to go over to another Cottage to help out. Mrs. Blaine paused. There was something about Daisy scrubbing her heart out on her knees for Jesus. Daisy was trying to do her best as Captain Rawlings had urged her: "Remember you are always an Army girl."

That night Daisy knelt on her knees beside her bed in the confusion and noise of her ninety or so bed-mates scrubbing their teeth at the basins and pulling on their night-shifts, the aides yelling from the nursing station, "Lights out, you girls, lock-up!" She tried to say the Lord's Prayer softly to herself before she forgot the words, to remember First Lieutenant Lovering and keep her in her heart. She folded her hands together and bowed her head just like she'd been taught. She sang to herself, "Jesus bids us shine with a pure pure light, like a little candle burning in the night...." Then she followed that with First Lieutenant Lovering's favourite line, something about "shadows stealing across the sky."

"Listen up, you sap-face!" Marcie's face was right next to hers, the next afternoon.

At once Daisy started to cry.

"You git down on them sweet little knees of yours and clean this shit." Big Marcie Evans from Group 22 on the ward kicked the slop bucket toward Daisy.

Daisy opened her mouth to say it "wasn't 'er job," because she was assigned to Mending in Ward Work. "'S not my job today, Marcie."

"Is your job now, see! Little fuck-face singing them sappy little songs to Jesus at night, 'Jesus fucking bids me shine,'" minced Marcie. The other girls tittered. "Well, you fucking shine them floors for me right now. And hand over yer pin money."

Sobbing, Daisy went into the dorm and put her hand under the mattress and pulled out a small cloth purse the girls had made her at The Nest containing her savings — a few dollars Captain had proffered for treats. She handed it over.

"Now git scrubbing," Marcie grabbed the mop handle. "Or you want this up your arse." She screwed the handle round and round in her hands before Daisy's horrified eyes. "Nice an' tight."

Daisy squeaked.

"I seen what you do with your pussy under the blankit."

Still sobbing, Daisy got down on the floor of the staff bathroom that had been assigned to Marcie for Ward Work and dipped the mop into a bucket of bilge-like water and began to swish the slime towards Nurse Chalmers' drains.

"Harder," Marcie sniggered. "So's I'll git a Merit."

Daisy knew then she'd better be quiet, very, very quiet and good and never answer back, as Jesus said. Then Marcie, and the staff, and everybody else would forget her.

Progress Sheets, Ward O-3.
August 30, 1959.

Daisy is a well-mannered 12-year-old girl. She keeps to herself.
Not aggressive or a bully. Able to look after her own needs.
Obedient.
M. Chalmers, Nurse Supervisor.

8.

DAISY COULD NOT SLEEP. It was the thought of the big-headed babies in their cots that kept her awake, she confided to Alice, as well as the restless shifting and loud breathing of ninety or more girls in beds stretched wall to wall up and down Ward O-3 in early winter, her first winter in Orillia, 1960. She still could not get used to the iron beds row on row, inches apart, or the geometry of the ward with its ceilings far away, the plaster stripping that could fall on her head. It was so far from the bedroom she had shared with Patsy and Isabelle. But she kept up her prayers to get her through the night, whispering under the blanket. Marcie Evans she now knew as the "Evil" that the Captain had warned her of; Marcie knew how to get a boy and even sneak out at night. She showed her tits to the male attendants in the basement and did many other very bad things.

There was low sobbing from the new admissions. The door to the corridor and bathroom was locked. The dull red night light glowed over the door. This was her new world that she now understood was forever, that no one, not even Jesus, could save her from. After seven months she had been promoted to Children's Dorm in her Ward Training, Nurse Chalmers had informed her with a tight little smile. She was to help the nursing aides with the babies all afternoon, as soon as she had changed out of her school tunic. Follow Miss Darcy.

There were always staff shortages. Nurse Chalmers knew there was but one Superintendent of Nurses, one Head Assistant, one Nursing Instructress, eight certified Nursing Assistants, and 246 Nurse's Aides for the entire institution of 2,600 patients. Dr. F. W. Snedden, the Inspector from the Department of Health, always checked over the Occupation Charts and Ward Records at inspection time. He approved Ward Training as good occupational therapy for the custodial patients who were destined never to leave the institution. Such training helped them expend their energy usefully. The high-grade girls (the few who would eventually earn probation) benefited as this work provided them with a means of earning a livelihood in domestic service. Nurse Chalmers filled in Daisy's records at the nursing station, to be handed in to Dr. Foster C. Hamilton, Superintendent, every night by 9:00 pm.

> Daisy Lumsden, Ward Training, transferred to work in Children's Dorm. March 1960.

Snow drifted across the white grounds and the trees groaned under ice, but Daisy hurried underground through the tramways she now knew — she could read the signposts. She followed Miss Darcy through the long tunnel almost a mile to the new Children's Dorm, built five years earlier in 1955. The low ceiling and stone walls of the tunnel were damp, and their shoes and voices echoed in clacking sounds. Sometimes you heard moans and muffled cries. Somebody was locked in somewhere. "None o' your business," said Miss Darcy. They passed a recess in the walls, or an odd window, with steel mesh across it and a gasp of sunlight that made Daisy long to escape.

The big-headed babies on the medical ward were terrifying at first, but only at first. Daisy steeled herself as befitting a Junior Army Soldier in Christ. Facing her was a small ward, with only four or five beds, cots and bassinets for the babies, and little tables for the ones who could self-feed. There was a Doctor's Office, a Nursing Supervisor's office, and a room she was not allowed near, said Miss Darcy, that contained X-ray equipment and an old 200-milliamp machine.

A few nurses in white with white headbands moved around anxiously. "We're short staff today again because of the storm," said one to Miss Darcy. "We need the girl in Babies."

Daisy had to carry the big-headed babies that had "water on the brain."

"Poor devils won't last long," said Miss Darcy, nurse's aide. Then she lit up a cigarette.

For her first task Daisy had to change their poopy diapers and mop up their sleepers. Then she had to carry them when they cried, and burp them over her shoulder, which was often.

"I could hardly hold 'em in my arms," Daisy remembered. "I was only a kid and my arms ached, their big heads would roll on their little necks. I was so upset, they all cryin' all day for their mammies," she added softly.

"Where's their mammies?" Daisy wanted to know.

"You're not here to ask questions, Miss Busybody."

They would not last long. Their heads would grow and split. She was horrified to listen to Miss Darcy. Nevertheless, no shunts for them. Daisy did not understand that these were the poor babies born after the Second World War — what else could be done with them other than to send them to Orillia to die? There was no money for all the babies born in Canada with hydrocephalus, so only those with the best prognosis received treatment. And yet, some lived into childhood in the hospital, due to excellent, devoted nursing care. Their nurses wanted them to live, to be happy in the dorm, to be taken outside in summer to the lake. Some children sat up and walked and talked and were bright. Some had tight bandages wrapped around their heads. You saw them around the grounds actually laughing and playing ball, their huge heads lolling.

But Daisy was frightened. "I was just a kid," she said to me. "I needed a mother myself, and I didn' have one."

Daisy applied herself assiduously to wash and change, burp and carry the babies, doing her best for Jesus, hoping to work herself up to Dining-Room Monitor and be able to say "Grace" at the head of the table in front of everyone.

"Don't be afraid, Daisy." That morning, she was to help Abbey feed the old women in Cottage L who were unable to go to the dining room. Her morning classes, which only amounted to an hour or so of daily instruction, were to be skipped. This was more important; they were short of staff again and needed help with the difficult ones.

"You'll just carry trays and wash dishes."

Cottage L was one of the oldest Cottages, designated for the older women. It sat next to the water tank and power house. Daisy often saw the old women — how long had they been here? — swaying about outside the cottage muttering to themselves, and picking their noses and scratching themselves in private places, gesticulating with their fingers and sometimes yelling bad words. Then an aide would take them by the shoulders and push them none too gently back inside. Daisy tried to stay away from them — they smelled — and also from the old men from Cottage B who had freedom of the grounds.

Cottage B, for older men, was on the other side of the power house. "They aren't going nowhere," Abbey said. Often they just sat on low benches on the grounds or on a low wall watching the younger patients digging the terrace gardens, mowing the vast lawns, or raking leaves.

"Hey there!" one old man called out eagerly as Daisy and Abbey hurried by Cottage M, carrying a mound of towels for L. He had a raspy, trembling voice. "Nice mornin' for little ladies."

"Hi there, Jake," said Abbey. He was one of the oldest residents; had been here for seventy years, she told Daisy. He remembered Dr. Alexander H. Beaton and his daughter, Janet. Daisy understood that Dr. Beaton was someone important and that that made old Jake important. She realized that Jake must have been a little boy when he came to Orillia, when it was the Asylum for Idiots, and had never left.

Shadows fell from the four big Cottages set in a rectangle: L, M, B and C dominating the grounds beyond the Administrative Building.

Abbey looked critically at Daisy in her frumpy over-dress, or "government service" dress as it was called, for indigents. "You shouldn't have to dress like that, Daisy. We workers complained to Dr. Snedden when he last come about the old-fashioned clothes you girls wear, so as to give you new, up-to-date clothes from town."

Abbey had had occasion to take a few young women from Cottage M into town to buy new outfits for them. "Just get cheap dresses from the thrift store or chain stores, for them," the Matron, Nurse Dinsmore of M had said. Abbey was determined that they would get the best, just like girls from the outside, and spent all the money and more on nice brassieres and something new called "pantyhose," flared skirts and twinsets, and even a bit of jewellery that the girls were allowed to wear, but only at the Socials and certainly not at Sunday service. "Immoral," said the Matron. "They're not here to look fancy for boys."

There was a covered verandah for patients and staff to walk from Cottage M to the other nearby Cottages. M patients did not need the tramways in winter or when it rained. Daisy could not wait to be promoted to M — it had its own beauty parlour run by the patients — but that wouldn't be until she was sixteen or seventeen if she continued being good and trustworthy.

Daisy was not sure what month it was; she only recognized seasons from the colour of the leaves or when branches were bare and icy winds blew up in gusts from the snow-bound lake below, or when it was hot and cicadas whirred somewhere up in the trees. Now it was fall again; it had come so quickly. The teacher in class had pinned pictures of a turkey dinner and a harvest to the wall and written "THANKSGIVING" on the blackboard, which they were to copy in their printing books and then learn the Thanksgiving song. Today the leaves on the trees and the bushes around Cottage L were burnished crimsons and browns, and filled with scarlet berries. "Is pretty."

They entered L. At once the stench hit her. Dr. Snedden, the Inspector, had noted in his report that many of the old women in the Cottage would not wear clothing such as pyjamas or nightgowns. Some had to be secluded because of dangerous habits and cruelty towards other patients. It wasn't the workers' fault, said Abbey to another aide, Miss Tucker. There was little that was not known about such reports in an institution like Orillia. Daisy understood from this that L was a bad place. "There was naked women lying around the dorm because they won't keep their nighties on," she confided to Alice that night.

"Just don't turn your back on them," Nurse Chalmers had warned. She was somewhat concerned with how the new nurse's aide was shaping up. Abbey had confided shyly that she liked working in the hospital, and that she was getting fond of the girls, "as if they were 'my' girls."

"Yes, well. We all feel that way at first, Abbey. But you'll learn different."

Cottage L was a long, rectangular, red brick building of three floors, and each floor had its distinct patients. They were on L-3, and the patients were to be fed from small side tables. Somewhat proud that she was being trusted — she was sure to be a Monitor after this — Daisy carried in the heavy laundered bed linen (none too clean by the Captain's standards at The Nest). "They drag them on the floor," said an aide.

Daisy put the sheets into a dirty cupboard at the side of the ward that was spilling with soiled cloths used as nappies for the incontinent who shit and peed themselves all day, complained the aide. It was noisy; yelling, shouting, and raucous laughter could be heard all the way up and down the chaotic ward. Women were quarrelling out in the hall where they had congregated on the floor, as they would not use the sitting room down the hall.

At once an old woman weaved between the beds toward Daisy. She was in a straightjacket, and strings hung at the back so that her hands could not reach them. "Please, please," she whispered, waving from side to side.

"Now none of that Mrs. Ellison, settle down," called a harried nursing aide sharply. Another old woman was tied up in sheets knotted at the back; she tossed restlessly on her bed, her wispy grey hair covering her face. Others lay naked on their beds, jiggling their shrivelled breasts in a most shocking way.

"You shouldn't be seeing all this," said Abbey. "You're just a kid."

"Come along, Mrs. Woods, let's put a dress on today," a faded flowered over-dress familiar at the institution, "and slippers," Abbey said sternly.

There was a small sitting room on the first floor below; a large dormitory crammed with beds, a Day Room, and a Nursing Office on the second floor; and, the most difficult patients were on the third floor. There was a large, dusty window overlooking the water tower. A long shadow crossed the Day Room and over the old bodies tied to chairs lest they fall, or slumped over side tables. Women who might perhaps have had children at some time in their past and now didn't know those children any more, thought Daisy, frightened. It was how you ended up.

Daisy held on tightly to her tin of Vim. She was in the utility cupboard scrubbing pans with a scourer at a tiny, stained sink clogged with slime she tried not to touch, a small cupboard that Inspector Snedden had also apparently, according to Abbey, found unsatisfactory. It was where dishes were washed by those patients deemed capable as part of their therapy.

Abbey was feeding the old women at small tables. "Come along, drink up your soup, Edna."

A nurse was at the station sorting out medications and labels. There was a sudden shriek, followed by a loud thud as someone hit the floor. "Here, get her, Elsie!" The aides were trying to force a dress on Mrs. Forbes. "She's a strong bugger."

"You'll have to go in the side room, Mrs. Forbes. Here, git her arms, Abbey."

That was the Punishment Room where Mrs. Forbes would be tied up in wet sheets, Daisy knew. She knew so much now.

Dr. Snedden, Government Inspector from the Department of Health, had drawn attention to the use of restraints and seclusion throughout the hospital in his report from 1956, frowned Dr. Hamilton, Superintendent at Orillia. Of course, Dr. Snedden had realized that allowances had to be made for the special class of patient at the Hospital who would likely never be discharged: "A considerable proportion are of low-grade intelligence, and many idiots and imbeciles are in residence in addition to those in the moron group." He added, "Some patients, too, are extremely deteriorated in their habits and behaviours."

Nevertheless, he had been distressed to find two such deteriorated young patients in seclusion in Cottage A-2, both boys suffering from a severe degree of rectal prolapse that they picked at constantly. He did not query further as to how their rectums had come to collapse. Restraining jackets had had to be used to control the boys' arms, the staff had explained, to prevent them from picking at themselves and causing bleeding. There was also the matter of finding a box under a mattress in Cottage B (males) that had contained three padlocks and keys. Rectified at once.

In Cottage L, however, he had come across three old women patients in seclusion, two of them since 1954 and 1955, written in as P.R.N. orders "with no indication of a time limit." P.R.N. was supposed to be temporary treatment, as opposed to permanent, given in times of crisis, as staff were surely supposed to know, Dr. Snedden had pointed out. Dr. Sneddon wrote in his report that "I do not consider this is a good procedure, and feel that all patients in seclusion should have a definite time limit put on their seclusion order as signed by the physician. This prevents undue seclusion."

Of course, Dr. Snedden had little concept of the realities of dealing with 207 low-grade senior women locked in wards (such as L-3), frowned Dr. Hamilton, Superintendent. One of the women in seclusion on L-2, for instance, was a chronic window-breaker.

Dr. Snedden also drew attention to the stench of urine throughout the wards in the Cottages and noted that some dormitories were too tightly packed in. For example, on L-3, he had come across 100 older female patients in the dormitory, some of whom simply could not keep their nighties on, even tearing them to shreds, as explained to him by the staff.

And so the complaints had continued. Dr. Snedden had found a patient in the Infirmary, Section 4-B (male division) locked up in a storage room, supplied with only a mattress and spring and bedding. Old safety razor blades, table knives, scrub pails, and other equipment had been shoved in a bathroom cupboard in Section 5-A. Yet again, pieces of a broken mirror were in the bathroom in Section 5-B; also dirty spoons, dirty pails, and dirty shirts were in the cupboard. Also, in Section 4-A, in the medicine cupboard, he had found external and internal medications mixed together and wrote, "This is not desirable."

As to the use of "restraints" — for instance, sheets and chair sheets tied in strips to bind difficult patients — it was an ongoing issue in the institution. Dr. Snedden had tried to be objective, for when one considered the "acute deterioration and behavioural manifestations" of some of the low-grade defects, one hesitated to criticize, he said. Occasionally, a disturbed woman in Cottage M, for instance, would have to be put in seclusion in a Punishment Room; and admittedly many low grades in the Infirmary were in straightjackets for their own protection. But on the whole, Dr. Snedden had been satisfied that "excessive restraint and seclusion" was not being practised in the hospital.

The report was doomed, of course, to go the way of all Inspection Reports as Dr. Hamilton well knew — filed away in a drawer in the Department of Health in Queen's Park to be ultimately forgotten.

Had not Dr. Lionel Penrose, Director of Psychiatric Research for the province, complained of the excessive use of restraints in his inspection report of Orillia for June 1940, after observing two paralytic patients under restraints in bed? "I do not believe it necessary to wind the bedclothes around these patients the way it is done here." He had seen two cases of fractured femurs due to injudicious lifting of delicate patients from their beds. Ignored. Not followed up on. Lost to the exigencies of time.

That is, until the day that brash young reporter, Pierre Berton, of the *Toronto Daily Star,* came to visit after Christmas, the last week of 1959.

9.

MR. BERTON, who had initially been welcomed at the Orillia Hospital School, all the nurses clamouring for his autograph, had written a scurrilous account of the institution in his column in the *Toronto Daily Star* on January 6, 1960, entitled, "What's Wrong at Orillia — Out of Sight, Out of Mind."

Berton had come with friends Gerry and Betty Anglin who were returning their twelve-year-old son to his Cottage B, (admittedly one of the oldest and most dilapidated Cottages in Ontario Hospital School, conceded Dr. Hamilton). Shocked, Berton described the overcrowding in some of the older Cottages and Wards — beds jammed together head to head, playrooms and classrooms used as dormitories. There was but one single washroom for 64 patients in one area, he reported, and one wash tub to 144 people in another. Though he praised the "newer" Cottages as well-run, he hinted at "atrocities going on" in Orillia. "You have been warned," he admonished his readers, likening the institution to a Nazi war camp, "though it was no Belsen," he conceded. Dr. Hamilton trembled.

Improvements would mean higher taxes, Mr. Berton pointed out. "It's easy to blame the government."

The Orillia *Packet & Times* at once retaliated with a glowing account of the annual Christmas Concert at the Ontario Hospital School, or OHS, which it described loyally as "the most exciting time of the year ... a world full of the spirit of goodness and expectation," as well as the wonderful display of the patients' handiwork in crochet, knitting, tatting, and baking.

There followed a spate of unsavoury publicity. Donald MacDonald, MPP for York and leader of the CCF — a socialist — arrived post-haste and called Orillia a "hell-hole" and the Cottages mere "buildings for human storage" and a clear "fire hazard" (indignantly refuted by the Orillia fire inspector despite the fire to one of the Cottages in 1960). MacDonald reported that dormitory after dormitory was just a mass of beds — one children's ward had only one nurse on night duty to 124 children. Dr. Hamilton was not certain whether it was MacDonald or Dr. Morton Shulman — another troublemaker and a member of the Opposition at Queen's Park — who had made claims of children locked up in "cot-cages." (Staff claimed the children were let out for feeding, toileting, and a break. There had always been "crib-cages" used in Europe, said Dr. Hamilton gruffly.)

MacDonald demanded an investigation. It was taken up in the Throne Speech, and when Premier Leslie Frost angrily defended Orillia in the Legislature, claiming that the Province of Ontario had "the most imaginative" treatment policies in North America for the mentally ill, Donald MacDonald actually hummed aloud, "Tra-la-la."

The Ontario Minister of Health, Dr. Matthew Dymond, responded indignantly to MacDonald's "usual exaggerated manner" concerning his claims of floors "impregnated with human excreta." "Ontario Hospital School is clean and well-tended as any in the province," he declared. "It is completely wrong to say the patients are neglected."

Lloyd Letherby, MPP for Simcoe East, accused the *Toronto Daily Star* and the *Toronto Evening Telegram* of "getting down in the gutter" to increase circulation. Had Mr. Berton and Mr. Macdonald really expected to see a "roseate vision" of "cosy vine-covered Cottages inhabited by shining-faced, happy children attended by hundreds of motherly nurses?" queried the editor of the *Telegram* dryly.

It was all a political racket, and everyone knew it, snorted Dr. Hamilton. He was always being pressured to take in more patients by the parents. It did not seem to matter whether there were any beds, he cried.

Nevertheless, there had been a fracas in the Legislature. A new institution was promised. It would be built in a cow pasture of 254 acres at Cedar Springs, near Windsor, for 1,200 patients, so as to relieve the pressure on Orillia. The Ontario Hospital School in Smith's Falls, later Rideau Regional Centre, outside Kingston, the biggest in the Commonwealth, had already been built in 1951. Intended for a population of 2,400, its size had been opposed by parents rebelling against giant institutions — it had a central corridor a third of a mile long — and now housed about 1,000.

Building a new institution, rather than transferring people to Smith Falls, which was operating only at half capacity, was favoured as it created jobs for the unemployed in these towns; Orillia, Smiths Falls, Cedar Springs all relied on the institutions for jobs. Besides, there never were enough institutions for the mentally retarded population (128,000 by 1970).

Donald MacDonald — that Bolshie — again protested in Parliament that big old-fashioned institutions like the Ontario Hospital Schools at Orillia and Smiths Falls were a thing of the past, though economical (the same services were needed for a small institution as a large one). The government thus agreed to establish a new small Children's Psychiatric Research Institute in London, with Dr. Don Zarfas, a psychiatrist, as its first Director. Don Zarfas, son of Mr. Frank Zarfas, the former steward at Orillia under Dr. J. W. S. Horne's superintendency, was always a bright boy, full of promise.

That summer, in 1960, the two oldest Cottages in Orillia, L and B, were torn down and the patients were transferred temporarily to the old T.B. sanatorium at Gravenhurst, known as the Muskoka Cottage Sanatorium and to Edgar, another small institution in the Muskoka area. Some of the old women refused to budge. Cottage L was their home, they shouted in panic.

Construction crews, bulldozers, and pneumatic drills pounded the peace. Wooden forms were laid out and filled with concrete, before the bricklayers began. Foremen stood around with blueprints in hand. Attendants struggled to keep the lines in order as the boys crossed the grounds; many of them, especially the higher-grade ones in Cottages D and C, now wanted to be labourers and cement mixers (afterwards, gangs of patients cleared away the rubble). In Ward O-3, Daisy made every effort to do her best. Clouds of dust drifted through wards and dorms, under beds and in cupboards as she struggled to keep up her scrubbing and scouring. She looked out wonderingly as old Cottage L went floundering to the ground in a rush of dust. What had happened to old Mrs. Woods and Edna? Gone. "To Graven'urst," said an aide.

Now the Ontario Minister of Health, Dr. Dymond, had arranged for Fletcher Film Productions to come into the Orillia and make a documentary on the place called *One On Every Street*, meaning one retarded child could be found on every street in Canada. Dr. Dymond himself was to appear in the film at the end and give a speech. Orillia was not "to be prettied up," he ordered. Nevertheless, patients' faces and heads were scrubbed where possible, given the limited number of bathrooms, showers, and hair-brushes. Their clothes were also ironed for the Sunday service scene. There was excitement in Ward O-3. Daisy understood they were going to be film stars. Nurse Chalmers had a new perm and the hem of her skirt taken up a tad.

Daisy and all the patients at the Hospital watched a special showing of the movie in the gym after it was shot. In the opening scene, an actor playing a thoughtful doctor told a pair of sobbing parents whose little girl had just been diagnosed as "retarded" that there were 500,000 such children in Canada: "You are not alone." Some 2,600 of them were in Orillia, to 900 Staff.

The narrator, Allan McFee, went on to explain that an institution was a place where the retarded could be happy and "understood." There were three categories of intelligence, he intoned: mild, moderate, and severe. There was a quick shot of some severely retarded patients coming through a dilapidated doorway, a mixture of young and old men. Some of the old ones had huge goiters swelling in their necks like balls stuck in their throats. "Thyroid problems," murmured Nurse Chalmers to Abbey as they watched, enthralled to see their lives on screen. No one seemed to wonder how cretinism could still exist when Dr. Helen MacMurchy had reported back in 1905 that cretinism was a thing of the past with the discovery of thyroid deficiency and its treatment.

One young man in his teens with an enlarged head turned his face to the camera and smiled, showing horrid, pointed teeth. Daisy gasped in her seat in the audience. Were such people sharing the Cottages and Wards with them? She felt so sorry. The Captain had said nothing of these people — where were they kept? They seemed to be underground in a basement somewhere, in a special Ward relegated only to them. The music had changed and the narrator lowered his voice to say that these were the "hopeless ones."

"Sometimes the surroundings seem to have aged with the patients," he said, almost apologetically. Some sort of comment seemed requisite to explain the peeling plaster and holes in the walls of the room where the severely retarded men now sat ravenously attacking their food in bowls. There was another quick shot of a child sitting in a wheelchair, in restraints, only too familiar. Dr. Dymond wanted an honest portrayal. The soft cloths wound around her arms were so she would not hurt herself, assured the narrator: "Some will never learn."

Daisy recognized Gloria Nettle in the Sewing Class scene; a row of girls plied their Singer sewing machines, as an attendant and instructress stood in the background. "I knows her!" Daisy cried out. There were shots of other occupations and trades — boys were shown tapping shoes in Cobblery — "Makes them content" — hammering wood in Wood Shop, and milking cows on the farm. "Time has little meaning for the severely retarded," the unseen narrator intoned again. "Mentally they will always remain children though in the bodies of adults."

The camera glided over a group of young boys and girls in Scouts and Girl Guides, a program run by the institution. Daisy had not remembered there was so much activity going on. Another shot of hundreds of patients at Sunday service showed the older girls, likely from Cottage M, all prettied up with curled hair, and the boys wearing dicky bows with their hair slicked to the side. "*Jesus loves me and I know I love him*," sang the choir, and then you saw them all bow their heads to say the "Our Father" prayer. Abbey had her eyes shut tight, but Nurse Chalmers kept hers open a tinge to check on the others as they mumbled through: "An' forgive us our trespusses..."

Dr. Dymond, Minister of Health for Ontario, now appeared at the end of the movie. "Will you allow your conscience to ignore what you have seen and heard?" he cried in a soft Irish lilt. "These afflicted people live in the same world as ourselves," he concluded mournfully.

It was some time before Daisy understood he meant her.

10.

TWO MORE GIRLS WERE ADMITTED to Orillia in 1961 from The Nest, her old friends Patsy and Isabelle, so she must be fifteen, Daisy thought. They had been in Grade Eight at William Burgess Public School, bright teenagers, as Captain Rawlings well knew. Isabelle would be sure to be a star in the upcoming Christmas Operetta at Orillia with that singing voice of hers. What else could be done with penniless girls from broken homes due to violence and drugs, too old for adoption, other than placement in Orillia, Captain Rawlings had reasoned. At least the girls had been given a good moral grounding at The Nest (both had reached Third Year in Bible Study and received their Red Seals for "Courage"). In the Ontario Hospital School they would at least get vocational training.

Both girls, upon admission, were placed by Dr. Serson at once in the highest academic group in Upper School.

Daisy was allowed to help them settle in. "I know how you feeling, Patsy an' Is'bel, is a shock but I'll help you. We can say our prayers together at lights out like what we done before," Daisy had said eagerly. There was "before" and "now" — two dimensions of time in Orillia, which Patsy and Isabelle would have to learn.

"I don't want to stay here!" said Patsy defiantly, near tears. She missed her long black hair, the thick plait. Her neck felt naked. Isabelle's long blond curls were also gone for now. Both girls were shocked and frightened at having their hair shorn after the very public tub bath, yet another humiliation.

"Is for to stop nits an' lice," Daisy explained soothingly to the horrified girls. "It'll grow agin, Pats 'n' Is'bel." She did not add a crucial bit of information: "Only to the neck is allow."

The two girls still wore nice dresses from The Nest, lovely stockings and slip-on shoes. They were shocked when the Matron, Nurse Chalmers, wearing a uniform, made them remove their clothes, which she then labelled and tagged with their respective names, as well as the name of parent or guardian (CAS of Toronto), and maddeningly put away to "keep nice for visitors." They were to put on institutional wear for Ward Work, like everyone else. Daisy helped them choose the drab dresses that Patsy and Isabelle soon realized had been worn by other girls the previous day.

"I'm going to let the Captain know about this!" Isabelle's lips trembled.

"Won't do no good, Is'bel. They reads your letters an' changes 'em."

The frightened girls kept close to Daisy, terrified of the Punishment Rooms. Patsy tried not to look when she saw a girl laced up in a straight-jacket swaying towards her. "Ugh, oh-h, ugh!" choked Patsy.

And Isabel began to cry, taking in the sight of all the rocking girls with their trembling mouths lying on the floor. She forgot about her pledge to serve others for Jesus. "They're all *retarded!*" There had to be a mistake. But Captain Rawlings never made mistakes.

Daisy asked Nurse Chalmers if the new girls could have beds next to hers, and move Alice away. Nurse Chalmers hesitated. But Army girls from The Nest were potential valuable workers as had been proved. She nodded, and the delighted Daisy showed horrified Isabelle and Patsy their "beds."

"But how can we sleep with all these people in the room?" asked Isabelle.

Patsy was more frightened of the nursing aides. "They *hit* that girl," she cried.

That night, the two girls lay next to Daisy trying to understand that this might be *forever*. In the long humid ward, with 90 or more beds crammed in — Ward O-3 had had to be divided into three rows and two aisles for the overflow — they felt constricted in a strange darkness, these beds filled with strange girls. There was an eerie hooting.

"Oh, what is it?" cried out Patsy, sitting up in bed; it was coming through the walls and windows.

"Is just an' owl," soothed Daisy.

"Quiet back there!" called a voice.

Patsy didn't like that the nurses' station was in the centre. It was like they were spying on you. The two girls had been shocked at bedtime, and had not wanted to pull down their knickers in front of everyone to go to the toilet. The aides had been bemused. "Oh-h, *you will.*"

And, of course, in the end, they had.

"You gotta learn th' ropes," warned Daisy, knowing this was a test from the Captain. But how to explain Attendant Gormley's sudden, harsh shout: "*Beds!*" one rainy afternoon in the Day Room.

At once the 90 or so girls of Ward O-3 scuttled under the rows of iron beds in dorm. "Oh-ugh-oh, what's happening, Daisy?" cried Patsy and Isabelle, rolling under a bed next to Daisy. They were on the floor, everyone was.

"Jus' keep yer hands an' feets in, don't ask," hissed Daisy, frightened.

Attendant Gormley was coming up the aisle, banging a broom — *crack, crack* — on the tiles. "Everybody's feet in, or else!" she shouted. She had had enough for one day. She whacked a foot sticking out under bed 20.

"Agh!" screamed the girl.

Patsy whimpered, cringing into a tight ball, making herself as small as she could under the bed, her head hitting the underneath mesh, which was filthy. She held her breath in terror as the attendant stomped by. Isabelle had her eyes shut tight, praying to Jesus to get her through this. This was a madhouse.

"And you'll stay like that 'til I says! Don't want a peep out of any of yous," yelled an exhausted Miss Gormley.

Mildred Chalmers paused wearily from record-keeping: patient progress sheets, clinical records, menstrual charts. Her dress stuck to her back in large wet patches. Ward O-3 was hot and humid and her office was no exception, especially at night as the heat upstairs was more intense than in the lower wards. Two ventilation shafts and ceiling fans, recommended by Inspector Snedden a few years earlier had, of course, not materialized.

She went to the staff bathroom and peeled off her dress. Her middle-age flesh seemed to slump and flop as she crossed the floor to the shower stall. She hung up the soiled white uniform and bib to dry on a twisted coat hanger, then looped it over a bar in the one shower stall, often used as a change room. The nurses also used the shower stall and toilets as both a utility room and a closet. Other damp uniforms hung limply against the mildew. Abbey was sitting urinating on the toilet in full view as there were no doors to the stall. It was no different from the situation in the patients' dormitory.

Nurse Chalmers pursed her lips. She knew from a reliable source as supervisor that Inspector Snedden from his government office in Toronto had reported in his Annual Inspection Report five years ago that the nurses' accommodation in Ward O-3 was "rather disgraceful."

Early June, summer in Orillia. The sweetness of freshly cut grass mowed by the boys in Cottage C scented the air, until the stench of the sewerage pit wafted over as the wind changed direction, something that had been complained of in superintendent Mr. Downey's time back in the1920s. Perhaps that was when Daisy wrote her letter to Junior Captain Lovering, remarkable for a girl with an I.Q. supposedly deemed 54 and thus deemed at the "imbecile" level, which was lower than being deemed "feeble-minded."

No one questioned Daisy's I.Q. or thought it odd that someone considered an imbecile could read and write.

The letter covered two pages in the childlike, round, cursive script she had learned in academic school. That would be in writing class when she'd been promoted to Group 24 and then 26. Some of the sentences were obviously dictated or revised by the staff who checked every letter sent out of the institution, as Daisy knew. You were not allowed to say what was going on, "or else!" Daisy warned Isabelle and Patsy. A year had passed since they had arrived, but Daisy still had to remind them that letters received were also read first by the staff and destroyed if they did not approve of them. Daisy wrote:

> *June 5 1962*
> *Dear Captain Lovring*
> *Just a few lines to say hi to you. How are you I am find I am soor for not writing you for along time so I got to write to you. How is the weather in Toronto the weather up here is some times nice and some times cold. I hope you will come and see us. May I please have a picture of you me I will give you a picture when I get one. I hope to hear form you. Pasty and I and Isbel Lee are in the same bed room together Isbel said hello to you and so did pat to said hello. Tell all the Staff I said hello to them for me Please. I am trying hrd to be a good girl I got a new watch from abby and a dress and some other things to and pasty got*

some new clothes and a watch to when we go to town again we will be getting summer clothes to wear. I still rember the pray I sing it ever night before I go to bed me and pasty and isbel Lee said it together. I better go now so good by for now may the good Lord bless you and keep you for ever more p s write back to me soon
Good by for now
Love
Daisy Lumsden

As Daisy waited and waited for a reply, she scrubbed out wards and laundered in earnest the babies' diapers every afternoon, so that Junior Captain Lovering would be proud. In the mornings she pestered Miss Galbraith in the schoolroom for news of mail.

Then one morning, a full year later, the teacher handed her a letter, already opened and read, of course. It was from Captain Lovering. Daisy trembled in anticipation.

"Do you need help reading it, Daisy?"

Daisy quickly pulled it to her chest. "No, thank you please, Miss Galbrit."

It was marked "June 26, 1963." And addressed to her, Daisy: *Miss Daisy Lumsden.*

"*Dear Daisy,*" Junior Captain Lovering had written. Daisy was thrilled. Junior Captain Lovering had not failed her. She was loved. Memories of cuddling in Junior Captain Lovering's arms over a cup of cocoa flooded Daisy's heart. The letter went on to say how pleased Captain Lovering was that Daisy was "getting along well." She too talked about the weather in Toronto, as Daisy herself had been taught by Miss Galbraith, "It's always appropriate to mention the weather." Junior Captain Lovering said something strange, that it was "almost too warm for comfort."

"It sounds as if you and Isabelle have a very good time together," she continued. Daisy sensed that Orillia sounded like a holiday camp to dear Captain Lovering. For a moment she felt confused. Choir, picnics, and shopping trips into town was not what she really meant, not what she wanted Miss Lovering to understand, but that she missed her and her Dada and longed to be back at The Nest.

"Colleen is going on holiday," continued Captain Lovering. "The Thomas children will be going to visit their father for a few weeks..." Did Constance Lovering understand the significance of such words?

Daisy felt a wave of sadness. Would she ever see her own Dada again?

The letter ended with the words: "I am being married on June 30 so I will be leaving the Home. God bless you, Daisy..."

11.

"DAISY IS A SNEAKY, SEXY GIRL and has to be watched around boys," Nurse Chalmers recorded in the Ward Progress Sheet that February day in 1964. "Lazy in Ward Work and untidy about self."

The change in Daisy Lumsden could be traced back directly, of course, to that fateful visit home over the previous Christmas, in 1963, that Nurse Chalmers had strongly opposed. The mother, Mrs. Lumsden (a virtual imbecile bordering on idiocy) had appeared at the door of Ward O-1 downstairs unannounced, without due notification, yelling obscenities and demanding it was time her daughter Daisy was let out as she was sixteen (she knew the law) and they couldn't keep her locked up in that prison forever. When argued with — the Lumsdens had been given the visiting rules — she had told Nurse Chalmers to "stick 'er thermom'ter up'er arse." This last comment had been struck through in the records, possibly by Nurse Chalmers herself. Nurse Chalmers had slammed the door, whereupon Mrs. Lumsden had thrown herself to the ground, beating her fists on the tarmac, tearing at her clothes, and exposing her dirty pink brassiere. What was one to do with such a woman — throw a bucket of water over her?

"She's 'aving fits," Mr. Lumsden said meekly.

Nurse Chalmers had objected. But Superintendent Dr. Houze had demurred. The CAS of Toronto had granted probationary access over the phone to Mr. and Mrs. Lumsden for Daisy to go home over Christmas, as was their parental right. There had been no trouble before on visits on the odd occasion she had been allowed to spend the weekend when she was younger, and Daisy was a sweet-natured, obedient girl, and a good ward worker.

"Precisely," Nurse Chalmers had said.

Daisy had returned obviously distraught. Something had happened, something serious. "Did anybody touch you? Did a man do anything to you, Daisy?" Nurse Chalmers had shaken her. But Daisy stayed curled up on her bed and would not move. Tense, moody, and irritable, the girl complained of pains in her stomach. Too, there was blood on her nightie though her menstrual period was not due. (Nurse Chalmers had checked the Menstrual Charts in her office.)

Nurse Chalmers sent her at once to the Infirmary. During the physical examination Daisy had apparently broken down, and confessed to Dr. Serson that she had been forced to have sexual intercourse "all weekend" by her mother with her mother's "boyfriend," a man she'd picked up outside of 999 Queen Street (the Queen Street Mental Health Centre, as it was called then). Her mother had given her drugs, she claimed, though she could not name them when asked, and could only guess they were her mother's sleeping pills. She also insisted that she had had intercourse "lotsa times," and that her mother had paid her boyfriend to do it. "She took off my clothes, I couldn' struggle I was too drugged up, and she paid him money to have sex with me."

Of course, it was obviously the other way around. Mrs. Lumsden had pimped out her daughter. Not the first time this had happened with their girls and no doubt not the last. Nurse Chalmers pursed her lips.

Daisy had known from her training at The Nest that what the man was doing with the thing between his legs was bad, very bad. Afterwards she had smelled the rotten, fishy smell nothing would ever wash away — his spunk. Daisy had struggled, she had wept: "No, Mommy, no please!" But he had done it anyway and *she* had helped, pulling Daisy's legs up over his shoulders. She had gagged, then shook from all his jerking, his hairy bum going in and out, up and down. "Dada!" she had screamed. But of course he was at work, the night shift at Christie's Biscuits.

She stayed huddled under the blanket all weekend — day after day, and between the times the man came back. She could not eat or sleep. She had to drink in the end, and the pills were in it she knew. The next day was Christmas; snow was falling against the grimy window and bells were ringing through the city streets.

She had hurriedly pulled on her skirt, sweater, shoes, and black stockings that Monday morning, then caught the bus back to the Hospital School in Orillia where she was met by an aide. She trembled, yet was glad in a dull sort of way to see the lights above at O-3 dorm winking through the dusk.

"Are you sure, Daisy...?" Dr. Serson had hesitated a moment on the examining table, creating a silence at the heart of things Daisy did not have enough words for. Dr. Serson did not know what to make of what he called her "story."

"She sticks to her story," he wrote in her record.

How much credibility should one give to these claims? Daisy was, it had to be borne in mind, an imbecile, mentally retarded, he frowned to himself. And so there had been no follow-up. How could there be with a mother such as Ella Lumsden? No torn hymen was acknowledged, or bruises noted; no vital sperm swab was taken to be sent to the laboratory for proof. If she had been raped all weekend as she claimed, sperm must surely have still been present in the vagina and cervix. But how valid was an imbecile's's memory? It was pointless for the hospital to take action, superintendent Hamilton hedged.

There was a hurried consultation as to who had given permission for the visit, knowing the parents were deemed "unsuitable," the mother virtually dangerous. Best to pass over the incident. Besides, who would they take action against? A nameless man? An unpleasant shadow of slum life. Daisy was now safely back under the protection and strict standards of Orillia, thought Dr. Serson and Superintendent Hamilton, which was why segregation of the mentally retarded was so critical.

The Lumsden girl would, of course, have to be removed from school. She certainly was no longer the "quiet senior girl" liked by teachers and staff, fond of reading, cooperative with workers, neat about herself. She had sung in the choir and been a Girl Guide. Miss Gormley, teacher of Group 28, had reported that Daisy would not remain in the classroom but spent her time "in the basement with the boys."

"You will now be a full-time Ward Worker," said Nurse Chalmers grimly.

"As if I care!" cried the new Daisy, her blouse loosely buttoned, mouth reddened with lipstick. "I never learned nothing in school, anyways."

The class records, however, showed a remarkable advance in three years from Group 20 through to Group 28. Daisy was reading at a Grade Five level in some subjects. She had recited the first verse of "In Flanders Fields" more or less correctly up on the stage on Remembrance Day: "In Flander fields poppies all blow / Between th' crosses, rows on row..."

"Why're we locked up here like prisoners, we ain't done nothing wrong! Why can't we be with the boys like normal teenagers?" she flashed.

"Because you're not normal. And you can wipe that muck off your face."

She had lain in bed in the dorm, at first, refusing to budge. Everything hurt down there where the Captain had said was a girl's treasure, to be kept pure for Jesus, something she no longer was. Daisy wept in secret, fearful of Patsy finding out, or Isabelle. Isabelle was now a Monitor — well, of course, after singing that lovely solo at the Christmas pageant before the Mayor and everyone — another Nest girl making Captain proud.

Now she turned her back to them at bedtime.

"Hey, you really give it to Chalmers, kid," said Marcie at break.

"You gotta smoke?" Daisy challenged, though she could not even inhale, and always choked.

"What's it worth?"

"Whatever it take," said Daisy, suddenly excited.

"After what happen I thought who cares? I might as well have some fun in that place. Me an' Marcie Evans used to sneak off down to the basement and meet boys in the Smoking Room, regular, boys like Eddie and Steve," Daisy recalled to me. They sneaked down the backstairs and through a door a male attendant unlocked just for Marcie. Daisy did not ask why; she now knew.

She felt a surge of power. She did not have to do what the nurses said. She was over sixteen a year ago, which made her seventeen, going on eighteen, said Marcie. "You ain't a Ward no more, Daisy."

Marcie lit up a ciggy, tossing the match to the floor. "Let the fucking place burn down!"

Daisy smiled at me, remembering: "Oh, I liked the boys all right. Hell, I was just a normal teenager! That was all I thought of, trying to talk to the boys, you know."

And she and Marcie did. They whispered and passed notes in school behind the teacher's back before Daisy was thrown out. They also made signs with their hands in Sunday service. Crossed hands meant, "I love you." Yes, there were all sorts of little opportunities here and there, despite segregation, to talk, to touch briefly, to promise to be some boy's girlfriend, and to marry him. Marcie showed her how to sneak the keys off the hook at night when the aide was sleeping a restless exhausted sleep, to tiptoe down the backstairs lit by dim lights to the underground and to waiting boys.

Every morning, the nurse gave out tobacco and rolling papers to the older patients who wanted to smoke, right after recess; you had your own tin with your name etched on it and nurse called out your name. Daisy and Marcie joined Eddie and Steve regularly for a smoke at break. Steve was Marcie's boyfriend and Eddie was now Daisy's. Both boys were from Cottage C and were older. They had been in Orillia for a very long time, longer than they cared; almost forever.

The stuff Eddie told them! He had been "gang raped in the arse" he said, by older men in the showers, predators, on his first week in Cottage B, before they pulled it down. Daisy had not known boys could be raped. She did not ask for details. Eddie looked upset.

He was only fourteen when it happened, and they was much older than him and had big cocks hanging to their knees, he said, his eyes scrunching up. He had been pushed against the tiles, the tile walls in the communal stall. The older boys, some of them men, grabbed at his cock. He had not known what was happening at first. He had started crying. Then they had pushed themselves into him, one after the other. When one was done, another was on him. He was sobbing and hollering for an attendant, but that did not stop the men. "I was all torn up and bleeding but the showers washed it away and stuff. The attendants didn' do nothin' ter save me. They didn' like seeing the men jerk off all the time over the beds so they looked away, you was on your own. Unless they wanted some themselves," he added bitterly.

That was the time he had gone to the can in the middle of the night in the short little nightshirt they gave you that only went to your knees. The night attendant followed him. Laid him over the bench in the Day Room in the dark. "But first I had ta take him in my mouth and swaller 'is jiz. Then he did it to me from behind like, 'til he finish, the fucker son of a bitch."

Daisy's hands jerked to her face in horror. She was hearing truths she had never suspected.

"He didn want me doin' it to nobody but him," said Eddie obliquely.

Steve broke in. "Tell her about morning lineups, Ed."

"Oh them. They makes you stand in a line naked, you're just out of bed, and they call you 'fuckin' retards' and one pull your balls."

"Ugh, he deserves to rot in hell!" cried Daisy, puffing desperately at her cigarette and coughing and sputtering with each drag.

"No. No! Not men! *Women*. The women attendants pull our dicks and give us hard-ons. They're worse than the men in how they get their jollies."

Marcie gave a short, harsh laugh.

Eddie was eighteen, a man. Forgotten by his family on the outside a long time ago, he mourned softly. His dad had come to see him once when he was six or so in the Children's Dorm, and had never come back; his mother had never come, not once. Abandon him, that's what. When they got out of this place he was going to marry Daisy, he promised, and they would have a place of their own and babies. Mr. Deane said he was doing good in woodwork. Mr. Deane was the instructor, a good fellow, one of the best. But some of the attendants on their Ward beat them plenty, he said. Once, they put his head down the toilet bowl and flushed it, all because he did not eat one day. There were good attendants and there were bad. They had this other punishment in two lines facing each other down the corridor and when it was your turn you had to get down on your hands and knees and push a rubber along the floor with your nose. "Eat dirt," the attendant would say. "Eat worms, boy."

"Yeah, an' that's not half of it." Eddie took a deep breath, and dug his cigarette into the sofa. "There was the *pervert.*"

Daisy listened attentively. She wanted to know everything, especially about a pervert. Something was opening up in Daisy's heart she had never suspected about the Good and Evil that the Captain at The Nest had divided the world into. She longed to tell the Captain about the evils done to these boys. The world seemed to swing in reverse.

"Yeah, well, Hicks," Eddie's face tightened, "he takes the girls too, him and Charlie Duggan from G, down behind the boathouse and to the far end of the beach on Thursday cook-outs and — you know — does it to them. They says, "You tell anyone and you know what you get." Daisy shivered, for she knew only too well; she had seen what wet sheets did when those old women mouthed off.

"But it's what he makes 'em do on Ward Work that's *perverted!*"

Daisy's eyes widened, but she had to hear it out. There was no end to this evil. She knew that male attendants sometimes helped out on women's wards, as their strength was needed to hold down difficult women or ones having seizures. But it seemed Mr. Hicks made the girls he was in charge of open their blouses as they scrubbed the floor. This way, their tits hung out as they leaned over. "And then he jerked off inside 'is pants."

Daisy nearly choked, puffing madly on her cigarette. Marcie gave another harsh laugh.

"An' don't he like little boys, too. Tell her, Ed."

"Yep, they played with them too, took 'em down the basement." There were little recesses, rooms here and there in the walls of the tunnels, and that's where they took them, so nobody could see or hear what was going on. Then Eddie, who had been promoted to "shepherd," in charge of helping new boys on the dorm, looked after them when it was over. He told them to stop crying. He mopped up their tears and got them some different underwear, as some was bloody, he said. He did it because he was a monitor, a "shepherd," "an' a shepherd looks after 'is sheep."

How much of this testimony could one believe, coming, as it were, from mentally retarded patients? These stories, incidents, and remembrances represented the truth that they clung to. And yet, why should one not believe them? There was the truth of the officials, of the staff and of the professionals; then, there was the truth of those who lived it on the inside, on the Wards.

12.

IT WAS 1964. After five years in the institution, Daisy had a good understanding of the layout of Orillia, of the six remaining Cottages, the Administration Building overlooking the terrace, the Superintendent's Cottage nearby, the old and new Infirmaries, the Children's Dorm to the south, and the Vocational and Occupational Work-Shops, Laundry and Sewing, to which she was now transferred. She even began to acquire some practical knowledge that she appreciated. She would not admit she *enjoyed* Orillia as she was still locked up, but she learned to do four-needle knitting, and even knitted a turtleneck sweater for herself.

Sewing Class was a different matter. It was institutional labour, as Daisy explained to me. "Oh, it was hard on your fingers, pressing all them dome fasteners into hun'reds of babbies' bibs and rompers. And then cutting out them straightjackits, the canvas so hard to get the needle through on the sewing machine."

The Singer sewing machines stood in a row in the long, dusty, and high-ceilinged room at the rear of the Administration Building. The girls sat in a line guiding the material through and peddling with their feet. First you laid the coarse, stiff cloth on the cutting board over a pattern of thick beige paper, and then you cut with the shears around the blue dotted line hoping to God you did it straight, said Daisy. You got it from Mrs. Jebb if the pattern tore.

"But Daisy," I cried, butting into the story. "You mean to say they made you *sew your own straightjackets?*"

Daisy blinked, then her face broke into a slow smile. "Yeah. Well, fancy that. Oh yes, that was very bad of them." Daisy continued. "There was boys in Laundry, so I liked that. They lifted all the heavy, wet sheets and stuff outa the machines with their muscles and into the big dryers; it was heavy work on account of the wetness. And we did the sorting an' folding. And we'd sneak off."

Daisy had also now realized how easy it was to evade the staff. That, in fact, the nurse's aides and assistants she had once so feared were busy, overworked, often fearful of the patients, and hardly able to control the hundreds of girls and women on all the Wards and in Day Rooms or wherever they had space. By the mid-1960s, thousands of patients — roughly 2,600 to 2,800 residents of all ages, with varying medical needs — lived in Orillia. Daisy was aware of the long lines of people being shepherded from place to place by older patients standing in for the attendants and nurse's aides who were too occupied and distracted to move the lines back and forth between the Wards/Cottages, the school, and the workshops.

A new building, called the Pavilion, was being built on the grounds after Pierre Berton's article had appeared in the *Toronto Star* and they had torn down Cottage L and Cottage B. It was to be named after a former superintendent, Dr. Bernard T. McGhie who had been Superintendent of the institution when it was Ontario Hospital, before it was renamed Ontario Hospital School in 1936. He had been Medical Superintendent from 1928 to 1930 and was now Deputy Minister of Health. He had once said that the "mentally retarded differed only in degree and not in kind from the normal and superior," something Daisy may have agreed with in her own way. More bulldozers and crews of workmen flooded the grounds. Wooden forms were laid out and once again poured with concrete. The nurses and attendants had to hurry their groups of patients, excited by the flurry of activity that surrounded them, around the grounds for safety.

Daisy put it to me succinctly. In the mid-1960s, "There was just too many of us."

So she and Marcie easily sneaked into the Socials on Saturday night in the gym, called the "ballroom" though they certainly were not on any Honour Roll, but who was checking?

"*One two three o'clock, four o'clock rock!*" Some of the kinder nursing aides had brought albums from home. They were expected to square dance as directed by the counsellors, or waltz as best as they could master such complicated steps and manoeuvres. But the kids preferred the new music. The girls were dressed in bobby socks, twinsets, and flared tartan skirts of the 1950s — "best" clothes set aside by staff for such an occasion. Oh, it was wonderful to be in nice modern clothes, thanks to some of the kinder staff who had fought the administration on behalf of the girls for these "modern" clothes. The boys were dressed in "good" pants and open neck shirts, their hair slicked to the side.

Marcie hurled herself about the floor with Steve, jiving and twisting, and soon others were following. Daisy was being swung almost over Eddie's shoulders in a move he said was the new "rock 'n' roll." Soon others were jumping around the floor, leaving their Orange Crush and potato chips to the side.

"Incorrigible!" Nurse Chalmers tried to call out to them across the floor.

"One, two, three o'clock, four o'clock, rock / Five, six, seven o'clock, eight o'clock, rock / Nine, ten, eleven o'clock, twelve o'clock, rock / We're gonna rock around the clock tonight."

This was a good time at Orillia. Even the attendants and nurse aides smiled. There were side tables piled high with cookies and soft drinks and potato chips, nothing too stimulating. Some of the girls got easily excitable. "Dances provide a admirable means to work off excess unwanted stimulations and prevent masturbation in the male population," Mr. Downey, a Superintendent in the 1920s, had once declared, as Nurse Chalmers remembered. She was serving soft drinks and keeping an ever watchful eye. What was that Daisy Lumsden doing throwing herself about the floor like that? She was supposed to be in the Day Room watching television.

It was the same at Sunday service in the gym the next morning. Daisy and Marcie Evans were giggling and winking at boys across the aisle, paying absolutely no attention to Army Chaplain Officer Dinsmore of the Salvation Army up at the podium. As Miss James in the school had said of Daisy: "She has found friends."

Thousands of quietly behaved patients with solemn faces listened as Army Chaplain Officer Dinsmore started them in prayer, some of the older patients rocking and moaning in their chairs. The Superintendent and his family sat up front, and the aides and attendants stood against the walls or sat near the aisles. While the Orillia Band played, the voices of the choir in plangent tones carried out beyond the shatterproof windows: *"I'll be a sunbeam for Jesus and shine the whole day through..."*

Army Chaplain Officer Dinsmore, dressed in his dark uniform with gold Army stripes, cleared his throat and urged them to love each other as

Christ loved them, and to live lives "that were ever pleasing in His sight."

"Yeah, right!" snarled Daisy later, back in the dorm.

"Where was Salvation Army when I was left in this place?" she had cried loudly — too loudly. "I was just a kid, I wasn' even menserating. I was terrified, I didn' know where I was or why I was here," she ranted. "'No ponytails!' they says. No lipstick, no earrings, no jew'lry at all, no nail polish, nothing!" screamed Daisy. "This is worse 'n' jail!"

Clearly this girl was out of control. An aide signalled another to get Nurse Chalmers. Nurse Chalmers took in Daisy's flushed cheeks and lipsticked mouth (against the rules of the Sabbath) and her careless, "sexy" attire. Daisy had certainly precluded any hope of ever being Dining-Room Monitor, she said sternly, a privilege she knew Daisy had always coveted.

"Who wants to be a fucking monitor anyway?" Daisy flashed back. "You don't git no money for it. Is just a way to suck us into doin' all the frigging work."

Nurse Chalmers stiffened. This was dangerous. The success of the entire work system of the hospital depended on the labour of willing patients striving to earn certain privileges and rewards, believing it an honour to progress from level to level. Girls were looking at the staff, confused. How much did they understand the significance of Daisy Lumsden's words? There was a sudden shriek from somebody, somewhere, then a thump on the floor. Someone was being dragged to the Punishment Room or, as it was sometimes called, the Side Room.

Daisy went on recklessly. "I was just a kid an' I was sent to Cottage L ter help out among all them naked old women. I could of bin stabbed with a knife in that utility cupboard, nobody care! I had to do all the fucking shitty work while the aides sat aroun' frigging smoking an' taking breaks," she shouted passionately.

"Hey, this one's got a mouth on 'er!" cried an aide.

"Watch yer language!" added another.

"So, what you gonna do about it?" Daisy challenged.

"You're goin' in the cooler!" said Nurse Chalmers through pursed lips.

And that was not all, noted Nurse Chalmers. One wintry morning Nurse Turnbull discovered Daisy Lumsden upstairs smoking in bed with Marcie Evans (an unsavoury girl who had once worked the streets of Toronto), instead of scrubbing the floors of the Infirmary: "Caught in bed by Miss Turnbull with Marcie Evans (Case #4960).

They had claimed it was cold," Nurse Chalmers reported on Daisy's Ward record.

It was time for a conference on Daisy Lumsden.

There was no doubt in the minds of Dr. Serson, Dr. Vera Binnington (who had been consulted on the case), Mr. Gooding, the hospital psychologist, Nurse Chalmers, and Head Nurse Tait (Ward O-1 and O-2, in regular contact with the patient) that something had to be done about Daisy Lumsden. Prior to the visit home in Toronto from December 21, 1963 to January 2, 1964, Daisy Lumsden had been a pleasant, quiet, and cooperative girl, particular about her appearance. She enjoyed life in Ward O-3 and benefited from the academic school program. The "Social Reaction" section of her Patient Progress Sheet cited her as being accepted as an equal by her peers, not quarrelsome or cruel, and showing no tendency to elope. "Cooperative and clean about herself" — the highest praise.

On her return to Orillia, as noted in her Clinical Record, she had appeared at once to Nurse Chalmers as "emotionally upset, exhausted, and withdrawn." Nurse Chalmers here wanted it recorded that it had been against her advice as Supervisor that Lumsden be allowed home on probation as the history of the entire family "left a lot to be desired." Nurse Chalmers, suspicious, had sent Lumsden to the Infirmary to see Dr. Serson.

At this point in the discussion, Dr. Serson, supported by Dr. Binnington and Mr. Gooding, referred to certain sensitive details in the Clinical Record, now passed around and read by all. During the course of the routine physical examination that took place after Daisy had returned to Orillia, Daisy had burst into tears, claiming that her mother — a terrible woman — had removed Daisy's clothes after drugging her, and then paid her boyfriend to have sexual intercourse with her. This happened frequently over the Christmas visit. The above statement had been repeated by Daisy in the presence of witnesses, specifically Superintendent Dr. MacLean Houze, who had taken over as Superintendent after Dr. Hamilton in 1961.

Since then, Daisy had been removed from school as a result of her sexual advances to the boys in the halls and in the basement, actions that could no longer be tolerated, explained Miss Tewson, the teacher. She had "reached the end of her academic ability," wrote Miss Tewson, even though Daisy's school report cards up to then had shown 70+ marks.

Daisy had been promoted in only three years from Group 20 through 22, 24, 28 and recently to Group 32, and she had achieved Grade Five level in arithmetic and writing. She was now transferred to Cottage M for older female patients, and relegated to Laundry and other Ward Work, which included sewing and knitting, for Vocational Training. Of course, it went without saying that Daisy would no longer be considered for probation, or be released into the community. She was incapable of earning a livelihood at this time.

As well, the parents, particularly the mother, Ella Lumsden (*née* Hewitt), a former patient, were a continual source of aggravation, with their repeated interference, constant phone calls, and threats both verbal and written. Something would have to be done about them, too.

"If the parents were only to desist in these respects and be cooperative, we feel that Daisy would have a chance to complete sufficient training here and enjoy what Orillia has to offer and even perhaps be placed at some future time back in the community," remarked Dr. Binnington.

There was also the question of her friendship with Marcie Evans. Details were given.

It was generally agreed that Daisy Lumsden was now a moody girl who caused a lot of disturbance on the Ward and at work, and had overt homosexual tendencies.

"She also cannot be trusted where boys are concerned."

Recommended: Mellaril, 100 mg. daily for the "homosexual tendencies," duly recorded in her Clinical Record. The drug Mellaril (Thioridazine), an antipsychotic, was cited by Sandoz Pharmaceuticals as "assisting the physician in the control of the problem child," stated Dr. Serson. "*Mellaril, the safe, effective tranquilizing agent for agitation, excitation, hyperactivity, nervousness, tension, anxiety, temper tantrums, belligerence, sleep disorders, behaviour problems in school, at home, and at play...*" went the Sandoz promotion. Of course, even at beginning doses of 100 mg. the Mellaril medication would have to be monitored regularly since one side effect was affected eye vision. Daisy's eyes were henceforth to be checked out regularly at Dr. Fournier's Optometry Clinic, who recorded "eyes healthy."

Meanwhile, a caution was put on Daisy Lumsden's file: "NO VISITORS."

"Wha's this for? I ain't swallerin' nuthin'!" Daisy trembled in line after breakfast — "meds" time — in the O-2 dining hall. A row of girls stood quietly after their porridge, walking one by one to the nurse at the top of the dining room. A table containing vials of pills of varying colours — blue, yellow, and white — stood in rows with the girls' names attached.

"Open. Swallow."

A tumbler of water was proffered by the monitor. Daisy shook her head and clamped her mouth tight. "Enough of that Lumsden. Or else!" said Nurse Chalmers.

"Hold her down, Esme."

A straightjacket was brought from the Day Room.

"Na-a-a," cried Daisy, at once terrified, opening her mouth wide.

Nurse Chalmers winked at Esme Dunn, a nurse-in-training. "Always works."

13.

THERE HAD BEEN THREATENING PHONE CALLS from that Mrs. Lumsden again, down in Toronto, claiming the institution was a drug house and accusing them of forced labour. Where *did* she get her information? wondered Dr. Houze, Superintendent. On September 9, 1964, Dr. Binnington had reported in the Duty Book that Mrs. Lumsden was the only one who gave any trouble regarding her daughter Daisy not being able to go out of the Cottage. "Is seeing her lawyer."

Dr. Bartley, on shift October 10, 1964, had noted in the Duty Book that Mrs. Ella Lumsden, mother of Daisy Lumsden (Case #65043) of Cottage M, had phoned at six p.m. and made disparaging remarks about the Hospital. "She did not sound as though she was of good intelligence."

Of greater concern was an incident recorded in the Duty Book by Dr. James. A lawyer's secretary had phoned to say that Daisy could go home. No mention of was made of who the "lawyer" was. She had finally hung up with the statement that "Daisy and her clothes had better be ready in the morning." Cottage M was notified of the parents' (presumed) intention.

And now this letter. Dr. Houze, who had taken over as Superintendent after Dr. Hamilton, stared in disbelief at the document in hand. Mrs. Lumsden — good God! — had somehow got herself a lawyer in Toronto, a Charles Farquar, Q.C., on Bloor Street, who had actually issued an Indication against Dr. Houze and the Hospital, and a writ of *habeas corpus*, claiming the Lumsdens were being denied custody of their child and that Daisy was being held unlawfully against her will.

One had to tread carefully with such threats, and not necessarily dismiss them, keeping in mind, of course, that Mrs. Lumsden was an imbecile and former patient. Nevertheless, she could be dangerous. She had already complained — the nerve of the woman — to the CAS of Toronto *and* the Juvenile and Family Court in Toronto, and even the local MPP for York, Donald MacDonald, a member of the CCF and dangerous.

Dr. Houze read once again, in disbelief, the Indication. Mr. Farquar, on behalf of his clients, Ella and Ernest Lumsden, wanted the release of their daughter, Daisy, and her return home.

> I understand that previous requests by Mr. and Mrs. Lumsden have been rejected by you without any good and sufficient reason, except that the patient appears to be "boy crazy." I am enclosing a Direction signed in this office by my clients authorizing you to make a full disclosure to me of such reasons as you might assign to any court..."

The Indication went on to direct that Daisy be discharged from the Hospital commencing December 21, 1964, or alternatively be permitted to visit her parents over Christmas, 1964.

> The Indication advised that the Medical Superintendent, Dr. Houze, of Ontario Hospital School, Orillia, provide a detailed report of the mental and physical condition of their daughter, and this shall be your good and sufficient authority for so doing.

A copy was being forwarded to the Honourable Matthew Dymond, Ontario Minister of Health.

The letter was signed: "Ernest Lumsden," followed by a scrawled, ill-formed "X" by Ella Lumsden. Written next to this dubious signature was a statement from a witness concerning the "X," and Ella Lumsden's mental capacity: "The said document having been read to her and she having appeared to fully understand the same."

Dr. Houze knew a careful response was required, especially considering Mrs. Lumsden's entanglement with that troublemaking Donald MacDonald down in Queen's Park.

He took up his pen. Charles Farquar, Q.C., needed to understand the true identity of his clients, Mr. and Mrs. Lumsden, both designated mental defectives. According to the records, Ella Lumsden was an "Imbecile" (I.Q. 45), and Ernest Lumsden had been certified "Backward."

Mrs. Lumsden herself was a former patient at the hospital from 1936 to 1939, and was noted to have a mental age of six years old at the time. As a result, she could hardly, Dr. Houze pointed out, be capable of providing proper care and supervision of a teenage girl like Daisy, whose mentality was only somewhat superior to her mother's.

Moreover — here Dr. Houze hesitated, but decided to proceed despite the word "CONFIDENTIAL" stamped on the file — this was a crisis: Mrs. Lumsden had actually sexually abused her daughter, Daisy, during Daisy's probationary visit home over Christmas, 1963, when the patient was age only sixteen. She had made her daughter "strip and have sexual intercourse" with her boyfriend while the father was at work on a night shift. Under the circumstances, Daisy expressed no desire to ever return to the parental home. In fact, concluded Dr. Houze, on no account would the Hospital ever release Daisy Lumsden to her parents. She was better off in Orillia.

Mr. Farquar's reply was, understandably, more subdued and conciliatory. He realized he had been put in an awkward position concerning the Lumsdens, which implied a certain betrayal of confidence on Dr. Houze's part. Mr. and Mrs. Lumsden were, of course, unaware that private records had been disclosed to him (the Lumsdens no doubt had little idea there *were* files about their small lives and histories) though it was obvious their permission as "subnormals" had never actually been requisite. Mr. Farquar was not sure of the ethical implications of all this as yet.

"The task of advising the parents of the child is not an easy one," he wrote to Dr. Houze cautiously, as an opener, thinking of the paragraph of Dr. Houze's letter concerning the parents' imbecility and sexual indiscretions. "I realize it would be inadvisable or even dangerous for me to disclose some or all of this information..."

He pressed on. "However, having the same on my file would assist me in conscientiously advising the parents who have been sent to me by an Officer of a Court in Toronto. These parents have paid me a small retainer, which I cannot return to them without arousing their suspicions."

He concluded by asking if Dr. Houze would be kind enough to at least allow the release of Daisy Lumsden home for the Christmas holidays or for a visit with her parents.

Dr. Houze's reply was now swift and confident. Even a visit would be determined by himself alone as Superintendent, and he deemed this not possible, not ever.

He wrote decisively now providing further details of the Lumsden family history — ten surviving mentally deficient children on Mr. Lumsden's side, and eleven on Mrs. Lumsden's side. It was impossible to release Daisy to such relatives, especially now that she'd been promoted to the probationary Ward where she was happy, and starting to do well in her new Training Programme, which included Laundry and Sewing.

However, it being the Christmas season, it was Daisy's own wish to meet with her parents in the visitor's room of Cottage M, but this would take place in the presence of guards, he added. Who knew what these Lumsdens would do? There had been anonymous calls and threats to blow up the Cottage obviously at Mrs. Lumsden's instigation.

Dr. Houze added one final, surely telling comment, powerful in its implication:

> We have over 500 children on our waiting list who are most anxious to get in, and we are constantly going through our list in the hopes that parents or relatives will assume responsibility of looking after their children. However, we also feel that we must protect the child being placed in an undesirable situation. Trusting this will explain our position regarding this girl.

Dr. Houze spoke sincerely. Since they had changed regulations to allow children into Orillia under age six, the population had increased further, putting stress on the staff. Parents were desperate to have their child admitted — one father in Dr. Hamilton's time had even offered to bring in his own bed!

The annual statistics of Orillia's Ontario Hospital School were only too self-evident: in 1950, for instance, the population of the institution had been 2,400 and the number of patients discharged had been but 46; and, in 1960, out of 2,810 patients in residence, only 109 had been discharged (52 had died). In fact, by 1964, despite Pierre Berton's fateful exposé in the *Star,* the anticipated exodus of patients withdrawn by parents and the Toronto Children's Aid Society (which obviously must not have believed the accusations), had not taken place. In fact, the population had increased, bringing the total to its greatest of all time — 2,916 — a telling number that demonstrated just how many patients had been long disconnected from family who had handed them over or given them up as "wards of the Crown" and of the CAS of Toronto, never to appear in their children's lives again. Some patients were lucky enough to be visited regularly and faithfully by their parents or guardians and taken home for weekends and holidays, as there certainly were set visiting hours. Others were sometimes taken by kind attendants and nurses to their own homes in town for overnight and weekend stays, but most, as Dr. Houze knew only too well, were left to live out their lives in the Wards and Cottages of the hospital world that was theirs. As Dr. Dymond, Ontario's Minister of Health, cried in the documentary made of the Hospital in 1960, *One On Every Street,* these "unfortunates" were to be "pitied in the name of our Lord Jesus Christ."

So, it was not all the more remarkable that Ella and Ernest Lumsden—designated as an "imbecile" and as "backward" — pleaded for their daughter Daisy's release.

"I'm stupid," Ella Lumsden had once confided to Daisy. Ernest Lumsden, a modest and humble man, was always recognized by the officials who dealt with him as a reliable, "good father," to the best of his limited ability. They were a nuisance, of course, particularly Mrs. Lumsden, constantly interfering with the Training Programme in Orillia: "If only the parents would desist..." wrote one exasperated psychologist at the hospital.

But the Lumsdens persisted in making the journey, arduous for them up old Highway 11, arriving by bus at the hospital, all dusty and worn, petitioning for Daisy's release. "We wants 'er back, is our daughter," they said. This was a mystery of love and need for Daisy, despite everything about them, their failures, their mental defectiveness, their betrayals and weaknesses; they wanted Daisy in their lives, and would not forsake her to Orillia; perhaps, the heart of the story.

Yet never once remarked on in the records.

14.

THE LUMSDENS WERE GRANTED A VISIT on December 23, 1964, as was their legal right, for one hour in the afternoon in the presence of Dr. Gallagher, Supervisor Nurse Bagley, and a guard. Smoking was prohibited; who knew what Mrs. Lumsden might do with matches?

Daisy was consequently brought downstairs and encouraged to repeat her story. One could only imagine Daisy's shame, perhaps, and confusion enclosed in that room with the doctor who had examined her, and her mother. Mr. and Mrs. Lumsden looked excited, surprised, at the sight of Daisy in a new dress.

"You growed a real lady now, Daisy!" cried Mr. Lumsden shyly, embracing Daisy who at once began to cry, "Dada! Oh, Dada!"

Dr. Houze wrote triumphantly to Mr. Farquar of the visit, citing Dr. Gallagher's report that Daisy had stated in front of her father and mother that it was her own wish that she not go home for Christmas and that she did not wish to go home *at any time*. When asked why, she had stated that when home on a previous occasion, her mother had told her that she must have intercourse with mother's boyfriend. Daisy said that out of fear she had allowed this to take place. The father admitted that he had had knowledge of this fact. Mr. Lumsden was "meek as a lamb," in spite of what he had said he would do when he came up there. They were allowed to visit with Daisy for one hour in the visiting room in Cottage M.

"My father said it was a terrible thing she done to me and he was mad as hell," said Daisy loyally to me, forty-five years later. She would always stay loyal to her father.

"And I said to my husbant on my wedding night I'm sorry I'm not a virgin for you Joe, and he said, 'I forgive you, it wasn't your fault.'"

Mr. Farquar, Q.C., responded before Christmas with a piece of information of his own: a note written by Daisy to her grandfather, Henry Hewitt. She had passed it secretly to her father during the visit when the guard was not looking. And he had slipped it into his pocket — dear, meek Mr. Lumsden, trusted and esteemed. The note was brief, full of unanswered questions. Had she written to Henry Hewitt — "gran'dad" — because she knew by now he was the only one who could read and was therefore powerful, the one who might enable her release and might possibly take her in?

Dear Gran'dad,
Just a few lines to say hello. I want to come home.
I can't stand this place. I really mean it this time.
I bet to now.
Love, Daisy.

Christmas Eve, Daisy eloped with Eddie Green, Steve Henderson, and Marcie Evans.

It had not lasted long. "I couldn' keep up with them 'cause I was menserating," Daisy told me. She had forgotten to put pads in her purse. She was doubled up with cramps as the four sped toward Memorial Avenue after supper, owls hooting through the trees that lined the icy lake. It was a cold, crisp Christmas Eve night.

Strains of carols had drifted down as they ran behind the gym: "*Hark the Herald Angels Sing, Glory to the new-born King...*" What would happen? The boys knew how to escape the patrol guards on the grounds. They had planned everything. They were to catch a bus in town to Toronto. Boys had more freedom than girls, Daisy knew. They could go around the grounds, and had passes into town if they got Good Behaviour.

Eddie and Steve had already dropped bags out of the second floor window at the back of their cottage. The bags contained a change of clothes (institutional clothes would be a sure giveaway in town) and some bread and cake they had pushed in their pockets during supper. The girls had grabbed their smokes in the basement Smoking Room and sneaked out through a side door by the canteen at the end of the tramway. Smoking was allowed for a half hour after supper. They had met up with the boys behind the school door at the back of the Administration Building. They could hear the Orillia Band striking up, and faint cheers and clapping as they kept running up the road between tall trees. The Superintendent's house was to the right, then the darkness. The sky glittered with stars. The town lay fifteen kilometres somewhere down the road to their right. The boys knew.

Daisy fell as they reached the road — and freedom — her purse rolling down the culvert, her smokes and makeup and a dinner roll tumbling out. She got down on her hands and knees in the dark, fumbling to find everything, fearing the patrols. Marcie and the boys kept going as had been agreed: "Each fer 'isself." Daisy crammed everything into her bag and began stumbling down Memorial Avenue, the boys and Marcie distant shadows. On the other side of the road loomed farm buildings, including the barn where dead babies were buried, their ghosts hovering in the night air, alive.

Bewildered, she turned back toward the institution, stumbling down the drive, clutching her purse in the dark.

"There she is!"

"Who goes there?"

What happened next is vouched for only by Daisy, sworn on the Bible at her insistence. A flashlight suddenly appeared around the corner of the Nurses' Residence, Building 47. It lit up her face. "It's the girl," someone said.

"Where are the others? We know there's four of yer." One of the attendants shook her roughly by the arm.

"Take your frigging hands off of me!"

"Watch your mouth, you little bitch, or we'll clean it out for you."

She was escorted to the Superintendent's Office, hands clamped on each shoulder, where Dr. Houze, Nurse Biggs, Nurse Supervisor from Ward "O-2," and Nurse Chalmers of O-3, grim-faced, were waiting. Each nurse attendant and male attendant on duty at the time would be penalized and lose pay over this. "Here's one of 'em, sir."

Dr. Houze wrote something down in the Minute Book. "You're a very foolish girl and now you must face the consequences." The attendants took Daisy away.

"Where are the others?" Nurse Biggs cried when they were back in the Ward. "Tell us!"

"Dunno. 'Ow the frigging 'ell should I know?" said Daisy sulkily. She wasn't going to squeal on Marcie and the boys.

Nurse Biggs slapped her hard.

"Bitch!" cried Daisy.

Nurse Biggs shook her again.

"I ain't done nothing bad. I can live where I like. I'm not a Ward no more."

"That's what you think, smartass."

"Well, I came back, didn' I, you old sods."

She was dragged to the bath area, where an old tub stood in the corner. "Where's the others you run off with? Answer us! We know you know."

"Take yer friggin' hands off of me! I don't know nothing. I ain't going in there!"

Nurse Carswell was already running the water, ice-cold, and Nurse Chalmers had brought in the sheets. "This'll take the mouth off her," one of them said.

"Out of control..."

Daisy struggled. She dug her teeth into Nurse Biggs' arm. "Watch them teeth, Ethel! Little tom-cat!"

They had stripped her down. "I was menserating but it didn't make no difference," said Daisy, angry at the memory. Her belt and pad were pulled down; her brassiere yanked off. She was submerged in the tub "for hours," she later insisted.

"Hold her down, Ethel!" said Nurse Biggs. Nurse Carswell had torn up the sheet in strips, ready, Daisy recalled, agitated at the memory.

"They tortured me. I was rolled up tight in ice-wet sheets of cloth. I couldn' breathe I was so cold. They put me in a ice-cold tub of ice water — the cold pack treatment they calls it, an' me menserating. They didn' care."

"Where's Marcie Evans and Eddie Green and Steve Henderson from C? Where they going to?" The icy strips of cloth tightened as they held her down in the water.

"To T'ronto," Daisy sobbed. "On th' bus from th' station in town."

The nurses looked grimly at each other. Daisy was hauled to her bed; her arms pushed into a canvas straightjacket. An attendant pulled the laces tightly at the back and knotted them. Daisy was weeping as she lay on her front, her arms twisted behind her. She was left on her bed in that position for the entire night.

"That'll learn 'er," someone said.

She was eighteen.

How much of this was to be believed in the confusion of memory? Daisy would not have been immersed for "hours" in icy water. The time recommended for "water treatment," or hydrotherapy, according to the *Nurses' Handbook* was twenty minutes.

Hydrotherapy was a common therapy used on mental patients who were agitated, violent, and out of control, as a means to calm them down and prevent them from hurting themselves. Contrary to expectation, being wrapped tightly in cold wet sheets produced heat in the body and a dangerous rise in temperature that could cause convulsions if not monitored. Twenty years after the incident, the *Mental Health-Psychiatric Nursing Textbook*, written by nurses Cornelia Kelly Beck, Ruth Parmelee Rawlins and Sophronia R. Williams (and published by C. V. Moseby Publishing Company in 1984) cautioned student nurses that "wet pack" treatment was not to be used as a "punishment," which surely begged the question.

Yet why should Daisy *not* be believed? There was the truth of the record-keeper, and the truth of the patient. Nurse Chalmers had summed up the entire "elopement" episode in the Clinical Record in one sentence: "December 24, 1964. Eloped from Smoking Room during Christmas Concert; was returned later."

Ella Lumsden visited her daughter after the New Year. She had known at once. "What the 'ell they done to you?" she cried out in the visiting parlour. "They got you drugs!" Her mother had pushed her face close to Daisy's. It was a garish face, with too much powder and that gash of lipstick. So she *had* cared then.

"Oh, she knew they'd drugged me, I was all drugged up stupid," Daisy told me, her voice shifting, taking on Ella Lumsden's aggressive tone.

Her mother had whispered harshly for the guard not to hear. "Stick 'em up your cheek nex' time, don' swaller 'em, Daisy. Next time I come you pass 'em to me, secret-like."

"Speak up over there!" called the guard.

It was here Daisy recalled saying: "Can't I frigging talk to my own mother without you guys pushing in?"

"That th' secret," her mother had whispered. Daisy had no idea what the pills actually were, only that they were called "meds." She had no knowledge at the time that she was taking Mellaril, only that she was "drugged." She had not been told; it was not for her to know.

She was to pretend to swallow them, but push the pill with her tongue up into her cheek, and take it out later and hide it in something under her mattress. Keep them for her mother, Ella had whispered again. She promised to come back.

Ella Lumsden would then take the pills to the "Clarke Ins'tute of Psych'atry." And to her MPP, Donald MacDonald.

15.

MR. FARQUAR CHANGED TACK. For the first time, Daisy's right *as a human being* to choose where she wanted to live and with whom, was addressed. She had turned nineteen in 1965.

Charles Farquar was well aware that society's attitude toward the mentally retarded had been changing, not just in Toronto but around the world. Ever since the United Nations' Universal Declaration on Human Rights in 1948, there had been a gradual awareness of what constituted human rights among the public at large. In 1965, aware that public opinion was veering against institutionalization, the government had created a Mental Retardation Services Branch in the Ontario Department of Health, under the direction of Don Zarfas who had grown up in the Orillia institution where his father had been the steward under Dr. Horne. Zarfas was a fine psychiatrist, revered by parents. That same year, Dr. John Fotheringham, head of the Mental Retardation Outpatient Clinic on Grosvenor Street, part of the Toronto Psychiatric Hospital, was also looking at the effects of "home" versus "institutional" care on retarded children in a study called 'The Toronto Study," which covered the years 1965-66. Mr. Farquar knew that its purpose was to compare a "community" group of parents who chose to keep their mentally retarded children at home, honouring their right to be raised in their community, and an "institutional" group of parents who had put their children in Orillia.

It was an initial important step in professionals recognizing children's right to be with their parents at home and not be institutionalized, Mr. Farquar realized, something he could possibly cite in Daisy's favour. Some parents were now daring to question the validity of big institutions like Orillia and had formed an association to oppose government policy. Parents' rebellion had been set in motion, like most great movements, by an inconspicuous event. A grandmother in Toronto, Victoria Glover, had submitted a letter to the editor of the *Toronto Daily Star* back in 1949, which had electrified its readers. Claiming to be writing on behalf of "all backward children," Mrs. Glover pleaded for the government to provide a school for them in the city as Orillia was "always full."

"*If these children can be taught something at Orillia, why cannot a day school be put at their disposal? I am sure their mother would gladly pay for their transportation to and from school. After all, they are paying taxes for other more fortunate children's schooling*," she reasoned. She said she spoke for parents who wanted to keep their children at home "*from a sense of faith and hope in a merciful providence.*" She had pleaded that these were "*real parents, only asking a little aid and encouragement to shoulder their own heavy burden. God bless them...*"

The challenge had swept Ontario in an inexplicable way. The whole point was that Mrs. Glover's grandson had an I.Q. below 50 and was supposed to be up in Orillia. Only children with an I.Q. above 50 were eligible for the special education provided in Auxiliary Classes in the public schools, even though to Mr. Farquar this seemed arbitrary. Why *50*?

Soon, parents inspired by Mrs. Glover's letter, met in Toronto and began their own classes. Those indefatigable mothers started up a little nursery school in 1952 for their retarded toddlers in an old Victorian house at 46 Willcocks Street in Toronto. Miss Ethel Teasdale was hired as principal and teacher; she lived on the third floor. One year later, the Beverley Street School in Toronto opened its doors for mentally retarded children who lived at home, to provide them with education and training at their individual level. Mr. Farquar recalled the great stir this had caused; imagine parents opening a school for their retarded children! Parents out in Mississauga, beyond the Toronto area, followed suit later in the 1950s, converting an old house on Fifth Line with their own hands into a little school for their retarded children, which they called 'Red Oaks.'

More significant, Mr. Farquar realized, was the parents' rejection of help from the provincial Department of Health. They were putting aside the old "medical model," demanding their children be educated and serviced not under the Ministry of Health but under the Department of "Education," something that had been blocked in the early part of the century by Dr. Helen MacMurchy, Inspector for the Feeble-Minded in Ontario from 1905-1919, who had wanted the treatment of mental defectives to be solely under the aegis of the medical profession. They were not to achieve this until 1973 when the Hon. Robert Welch, Provincial Secretary for Social Development, issued a policy document on mental retardation that affirmed that retardation was a social and educational issue, and *not* a medical problem. Ultimate triumph would come in 1980 when the conservative government would pass the *Education Amendment Act*, or Bill 82, that guaranteed that school boards would provide special education programs for students with special needs. Irrevocably, the care of the "feeble-minded," now called the "mentally retarded," would pass from the Ministry of Health to the new Ministry of Community and Social Services, commonly referred to as COMSOC.

But these advancements were far off, something that Mr. Farquar only sensed. He was aware however that The Parents' Council for Retarded Children had been formed in 1948 and as had the Ontario Association for Retarded Children in 1950s (now called the Canadian Association for Community Living), followed by a Canadian National Association for Retarded Children in 1958, a year before Daisy had entered Orillia. These organizations had even begun a campaign to close institutions, putting out the slogan: "Placement Is Not the Only Solution." It was unprecedented. Mr. Farquar wondered if Daisy's parents had been influenced by this, and important people around them may have known about it too, such as Donald MacDonald, leader of the CCF, to whom the Lumsdens had turned to for help. No doubt MacDonald was aware of these parents' movements and associations, all of which the NDP would support.

But by the early 1960s , the parents had split into two opposing groups: the "community parents" fighting for closures of institutions and services at home, and a more conservative group dubbed the "institutional parents" who wanted their children retained in smaller institutions but with improved services and staffing. They had put out a slogan of their own in 1962: "Bricks Have A Soul — Staff and Volunteers." Daisy was in Cottage O at the time. Mr. Farquar wondered what Daisy would have had to say to that.

Of course, "Parent Power" was still but a small grassroots movement, Mr. Farquar realized, not yet given much credence by the government or administrators in Orillia. Despite parents' petitions that no more large institutions be built, the medical profession still believed they were the best place for mentally retarded people. Even Dr. Matthew Dymond, Ontario's Minister of Health, while sympathetic to parents' grievances, was still pro-institution, just smaller ones. Dr. Clarence Hincks, head of the Canadian National Committee for Mental Hygiene (CNCMH), concurred. The problem was the different concepts of "smaller." In some provinces this meant no more than 20 patients in a given facility; in others it meant a 500-600 bed institution (as opposed to Orillia that housed over 2,000).

And there was that social worker, John Brown, the Director of Warrendale, a set of group homes for troubled adolescents in the Toronto area. He was another agitator, according to Dr. Houze, and a bit of a crackpot, in his support of parents. Mr. Brown had once called psychiatry "the most vicious profession," and accused the Department of Health of running a "Children's Services Mafia" that passed children from professional to professional through what he called "the Toronto children's pipeline" in the most cynical way. Restraints, beatings, and isolation, he claimed, were "the order of the day." Mr. Brown believed in something called "unconditional love"; it was rumoured that teenagers in the group homes he ran out in Etobicoke were encouraged to suck on baby bottles — Good Lord! — as needed. But John Brown also believed in parents' involvement and empowerment, and returning children to their homes as soon as possible, something the public supported. He had been amazingly successful in his approach. And, as Mr. Farquar well knew, that was what counted.

Mr. Farquar therefore requested of Dr. F. C. Crawford-Jones, the new acting Superintendent, a handsome man apparently well-liked by staff and patients, who had been appointed following Dr. Houze's recent sudden death, that Daisy be allowed to come to his office in Toronto to discuss the matter of her release in private. "She is now well past the age of sixteen years and is, in fact, nineteen years of age and has the right to determine with whom and where she shall live, where she shall be employed, what religion she shall practise, etc." Daisy's parents and grandfather Henry Hewitt were willing to bring her to Toronto and return her to Orillia, explained Mr. Farquar. Henry Hewitt had kept in touch with his daughter Ella and granddaughter Daisy, despite Daisy's long committal in Orillia — by now six years — her entire childhood and adolescence spent in shelters and institutions. Yet their bond was intact, a recognition that Daisy was of his blood.

"I insist upon seeing Daisy alone in my private office for the purpose of obtaining her instructions. My instructions (from Mr. and Mrs. Lumsden) are to advise you that suitable accommodation has been arranged for this girl in her parents' home," Mr. Farquar said.

Mr. Lumsden now claimed he had a three-bedroom apartment in new Regent Park on Gerrard Street, which had been built around the old site, Sumach Street, where the Hewitts had lived for decades. It was occupied by only himself and Mrs. Lumsden. He had a steady job as a warehouseman at Smith's Transport where he'd been working for four months at wages of $90 a week, and would be able to support Daisy.

Mr. Farquar concluded on a legal note: "As you know, any action brought in this connection must be brought by the parents as 'next friends' of Daisy, who is still an 'infant-at-law.'"

Dr. Crawford-Jones' reply was immediate:

Sir:

The Lumsden home may be "suitable accommodation" but we have to consider the suitability of the overall situation before we can allow a patient to be probated or discharged. This is quite clearly spelled out in the Mental Hospitals Act, Chapter 236 under Part II, paragraph 7; and Part III, paragraph 14; Part IV, paragraph 25.... I would like also to draw your attention to Chapter 36, Part II, paragraph II (1)(d) which can be invoked if there continues to be interference by any persons that is detrimental to the patient's well-being."

Charles Farquar, Q.C.

Dear Dr. Crawford-Jones,

There has never been any doubt in my mind as to whether or not the Superintendent of an Ontario Hospital may retain a person who has been properly committed as a patient, if, in the opinion of the Superintendent, the patient is still mentally ill. Whether or not such illness exists is, of course, a question of fact and can only be determined on evidence before a Court of competent jurisdiction.

As to my taking instructions from an infant-at-law, there is no statutory or other reason to prevent my doing so.

In my long years of practice I have found that the Courts will always regard the desires of any person over sixteen years of age

> as to his or her place of residence. All of the above is of course, predicated upon the determination of the mental competency of the patient. In the letters on my file, there is no statement made by the late Superintendent Dr. Houze, or by yourself, as to the mental condition of Daisy Lumsden.
>
> I respectfully suggest that such an assessment be made by an independent party.

It was finally agreed that Daisy Lumsden would be brought down to Toronto for an independent assessment at the Toronto Psychiatric Hospital, Surrey Place; the results to be accepted by Dr. Crawford-Jones and his colleagues, and Mr. Farquar and his clients, Mr. and Mrs. Lumsden.

One could but imagine the excitement and delight of the Lumsdens over a bottle of beer in the Winchester that night. "Here's t' Mister Farkar!" Ella laughed, opening her mouth wide. Her lips were painted red, the colour she loved. "Daisy soon be 'ome!"

Dr. Adua Assaf of the Psychology Department in Orillia conducted the Hospital's own tests on Daisy before she left, as agreed between the Superintendent Dr. Crawford-Jones and Toronto Psychiatric Hospital. She found Daisy to be a "dull nineteen-year-old girl with little language, slow in her response." Daisy did not even know, for instance, how many cents made a quarter or a dollar.

She had been unable to detect any absurdities in the "Absurdities" pictures part of the I.Q. tests. But Daisy's idea of "normal" was based on six years of experience on the Wards of Cottage O, and helping out in L. Had Dr. Assaf ever tried to feed and mop up old women and demented old souls in that strange, hell-like place, Ward L-2?

As to Daisy's comprehension, Dr. Assaf noted she had been unable to answer the simple question, "What should you do if you find in the streets of the city a three-year-old boy who was lost from his parents?" What had Daisy, a long-lost child herself, made of such a sad question?

"I was all drugged up," Daisy said to me.

Indeed, no one seemed to consider that Daisy was still on medication — 100 mg. of Mellaril a day for "homosexuality" — and had been for the past two years, which may have affected her responses. She had entered Orillia with an I.Q. of 62, as assessed at the Toronto Psychiatric Hospital in 1959 (and an I.Q. of 66 assessed by the CAS when she was a temporary ward at age five) when the intern, Miss Carlton, had considered Daisy "bright looking" and "full of energy and zest." Dr. Assaf confirmed that day in 1966:

> Daisy Lumsden, age 19:
> I.Q. 42 on the Stanford-Binet scale
> Mental Age: 8.

This was never to change. Orillia was ever to insist on I.Q. 42, placing Daisy forever in the "Imbecile" range.

16.

DAISY SEEMED TO HAVE COME FULL CIRCLE. That May, 1966, she was entering the old Toronto Psychiatric Hospital at Surrey Place where her mother, grandparents, uncles, and aunts had been outpatients thirty-seven years before, in the 1920s and 1930s. Daisy was escorted into the foyer that was filled with boxes and piled furniture. The Toronto Psychiatric Hospital was closing and moving to a new location. "1966, the end of an era," someone said. The old building that was TPH was to be used for a Mental Retardation Centre, to replace the old outpatient clinic on Grosvenor Street. The psychiatric hospital itself was moving to a new building a few blocks west along College Street, to be called the Clarke Institute of Psychiatry, named after Dr. Charles K. Clarke, first Professor of Psychiatry at the University of Toronto in 1908. The new Institute was a streamlined building; the latest in modern architecture. It was eight storeys tall and had rows of oblong windows, so different from the humble TPH with its mellow brick and garden.

Daisy stood with Mrs. Bagley holding her travelling bag tightly; it contained her nightie, toothbrush, comb, one change of underwear, and a new dress made in Sewing Class in Orillia. She was to be placed in the Women's Ward, for at age nineteen she was chronologically a "woman," even if legally she was still deemed an "infant-at-law."

Daisy and her mother Ella always insisted that Daisy was sent to the "Clarke Ins'tute." Daisy's stay lasted six long weeks. She observed the tumult around her of staff in the process of moving from the old psychiatric hospital at Surrey Place to the new Institute on College Street. There was turmoil, tension, and excitement. There were decisions being made and conversations taking place all around her that she could not comprehend. Nurses were trying to determine whether to stay on at the new Retardation Centre or to go; salary scales, pension plans and other benefits were hot topics of discussion. Rooms and corridors were filled with boxes of vital files and records to be transferred to the new offices in the Clarke Institute of Psychiatry (all other records were being stored with the Ontario Ministry of Health). The files of patients past and present were taken in vans along College Street to the new hospital where personnel were ready to file them appropriately. Daisy heard "Clarke Institute" and "The Clarke" over and over — a mystical name full of potent significance, perhaps leading her to believe that was where she now was.

"They was good to me at th' Clarke," she always insisted to me.

Perhaps Ella Lumsden sensed, too, in her instinctive uneducated way, that the "Clarke Institute" was the place of power, the new focus, the place to where you took Daisy's pills, the ones she had been given in Orillia. She had told Daisy to stick them in her cheek and then hide them under her mattress. Ella had a handful that she had collected on a subsequent visit to Orillia.

Daisy had little idea why she had been brought to Toronto. No one in the psychology department in Orillia, nor Superintendent Dr. Crawford-Jones, had thought to consult or inform her. She did not know it was her right to know. She had simply gotten into the van with her bag packed, hoping she was leaving Orillia for good. Dr. Stanley Miles and Dr. Jim Peachy, two psychiatrists, greeted her in the foyer and said they hoped that Daisy would soon settle in and be at ease. Dr. Peachy was young and wore a pink shirt. He had smiled. Daisy had been confused and wanted to cry.

Dr. Miles explained to her she was now in the Toronto Psychiatric Hospital so that she would understand where she was. He even explained where it was: on Surrey Place off of College Street, which was a main street in Toronto that intersected University Avenue, near Queen's Park. It was in the heart of Toronto and its great hospitals, and close to the Ontario Legislature, said Dr. Miles. Though the close proximity of the government at Queen's Park was something that Mrs. Lumsden should perhaps not necessarily know. He had already been warned of the Lumsdens' impending *habeas corpus*. It seemed Mrs. Lumsden had threatened to blow up Cottage O.

He had met Ella Lumsden that very morning in the foyer, accompanied by her husband, Ernest Lumsden, and Mrs. Lumsden's father, Henry

Hewitt, Daisy's grandfather. She had gripped his arm in a disconcerting way in the Admitting area, and thrust some grubby-looking pills into his hand that she said were straight from her daughter Daisy's mouth up in Orillia.

He had tensed, the white pills squished in his palm (he had made a mental note to sanitize his hand), assuring Mrs. Lumsden they would do their best, in keeping with the new kindly approach to patients and their families fostered by Dr. Stokes. Dr. Aldwyn Stokes had succeeded Dr. Clarence Farrar as Director of TPH in 1947. He had wanted a new openness and consideration shown towards patients, for according to Dr. Stokes, the patient was in the "real" world and psychiatrists must be willing to open up and enter that world. Dr. Stokes, of course, was a man ahead of his time, which was what had made TPH such an exciting place to work in.

Dr. Miles had tried, therefore, to ignore Mrs. Lumsden's somewhat dirty, chipped nails splashed red with polish, digging into his arm. For even more disturbing was Mr. Hewitt, Daisy's grandfather, an obviously tough working-class man, now seventy. Mr. Hewitt had cried loudly in an anxious way that he "didn' want no lobot'mies done on 'is gran'daughter, Daisy," a procedure Mr. Hewitt had read about in the newspapers (decades ago, surely). "I dun't want no 'oles drilled in 'er 'ead, Doct'r Miles."

Dr. Miles and Dr. Peachy had quickly drawn this family into a small consulting room off the public hallway. "We won't be drilling any holes in anyone's head here, Mr. Hewitt," Dr. Peachy had assured.

"I know 'bout them lobot'mies done here," Mr. Hewitt had persisted. He had small, hard eyes like bird's eggs.

At once the atmosphere around the coffee table had changed. Indeed, the hospital had been *the* place for leucotomies, or lobotomies as they'd been commonly called, in the 1940s, but were now a thing of the past, cast aside and forgotten. The discovery of Chlorpromazine, a wonder drug for those suffering from schizophrenia, had obviated the need for lobotomy; and it had thus gone out of style.

The Toronto Psychiatric Hospital had been famous at one time for lobotomies. Prospective patients had been brought in from all over the province, patients who, afterwards, had foreheads bearing the telltale stitches, bound in bandages. These patients had received the "Great and Desperate Cures," as psychiatrists once called it, believing it to be so. But TPH had proved too small a hospital for the increasing demand from patients' relatives. Consequently, Dr. Kenneth G. McKenzie had performed hundreds of the operations at Toronto General Hospital. The Toronto Psychiatric Hospital then became a place of recuperation after surgery up until 1949. It was Dr. Stokes in the 1950s who had expressed concern about what he had termed "operations performed indiscriminately without regard to proper medical judgment." Dr. Stokes was regarded fondly by students and colleagues.

Mr. Hewitt was struggling to recall something, something important from the past — although was anything ever truly "the past?" Distant wards in the hospital, high up ... a memory of a circular wooden staircase winding upwards to locked rooms somewhere for the violent ones... "We was here for th' boys once," he hesitated. He recalled the old psychiatric hospital in the 1920s and, further back, the "feeble-minded" clinic in the Toronto General, and, even, Dr. Clarke himself who once examined him; a sense of his being at the heart of history. Dr. Clarke he recalled only as a heavy-set man with a reddish moustache. Dr. Clarke had not locked him up. He had allowed him to go home, back to Florrie and the kids. Dr. Clarke had said that Henry Hewitt was not nuts.

It was unexpected. Dr. Miles sighed. This was what happened when you gave freedom to patients and their relatives, and tried to enter their world, he thought. This Mr. Hewitt was a discomforting reminder that he had met, indeed known, the great Dr. Clarke after the Great War. His experience in this system thus extended far beyond Dr. Miles's and Dr. Peachy's own experiences at the hospital.

"Doc'r Clarke, sir, he was agin'st restraints, took 'em away down in the asylum." Henry was not sure how this related to Daisy, only that there was some connection he did not quite understand as yet — and who could? — a subtle linking of past and present.

"Y-yes, well, Mr. Hewitt."

Dr. Miles coughed. Mrs. Lumsden looked about restlessly and said this was a fine place and Daisy could live there. Dr. Miles responded that Daisy would be well taken care of, and Mr. and Mrs. Lumsden were welcome to see Daisy's room on the Woman's Ward once she had settled in, to Mrs. Lumsden's surprise — for this was the new open approach to patients in vogue at the hospital, smiled Dr. Miles, allowing group activities that encouraged the psychiatrist to follow the patient's emotional needs: Milieu Therapy in action.

17.

DAISY'S ROOM IN THE WOMEN'S WARD contained six beds, for five other women and herself. Even though this was a mental hospital, the women didn't *seem* mental. One of the younger women, Sam, younger than herself, only sixteen, was from Rosedale — "in" she said, for bad behaviour and giving the old biddies trouble. "Biddies," of course, meant her mother and aunt. She laughed defiantly at Daisy. She had long, uncombed hair down her back (Nurse Chalmers would soon have made short shrift of that) and wore strange wooden beads round her neck. Sam, short for Samantha, was in for something called "Behaviour Therapy."

"Where are you from?"

She didn't want to say "Orillia," as it wasn't anything to be proud of, she knew. "I'm from ... a hospital."

Daisy was conscious of her too long, drab, institutional dress with its silly Peter Pan collar that Mrs. Demsey had had them cut out in Sewing Class, and her flat ugly shoes and bobby socks. Sam wore a short denim skirt above her knees, combined with a long loose top that hung down to her knees — and no brassiere. She was a "beatnik," she said, tossing back her long hair. This must be the fashion in Toronto, Daisy decided. If Sam could help her find some scissors, she could cut a chunk off the hem of her own skirt.

"I'm afraid scissors aren't allowed on the ward," said Nurse Wilkins.

"We've got to jam with Pebbles and Mel in the morning," yawned Sam. "Pebbles" was Dr. Charles Peebles and "Mel" was Dr. Philip Melville, Daisy realized with shock. Sam had used nicknames as if they were the best of friends.

"A conference, Daisy. We have one every morning for our clients in the sitting room to talk out issues bothering you," explained Nurse Wilkins kindly, as if Daisy understood. "You can express yourself freely here, Daisy." Daisy tried to understand that she was now a "client."

"Let it all out, man," said Sam polishing her nails.

The room was so wonderful. In awe, Daisy touched the bed with its fresh clean linen and pale pink counterpane — all four women had identical linen, so as not to show favouritism she decided. She had a real fluffy pillow. There was a small bedside table with a drawer and a little shelf below, just for her, for her "personal things," said the nurse mysteriously. Daisy was not sure Miss Wilkins was a "real" nurse since she did not wear a white uniform, no uniform at all that Daisy could see — no nurse's cap and band — and certainly not white rubber shoes. Instead, she wore a pretty short dress and casual sandals, but she did have a stethoscope around her neck.

There was an added luxury of a bedside lamp, marvelled Daisy, and a chest of drawers she shared with Sam. A long window overlooked trees and tall buildings; far below, was College Street. She glimpsed cars and a red streetcar and people walking about freely. That night the tall buildings shone with lights — it was so bright after the darkness of Orillia.

Most of all, Daisy marvelled at the bathroom with its *door.* "A door?" she murmured, touching it with pleasure. In this place, you got to pee and change your pad in private.

"Yes, Daisy, a door," smiled Nurse Wilkins brightly. She knew Daisy was mentally retarded; poor thing, not knowing what a door was. "*Door,*" she emphasized clearly, in a kind way.

And only one toilet and shower at a time.

"An' curtains round the shower stall," Daisy touched the plastic curtains that hung from the shower rod. Such curtains she had never seen before; they were beautiful, shining, and *clean,* and had a pattern of flowers and birds scattered wonderfully about. She smoothed the curtains with her fingertips and felt a pleasure close to adoration. To undress naked and shower *alone!* She could hardly wait her turn.

"Yes ... those are called *shower curtains,* Daisy. You pull them around the stall before turning on this tap. Dr. Melville moved heaven and earth to get them — and toilet seats — on the ward."

Daisy still was not sure about Nurse Wilkins, who was to be called "Janet."

She felt confused. She had already mistaken the cleaning lady for a nurse, thinking her white stockings and rubber shoes were a uniform. Some young man with longish curls who wore jeans turned out to be a doctor.

Yet she could not sleep at night in the beautiful room, even though the beds on either side were far away. She missed the beds pressing in around her in Cottage M, the girls' heavy breathing, their presence. There was no nursing attendant at a Nursing Station keeping watch. How would she know when to get up? There were no bells here, no nurse aide shouting down the aisle, "Git moving." The front doors downstairs in the foyer were locked at night, but by day they were open; the door in the women's ward was also left open and it led out to the corridor, so you could walk out into the street if you wanted. Daisy tossed and lay still again, listening intently to the sounds of her childhood in Toronto long forgotten, to the trams and cars and a long, high whine that must be a siren: Fire! Police! Ambulance!

Sam was painting her toenails a wild purple shade as she sat on the bed after breakfast, still in her pyjamas. She was on Largactil, she said, to settle her down. The other women were watching TV attached high up on the wall, *The Breakfast Show*; another, a hysteric, was reading *True Crime*. The older woman, Mrs. Drew, was having Shock that morning, and had to miss breakfast. Mrs. Drew had frizzy grey hair and pale, fluttery eyes. No one paid her any attention. "Fries your brains," she said to nobody and everyone. She kept repeating it over and over, and pressing her head her hands trembled. "Z-z-z-z-t, and you're done."

"Done *for*, you mean," muttered Sam.

Medications had been brought in before breakfast on a nice tray carried by a nurse aide, though she wore no blue uniform or banded cap that Daisy could see. "Meds!" she smiled brightly. The women shambled over. Daisy obediently swallowed hers though she was certain her mother would raise a stink.

"My ma will soon fix the doctors 'bout these pills," she confided to Sam.

"What meds you taking?"

"Dunno. Pills my ma said not t' swaller but stick 'em up my cheeks."

Sam let out a laugh. "Boy, Daisy, you're something, eh?"

This seemed to mean Sam liked her. Daisy smiled.

The men were upstairs on the second floor, but they were free to come down and have meals with the women, or watch TV, or play cards, or just smoke. Nobody stopped them. They did not roll their own smokes from tobacco tins, but everyone had real packets of Players bought from outside. And somewhere on the third floor, no one knew exactly where,

Mrs. Drew. was going to get Shock. She started to cry and resist.

"Now, now, it'll be over before you know it, Phyllis," said Nurse Willoughby.

"That's the problem," muttered Sam, in a tone Daisy understood was smart. Daisy could tell that Shock was not something Sam approved of.

"*Electric* shock, ECT," clarified Sam, when Mrs. Drew had been led away after being told to swallow a drink in a little white paper cup. She was agitated, begging for another chance.

"Z-z-z-z-z-t."

The women moved to the little sitting room off the bedroom now, excited, for cheery Dr. Peebles had arrived, wearing a flowered shirt today. He would be followed by Dr. Melville later, Sam's personal therapist.

"Wild, man!" screamed Sam. She sat cross-legged on the rug. Daisy stayed back near the corner, shyly. This was "rap" time. The women talked strange to Dr. Peebles whom they called, unbelievably, "Pebbles." They talked about their orgasms or lack of them, or when they felt they were "on the edge."

"I want it all the time, Pebbles!" moaned one woman. She also had long straight hair that fell recklessly about her face (combing one's hair was obviously optional here).

"Oh, I do too," said Daisy eagerly, wanting to be part of the group. Everyone turned around and laughed.

"Oh, Daisy!" Sam giggled.

What had she said? Once again, Daisy was painfully aware of her Orillia dress right out of the 1950s. She did not speak again, even when Dr. Peebles looked at her directly and asked, "What is your opinion, Miss Lumsden?" All she could do was shake her head.

Later that morning, while Sam was having a "rap" with "Mel" — Dr. Melville — she ventured out through an unlocked side door. She walked along Grosvenor Street past a hospital called Women's College, and turned down to College Street, a busy road with trams and throngs of people walking to work in the bright city sunshine. A street vendor was selling hotdogs at a stand on the corner. She reached University Avenue. More huge, heavy, stone buildings that looked like Orillia's Administration Building came into view. It was Queen's Park, the towering legislative buildings you would not dare go into. A flag hung on a pole; it was the old Ontario Red Ensign. She walked further, toward the lights.

There was a distant roar, thousands of voices were singing. "Groovy," said someone at the lights and a group of teenagers dressed like Sam surged forward on the green light. The girls all wore short skirts Daisy now knew were called miniskirts or minis. The boys had long hair and wore jeans and T-shirts and rows of beads or long medallions just like the girls. In fact, Daisy found it hard to tell the boys apart from the girls. She moved with them until they stopped and melted in with the crowd at the park, where boys and girls sat together on the grass, smoking strong, sweet-smelling cigarettes that looked like sticks you might pick up off the ground. Three young men with hair down their shoulders were playing electric guitars at a microphone, wound round with wires and outlets attached to a small van: "*Love, love me do / You know I love you / I'll always be true...*" One girl had one of her breasts pushed out of her open blouse, as she sat on the grass, feeding her baby in front of everybody. But no one seemed to notice thought Daisy, bewildered. A girl who had a baby in Orillia would never sit out on the front lawn suckling it. The babies were taken and buried behind the farm, Daisy knew, or put straight into the Children's Dorm; Nurse Chalmers would see to that.

"Disgusting," said a woman crossing the park. "Something should be done about these hippies."

Daisy repeated the new, important word to herself. Sam was a "hippie" as well as a "beatnik." She could hear bits of conversation all around her: "...should cut their hair off ... all these kids taking over ... should call in the army to take care of them...," but she wasn't sure what it all meant.

There was a statue of a man looking thoughtfully down the avenue. "MacDonald," she read, excited that she could make out the important word. But the avenue was long and endless, and she had no money — nowhere to go — no means of getting food or a room for the night. Where was Sumach Street and Granpa Hewitt and Ganny? She did not know; she did not know that Regent Park had been built. Frightened, she turned around and made for the lights. On the other side of the intersection, peering between more grey-white buildings she thought she recognized the dull gold brick of the hospital. She hurried along College Street and back around the corner to Surrey Place, alarmed but excited. She had been to a "Love-In"; she had heard a girl scream ecstatically. This girl also had her tits bobbing through a see-through top. Brassieres were out in Toronto, Daisy decided, so why was she wearing one?

The first thing that Dr. Miles noticed in the interview was that Daisy Lumsden did not seem to have any idea why she had been sent to the Toronto Psychiatric Hospital. Of course, it was doubtful that Dr. Crawford-Jones in Orillia would have discussed with Daisy the parents' threat of *habeas corpus,* and their claim that she was being held against her will illegally in the institution. Daisy was too limited intellectually to understand. The records forwarded from Orillia showed her to be a half-moron or moron, though her last I.Q. recently assessed as 42 by Dr. Assaf at Orillia put her in the "imbecile" range, a fact shared with the young student, Miss Woodcock, who sat taking notes to the side.

Daisy was also strangely convinced that she was in the Clarke Institute of Psychiatry, a notion she had gotten from her mother.

"I apologize for the confusion and mess everywhere in the hallways and offices, Daisy," Dr. Miles smiled, indicating the women's sitting room (and not an office, noted Daisy). The room was filled with boxes of files and office equipment awaiting transfer. "We're in the process of moving this month to our new building on College Street, the Clarke Institute of Psychiatry."

He glanced at Daisy, who that morning was wearing a dress that looked as if it had been hacked at the bottom by a saw. It hung above her knees in jagged edges, and something had happened to the collar around the neck, as if it had been ripped out of its stitches. He wisely made no comment.

"My mother took the pills to th' doctors here at th' Clarke an' made a big fuss about the bad things they done to me up in Orillia is why I'm here," challenged Daisy, her voice shifting to a heavy, grating tone like her mother's.

"You'd like to be off the Mellaril, Daisy?"

This was in keeping with the new approach at TPH of discussing a patient's meds with her, within reason, of course.

"Mell'ril? Was that the pills what I been swallerin'?" she asked. "I didn' know what pills it was. They never told me."

Dr. Miles was aware of the necessity of being loyal to his colleagues in the psychiatry department in Orillia and to exemplify this to the young intern, Miss Woodcock, busily taking notes in the corner. According to the Examination on Admission form, Daisy was assigned 100 mg. of Mellaril for "homosexuality."

"We agree you don't need them any more, Daisy."

"Tha's what my mother said. She said Orillia give us too much drugs. She said not t' swaller 'em but spit 'em out when nobody was looking."

Daisy had a vague sense of her mother's triumph, of something being exonerated, though she was not sure exactly what. Suddenly, she began to sob.

The sensitive issue of Daisy's relationship with her mother had to be raised, of course. The *habeas corpus* the mother had brought against Dr. Houze and the institution placed Daisy under "forensic" investigation. Dr. Miles thought it best broach the subject of her mother by bringing up the words "going home." Would Daisy like to go home after her release?

"Home?" Daisy asked through her tears. She had a memory of a room, her mother's china crashing down, a man...

"When you leave this hospital, Daisy."

"Oh, but I likes it here," Daisy put in quickly.

"Yes, but Daisy, you cannot stay here forever. This is a psychiatric research hospital not an institution."

Then it came out: her fear of her mother forcing sex on her. "She might make me 'ave the sex again..." This was the crux.

Dr. Miles glanced at Miss Woodcock, who wrote: "The patient expressed rather strong ambivalent feelings about returning to her mother."

In the Clinical Record, Dr. Miles was later careful to omit the actual word "rape" in Daisy's account of that Christmas 1963, noting that she insisted her mother had "paid a man to sexually molest her." He added, even more carefully from a legal point of view: "She claims she has been worried about this since that time and at the present." Of course, there was always the possibility that Daisy's mother *had* enjoyed watching her daughter, this sort often did. Dr. Miles shuddered.

"You'd prefer to return to the Orillia hospital, Daisy?"

Daisy sobbed even harder, and struggled for the words that could tell this kind man what she felt. "No, they makes you work hard all day with th' big-headed babies on th' wards an' doin' laundry, hundreds of sheets an' sewing all them dome fast'ners for the baby bibs. I get pushed round by the other girls an' get the blame."

Miss Woodcock translated this as: "She expressed dislike of the Orillia hospital — she had to work for long periods of time at different jobs, that other patients pushed and shoved her around but she did not know where she would like to go definitely."

"Maybe she be diff'rent now," said Daisy slowly, shifting back to her mother, between tears. But it wasn't just her fear of "sex" as it was something else. She tried to express her horror of her mother's "fits" and all it meant from so long ago, being a little girl and being really frightened, a past now so suddenly real, a past she thought she had forgotten. "She might 'ave fits..." Yet the idea of "home" she so longed for persisted. The idea of a loving mother, looking after her, persisted, too.

Dr. Miles made every effort to understand this.

She felt she would like to go home because maybe she — the mother — would be different now. Miss Woodcock dutifully recorded: "Daisy, however, expressed fear that her mother might have fits."

Dr. Miles glanced — a significant exchange — at intern Miss Woodcock. This was important. Mrs. Lumsden was an unfit mother. Daisy's admission that she feared a repeat of sexual assault by her mother meant that the *habeas corpus* could possibly be annulled.

Mrs. Lumsden was the key to the outcome here. She sat with her husband in the Visitors' Room, looking around in awe at the chintz curtains and matching chair covers, the coffee table — "Tha's a nice bit o' wood" — and at the doctors sitting casually in easy chairs. In particular, she liked Dr. Peebles's shirt, she said, and that she and Ernie were sitting in a lovely sitting room. She smiled eagerly at Dr. Miles. For the first time in her life, perhaps, Ella Lumsden was being listened to, her opinions and wants deferred to. Indeed, she was being given credence and certain respect. And it was significant how much she had to say.

Dr. Miles recorded in his Progress Notes:

> May 5, 1966.
> Today I interviewed the patient's parents.
> The conversation, to begin with, was concerning Daisy's present situation with regard to the Toronto Psychiatric Hospital and the Orillia Hospital. Mrs. Lumsden expressed apparent dislike for the Orillia Hospital and her concern that the patient not be returned there. (What Mrs. Lumsden had actually said was that Orillia was a "drug house" and the patients made to work in "chain-gangs.") She stressed that the patient is "not stupid," is able to do housework, to sew, to clean floors, and to cook, and therefore should be allowed to go home (or at least to have her own room). When questioned about Mrs. Lumsden's health recently and in the past, it was pointed out that she had fits, the last one about a year ago and has been on capsules, one three times a day and a little pill. Mrs. Lumsden appeared to be able to give me the adequate dosages with the number of capsules taken.

The seizures were also important as they affected Mrs. Lumsden's capabilities as a mother to take care of and protect Daisy, and, therefore, the outcome of the *habeas corpus*. Though it did appear that a doctor at the Mental Health Centre at 999 Queen Street had considered Mrs. Lumsden's "fits" to be genuine seizures and had put her on medication, one had to take into account the opinions of doctors and psychiatrists throughout her records who had invariably regarded Ella Hewitt's fits as "functional": "she appears to have 'seizures.'"

Dr. Miles had taken a quick look at the records from the Children's Aid Society, which showed a letter to Miss Prewse, social worker, in April, 1951, from the Assistant Superintendent Dr. H. F. Frank at Orillia stating: "Concerning Ella Hewitt, no seizures reported during her stay at the Orillia hospital."

"'S long as I takes the capsules an' drinks no beer, I'm good, Doc'r Mile." Mrs. Lumsden flashed a huge, disconcerting smile at the doctors, her lips smeared with bright red lipstick, her cheeks rouged. She was dressed quite appropriately, though, Dr. Miles noted, in a neat costume with fake pearls.

Dr. Miles turned his attention to Ernest Lumsden who seemed a well-groomed, well-developed individual with a tendency to stutter. "I-I'm off w-work at Smith Transport cause a th' th' truckers' strike," he began hesitantly. "But I got a sec'nd job, sir, wiv Gen'ral Steel Ware." He assured Dr. Miles he would be returning to work shortly.

"I can get Daisy a job at the Ontar'o Laundry jus' like that," cut in Mrs. Lumsden, snapping her fingers in Dr. Peachy's face.

"N-now, now, Ella," Mr. Lumsden put a gentle hand on his wife's arm. Mrs. Lumsden pushed this aside, insisting she could also get Daisy a job where her daughter Lizzie was working. "Aw, n-na, Ella," went Mr. Lumsden again.

"Fuck, can so!" cried Mrs. Lumsden exasperated. Mr. Lumsden at once fell silent.

Dr. Miles noted further that both the Lumsdens did not wish that the patient be returned to Orillia, which Mrs. Lumsden once again called a "jail 'ouse."

"What is your opinion of the Toronto Psychiatric Hospital?"

"It a fine, fine place," Mrs. Lumsden bent forward eagerly.

Mr. Lumsden nodded agreeably and said, "This the b-bestest. Daisy c'n live here, she be happy."

"But why Daisy not live at 'ome?" persisted Mrs. Lumsden. "We got a room for 'er ready."

One wondered what sort of home was in Mrs. Lumsden's head that she felt she had to offer Daisy in the circumstances, whether she fully comprehended the effects of the sexual abuse of the past on Daisy — not yet alluded to — and that Daisy had not lived with her parents since early childhood. She seemed to have spent most of her life in shelters and institutions.

Mrs. Lumsden again persisted, in that harsh grating voice of hers, that she could get Daisy work. She was getting somewhat agitated — her face was flushed, her teeth were clicking. Why couldn't Daisy live at "Lor'mer Lodge, with 'er younger sister Lizzie?" She grasped the sleeve of Dr. Peebles's shirt. A doctor who wore pink had to be kind.

Dr. Peebles shifted his arm (this was a woman who had threatened to blow up one of the Cottages in Orillia, according to the files).

"Lizzie is there in Lor'mer Lodge doin' good, Doct'r Pebbles, cleanin' an' such."

While Daisy had been in Orillia, Mrs. Lumsden and her husband had obviously made the effort to keep in touch with Lizzie. They were aware of her living arrangements, as well as her place of work, despite Lizzie's protestations to staff at the Lorimer Lodge and to Dr. Peebles earlier that she "didn't want nothing to do with her. She ain't my mother, I don't feel nothing for her."

Dr. Miles needed to make explicit order out of all this. He wrote in his Progress Notes:

> Both parents would not wish that the patient return to the Orillia Hospital. When asked about staying at the Toronto Psychiatric Hospital, both felt that this was a fine place, that she would be happy here and they would agree to this. However, Mrs. Lumsden is more adamant in that the patient come to live with her and she could not see why the patient should live in Toronto without living at home. Mr. Lumsden appeared to be more flexible in this respect.

Lizzie was being interviewed separately. She would provide another interesting dimension to the family relationships with the mother, thought Dr. Miles. She was a pretty, blond, bespeckled young lady of seventeen. He wrote in his Progress Notes that Lizzie was "friendly and cooperative."

"I didn't even knowed I *had* a sister," said Lizzie, blinking rapidly at Dr. Miles. She had an obvious horizontal nystagmus that was coarse, he noted.

Daisy did not wonder or question how Dr. Miles, as a psychiatrist, had been able to locate Lizzie so quickly at Lorimer Lodge.

Daisy, of course, was unaware of the existence of the confidential Toronto Social Services Index, a professional network that until the 1960s had relayed confidential information about patients back and forth between various agencies including the Children's Aid Society and the Toronto Psychiatric Hospital without the patients' knowledge or consent. In actuality, unknown to Daisy or the Lumsdens, this was a sensitive ethical issue that had been challenged by young, outspoken Morton Teicher, chief social worker at TPH in the 1950s.

Teicher, horrified by the abuse of patient privacy and confidentiality, wrote an article recommending its abolishment, in 1952: "Let's Abolish the Social Service Exchange," published in *Social Work Journal* in January, 1952, which had resulted in the Exchange being dissolved a decade later. However, links between agencies still continued as evidenced by the two Children's Aid Societies, Catholic and non-Catholic, exchanging information about the Lumsdens and the Hewitts.

Lorimer Lodge, formerly The Haven run by the Salvation Army Mission Service, now included mentally retarded women as part of its clientele, or young women considered in trouble with the law or out-of-control in the community. Many of the women were homeless. Lizzie had been transferred once her wardship was up with the CAS of Toronto at age sixteen; they had made these arrangements as Lizzie had wanted to live in the city: "It was dull up in Richmond Hill." There were movies and dances, taverns and "clubs" in downtown Toronto. Indeed, Lizzie enjoyed the nightlife Toronto offered; the Matron at Lorimer had reported her out after hours at a tavern on Parliament Street. Now Dr. Miles had inadvertently enabled the two sisters to reunite after a decade, something that Lizzie had not necessarily favoured at first. The long-lost sister she had allowed herself to forget up in Orillia: "What wa the use of thinkin' about 'er?" she said to Dr. Miles.

Daisy had stared at Lizzie at their meeting in the Visitor's Room. Here was Lizzie alive in Toronto all this time, carrying on with her life while she had been locked up in Orillia.

"'T'warn't fair," Daisy had cried.

Lizzie was cautious. She suddenly had a sister, which might mean having to pick up with her mother and father again. She had no idea why Daisy had been brought down to the Toronto Psychiatric Hospital, Dr. Miles noted, (no idea what a *habeas corpus* was) but thought it good for Daisy to return home rather than go to Orillia. She had a pert face with a tight expression, unlike her sister Daisy. She kept her slim legs with their pretty ankles crossed, her feet tight in thin-strapped high-heels.

"Would you like to go home, Miss Lumsden?" he asked slyly.

At once Lizzie stiffened. "Only for weekends"

Dr. Miles wrote in the Progress Notes:

> When asked whether she herself would go home, she said only for weekends because "They are not like my parents, only foster parents." She thought it would be a good idea for the patient to go to Lorimer Lodge or to live in a home situation as she is living in now (as a domestic in a nursing home).
>
> Progress notes re: Daisy Lumsden:
> May 12, 1966
>
> The patient Daisy appears quite depressed. She is also quite suspicious. During interview today she became quite tearful claiming that this hospital was only going to send her back to the Orillia Hospital. She fears this greatly. Actually the patient shows amazing insight into her own limitations and she would appear to see that this is possibly the best alternative that she has. With regard to her future, she firstly would favour going to live with her sister, Lizzie. When it was pointed out to her that this might not be possible, she began to appear more depressed. She seems not to show enthusiasm about going home with her mother; neither does she push for this. Generally, she shows impatience and anger that the question of her sexual relations of about three years ago continually is brought up. She feels that this would not happen again due to her mother's promise.

One wondered what this "promise" was, most likely concerning sexual abuse by any one of Ella Lumsden's boyfriends, but Daisy could not or would not say the words to Dr. Miles, only insisting: "She promise me, it not never happen again."

Such was the sensitivity of young Miss Ramage, the social worker, that it was Mrs. Lumsden herself who introduced the subject of her alleged sexual abuse of Daisy. She denied forcing her daughter to have sexual intercourse with a boyfriend.

Miss Ramage wrote: "She denies this and states the doctors up in Orillia are out to blacken her character."

Dr. Miles and Dr. Peebles had consulted the newly formed "Social Department" at TPH for a second opinion on Mrs. Lumsden, in keeping with the eclectic approach the hospital prided itself on. The Social Department was one of the few in Ontario, and was ahead of its time. It developed new skills in interviewing patients and their relatives. Miss Rita Lindenfield, Director, and at present on leave, was replaced by Cyril Greenland, former Head of Social Work at Whitby Asylum, who was of the opinion that patients should be "invited" to participate in interviews, as part of the new openness at TPH.

Certainly young Miss Ramage seemed to have Mrs. Lumsden's confidence. "Don't b'lieve them doctors up in Orillia. I ain't done no wrong."

But Mrs. Lumsden also claimed she had never been separated from her husband, which Miss Ramage knew not to be true. Mrs. Lumsden insisted that Daisy had told her she wanted to come home to live with her, which was not what Daisy had confided earlier to Miss Ramage. But then, Daisy had changed her mind. On May 9, 1966, she had suddenly said: "I just wish I could go home and then I would be happy." Obviously, another fantasy of "home" on Daisy's part, frowned Dr. Miles, a fantasy that Mrs. Lumsden did not have the wherewithal to provide, and that inexperienced Miss Ramage was too innocent to detect as yet.

Mrs. Lumsden reached out for Miss Ramage's hand with her own gnarled nail-bitten one coated with bright pink polish. "I can get Daisy a job at th' Ontar'o Laundry," she insisted.

One had to be cautious about this, Dr. Miles wanted to intervene with trusting Miss Ramage. Part of the trouble with social workers was that they tended to overly identify with patients; Miss Ramage was seeing the Lumsdens as people with common marital problems just like anyone else. But Miss Ramage saw Mr. Lumsden's faithfulness in this marriage and the faithlessness of Ella as only too familiar a scenario from the marriage counselling and advice columns of the circulars put out by Social Department.

Mr. Lumsden later confided in private to Miss Ramage that "some of the things his wife said 'bout Ontar'o L-Laundry wasn' true," and that they had separated many times. He had also told her that she spent nights out with other men, which had resulted in a hysterectomy, but that he was too afraid of upsetting her by pointing out the truth in front of her. Besides, all that was in the past.

Miss Ramage saw that Mr. Lumsden was the more stable one, and when Mrs. Lumsden became "overly excited and unrealistic," she wrote later, Mr. Lumsden "brought her back to reality."

In fact, Mr. Lumsden now confided that he had faced many problems as a result of being retarded. "It ain't a good thing bein' retard, Miss Ramage," which Miss Ramage felt showed great strength of character considering his intelligence.

"I kn-knows what it is t' be look down on and be retarded," he mumbled softly, "and I w-want to spare my chil'ren this, make sures they be train pr-proper vocashnally." Perhaps he had not been so opposed to Daisy being at Orillia, Miss Ramage surmised, and that he only wanted Daisy discharged to please and pacify his wife. Mrs. Lumsden was certainly desperate to get Daisy out.

Here Miss Ramage hesitated. Like all well-trained social workers, she admitted tentatively in her notes that, "There are many things I do not know about Daisy's relationship with her mother," further emphasizing that she had not seen them together. In addition, Mrs. Lumsden had confided to being "lonely." Miss Ramage had noted: "She was often lonely at night in her apartment while her husband was at work."

Mrs. Lumsden had looked anxious then. She was eager to make a good impression, Miss Ramage felt, but was not sure how to do this. In her report to Dr. Miles, she indicated that Mrs. Lumsden seemed to have little idea how much she was making a nuisance of herself by phoning reception and the women's ward constantly. She had promised to give Miss Ramage and the two doctors a "warm reception" when they visited her home and that she would serve them coffee and cake. (Dr. Miles was not certain about the cake aspect.)

Meanwhile, Dr. Peebles had looked into Lorimer Lodge, and the staff there reported that Lizzie had made "satisfactory progress," and that Mr. and Mrs. Lumsden rarely visited or interfered with her progress. Of course, Dr. Peebles did not know as yet that Lizzie had told her parents to fuck off and stay out of her life. Miss Ramage herself noted that Daisy had been well-behaved at TPH, but sad: "I feel she is often left out of conversation and activities because she is retarded." She wondered whether all the good training in the world at the Ontario Hospital School in Orillia could redeem the loss of family Daisy seemed to feel. Miss Ramage intimated as much to Dr. Miles.

The love Miss Ramage felt Daisy yearned for could not be fulfilled in Mrs. Lumsden. This was a complex tragedy that moved in circles, unspoken. But that Miss Ramage had inadvertently touched upon the loneliness at the core of Mrs. Lumsden's life in her empty apartment, all due to the loss of her children.

And so Daisy was to be returned to Orillia "until her time was up" in the institution in December of 1966, when she could finally leave, slated for probation in a place like Lorimer Lodge.

"I was betrayed. They sent me back. I never got to choose what I wanted which was to stay in T'ronto, nobody listen." But Dr. Miles had promised she would be released from Orillia into a halfway house, a transitional residence, in the new year, in January 1967, to prepare her for complete independence. It meant only a short stay back in Orillia once she left TPH, if she could only be patient, he urged.

Of course, there were objections from Dr. Crawford-Jones in Orillia. He phoned Dr. Miles reminding him of the Lumsdens' constant interference with Daisy's Training Program, and their harassment — the verbal threats, the abuse, the lurid phone calls — to the point of threatening to blow up the place. Daisy had, consequently, become belligerent, antagonistic, and difficult to handle.

On no account would they allow Daisy Lumsden to transfer to Toronto, not to Lorimer Lodge, certainly not to her parents' place. Whitby, yes. Possibly Cobourg.

18.

"OH, ME AN' LIZZIE HAD FUN planning our wedding!" That January night in 1967, the sisters had talked excitedly on the eve of their elopements, snuggled up on their parents' bed in the old apartment in Regent Park. Their mother Ella was watching *The Lawrence Welk Show* in the living room. The old rooms on Sumach Street Lizzie barely remembered; she had only been three when she was taken away. And yet, those old rooms hovered like a ghostly presence.

But Daisy remembered Sumach Street. She remembered her and Lizzie sneaking out in the early morning to lick the cream off the neighbours' bottles of milk left by each door. "Oh, there was hell when they found us out!"

And Lizzie grinned as if she did remember something.

No matter. For now they were getting married: Lizzie to Arnold Moggs and Daisy to Joe Potts who had originally been dating Lizzie. "I 'ad 'im first!" said Lizzie triumphantly.

She had been two-timing him with Arnold, Daisy explained to me, with a giggle. Lizzie was in love with Arnold (this was long before she called him a "bastard" and tried to split his head open with a hatchet, Daisy added).

Joe had come with Lizzie to see Daisy in the halfway house in Cobourg where Daisy had been placed on her release from Orillia at the end of December 1966, her time in the institution itself up at last. She was a patient on probation, just as Dr. Miles had promised, but still under the guardianship of Orillia until she turned twenty-one.

"Goodbye and good luck, Daisy," Dr. Crawford-Jones had said, and Mrs. Bagley and Nurse Chalmers had shaken her hand. But Daisy had not given Orillia even a backward glance as she set out eagerly for the

Halfway Home run by Miss Alice Morton, Director, in Cobourg. Dr. Crawford-Jones had been determined not to send this patient to Toronto under the aegis of her controlling, insane mother whom all the staff felt wanted Daisy home for her own emotional purposes.

Joe had started to come out to Cobourg alone by bus. They conducted their courtship in restaurants. "He took me out to nice places!" I could not help but notice how Daisy's face glowed at the recollection.

But Mrs. Morton was by then complaining to Orillia of Daisy Lumsden's "filthy language" (obviously learned at Orillia, but the irony of this was lost to Mrs. Morton) and that she "couldn't put up with it."

Daisy was also taught housekeeping and self-care skills. She had the job of cleaning the residence and a lady's house in town, and was given a small paycheque that she was taught to handle. She was paid once a month during training. They took her social insurance card and health card, Daisy explained to me. This was an exciting, scary time for Daisy; she was partly out in the world on her own for the first time in her life, and yet sheltered at night in the safety and community of the halfway house and its rules.

"You look like a institutional girl," Lizzie had said critically of Daisy when she came to Toronto on a pass one weekend. She surveyed Daisy's pudding-basin haircut. "Gives you right away."

Daisy had blushed. "I know Orillia is nothing to be proud of," she had mumbled. "It was a bad bad place."

Lizzie showed Daisy how to backcomb her hair. It had finally grown longer now that she had left Orillia, and she longed to have a beehive like Lizzie's.

Lizzie took a drag on her ciggy; she knew how to inhale. She had laughed when Daisy choked on hers. Daisy had never quite mastered inhalation at Orillia. "Hell, Daisy, how'm I gonna take yer to th' Isabella Saturday night?"

Now Daisy and Lizzie broke into giggles. They could hear the strains of Lawrence Welk from the living room; he was introducing some oldie on his show, a song from the dark ages of World War Two, their mother Ella singing along in a croaky voice: "*We'll meet again, don't know where, don't know when...*"

The two sisters had found each other and husbands (the same sort of men), back in the very neighbourhood of their parents and grandparents with its rented rooms and taverns.

Joe was a Catholic 'Home' boy; he had been in St. John's Home for Boys in Aurora, a terrible place, he said. Now, he had work cleaning offices, steady work.

Arnold was on the road, and earned good dollars. He had been in Orillia for a time. "And boy, can he tell stuff about *that* place!" cried Lizzie.

Lizzie had met him over a beer in the Canon House on Queen. She could not wait to get out of the grips of the staff at Lorimer Lodge. "Oh, it was a nice place and all that, Daisy, up on St. George Street; a very nice place." But Lizzie wanted fun, excitement; she wanted to stay out late at dances and at pubs down around Queen Street, where all the men were. There were lots of places to go: Supie's, the Royal Oak, and the Phoenix.

Lizzie and Arnold had already found rooms in a house in an old workers' cottage on Shuter Street, opposite the Methodist Church. Arnold said he loved her. Now Daisy was going to the Isabella Hotel with Lizzie. Two sisters out together on the town, free as larks, without their prospective husbands.

"What's the 'arm in it? You're only young once," said Lizzie. "But I stays faithful ter Joe," Daisy stressed that.

Daisy still did not know of the ways of city and clutched her purse close, click-clacking awkwardly in her high-heels down Jarvis, the most notorious street then in Toronto. Here was the underbelly of the city; here was where drug pushers, the pimps, the hookers and the peddlers surfaced after dark, an underbelly that Ella and Lizzie seemed to know so well.

That was when she met Eddie again. He was sitting alone at a table, glass of beer in hand. Daisy recalled talking to him.

"So, I went up to him and I said, 'Don't I know you from somewhere?' And he said his name was Eddie. I couldn' believe it, it was my old boyfriend I run away with from Orillia! I didn' give away from my name at first. I didn' want to say nothing about Orillia, or bring up Orillia. I never wanted to mention that place that I been in. I jus' asked him, 'Do you remember your old girlfriend?' And he said, 'I had a lot of girlfriends.' So I said, 'I'm Daisy.' And he said, 'Daisy?' And then I said, 'Daisy Lumsden. From Orillia.' And he said, 'Oh, aye. She ran away and got caught.' I said, 'Well, that's me. I'm getting married soon.' 'That's nice,' he said. I knew he wasn' interest in me. So I said, 'Nice seein' you again and all that, but it's goodbye. I love my husbant. I'll always be faithful to him.' Daisy looked at me firmly.

It was then that her mother Ella had come over to the table and said, "I see you've met a nice young man, Daisy. Why not bring him over to our table?"

Daisy remembered her mother one night, age forty-five or so, happy, sensual, perhaps pretty, dancing with abandon in the Isabella, along with her two daughters. "Oh, she did her thing all right, always jiggling out on the floor with some guy," Daisy told me.

And there is another story here, of course; the story beneath the story, glimmering under the surface. A story that the records can not be a witness to. Daisy never saw Eddie again; a glimpse of the past forever closed.

Suddenly, in one of those spurious acts like her original "elopement" from Orillia, Daisy decided she would marry Joe on the same day as Lizzie, in the registry office at City Hall, Toronto, through a Justice of the Peace. Daisy smiled at me. "Cost us twenty dollars."

This was her first act of independence in her entire life. She was still only twenty and under the guardianship of Orillia as a probationary patient, and Joe was nineteen; Lizzie eighteen and Arnold twenty. Lizzie wore a white sheath dress and cotton flowers in her hair. A second-hand ratty fur coat bought at the bazaar was draped over her shoulders. Daisy wore a yellow dress. They stood shivering on the steps of City Hall in the snow where their grandparents had stood newly married half a century before.

"Course I didn't have no fancy wedding gown, no veil or white dress, but I wore that yellow dress nice and clean," said Daisy to me somewhat quaintly, the old Salvation Army virtues she had learned in The Nest surfacing — cleanliness, godliness, simplicity — coming to the surface. These virtues had, perhaps, been her mainstay throughout her life.

Staff at the halfway house missed her at once on Monday morning. Mrs. Morton phoned Dr. Crawford-Jones in Orillia. Daisy called the staff later that day. "I jus' told them I wasn' *ever* coming back, I was married!" Daisy chuckled. She enjoyed recounting this part of the story for me, of showcasing her empowerment, and her sense of revenge. As a married woman, Daisy was no longer a ward of Orillia.

Staff informed Daisy they wanted "proof" before she was allowed to get her "things," by which was meant her pathetically few possessions in a shopping bag. "Show us the marriage certificate," demanded Mrs. Morton.

Daisy, accompanied by Joe, her "lawful wedded husbant," took the bus out to Cobourg and waved the marriage certificate at the staff as soon as she was inside the door. The staff said dryly, "Well, congratulations!" The girls pressed around Daisy, awed and excited at her ring, a cheap gold band from Woolworth's. Daisy was told to "get her things." Such was the end of her institutional life, and her former status as a ward of the CAS of Toronto and the Crown. No longer was she answerable to those in authority over her. It was the end of her childhood, if she did but realize. Perhaps she did.

"You too young to be marry, Daisy. Enjoy yer life first." Daisy recalled to me her mother's anxiety that wedding day in 1967.

"Well, I already *am*. So shut up."

Ella had then said, bewildered, "Well, I don't care what you do." Turning to Lizzie she'd cried: "*You're* not getting married, Lizzie!"

To which Lizzie replied, "Go fuck yourself."

"It's none of your business what we do," Daisy cried. "I love Joe, he's my husbant now, we got married this mornin', so shut yer damn mouth." She had continued passionately, "You didn't look after me when I was little, so you got no right to tell me what to do now." She had been put away at age four and a half, sent to live in the Shelter, then at The Nest, then Orillia, and now it was too late. Her voice rose: "You didn' do nothing for me when I was a kid. You wasn' my mother. You didn' *protect* me!"

The records had shown it. The records had revealed all. But in the retelling of this moment of forty years ago when she had been but newly released from Orillia at age twenty, Daisy's voice wavered. As we sat in her living room of her apartment in Toronto's Cabbagetown clutching the records, Daisy recalled again how she had confronted her mother for the first time, after the wedding. It had been a sort of revenge, she now realized. Ella had turned, confused, her watery eyes pale, fluttering like a bird's against the assault, the accusation.

Daisy hesitated. For had not the records she had so longed to read yet proved otherwise? The powerful records of her mother and herself, the terrible truths. She put them away, burying them at the bottom of a chest of drawers for the moment.

She was in her sixties, now. Her father long dead; her mother had passed away in a nursing home at age 82. Her illiterate, low-grade imbecilic mother who had fought for Daisy's release, braving superintendents, social workers, doctors and psychiatrists in daring defiance. And she had amazingly won out. For Daisy's sake. Daisy had to acknowledge this, she admitted. That her mother must have loved her, in her own, jumbled way. "She must of cared then, Thelma." Daisy sat and wept.

Daisy had some understanding, now, of the past, of her past, of Orillia, and of her family caught in a time during which decisions were made for them, particularly for her mother. Now Daisy wanted to know more, to open her mother's records and probe further, secrets still withheld — her mother Ella Hewitt's story. The young girl Ella, put away by her parents, Daisy's grandparents, Florrie and Henry Hewitt, as a "sexual delinquent."

Daisy sensed a betrayal. It held her. She recalled the words of a social worker who had cited in Daisy's own file, under "family history," the reason for Ella's committal at age twelve: "*Parents fear she will become a sexual delinquent.*"

What did that mean exactly? Was her mother having sex at *age twelve*? And where had Ella's parents learned to cite such professional terminology, one wondered. Her mother Florrie was deemed an "imbecile," and her father, Henry Hewitt, a semi-literate working-class man with only Junior 111 schooling in England. Perhaps the social worker had influenced Mr. Hewitt, interpreting his words for her reports and rewriting them in professional lingo. Or Henry may have heard the phrase bandied about by psychiatrists at the Clinic at the Toronto Psychiatric Hospital and grasped its significance, the unfailing key that would get his daughter ahead on the waiting list for Orillia: "sexual delinquent." Once again, the records would reveal the truth; the records would tell.

Ella Hewitt's family files might reveal so much more about her supposed "waywardness," not least the very social milieu that had created the idea of "feeblemindedness" in the first place.

And so Daisy got out her mother's records:

> Ella Hewitt, Case #5096, Orillia Hospital.
> CONFIDENTIAL. NOT TO BE DISCLOSED.

Like Daisy's, Ella's file amounted to over a hundred pages, packed with medical and psychological information, psychiatrists' reports, I.Q. tests, ward reports; information long withheld, faded with age, surely complex.

The vital "Family History Form 120" was at the front. Written dutifully and meticulously by a social worker at the Catholic Children's Aid of St. Vincent de Paul in Toronto, necessarily portraying her point of view, it would take Daisy back to the era of her grandparents, the early 1900s.

Young Florrie and Henry sailing for Canada in 1913. They had not yet met.

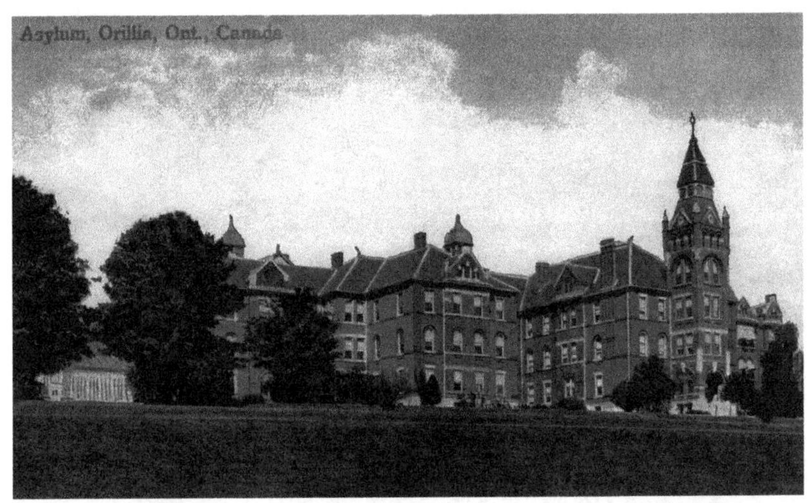

The Asylum for Idiots and Feeble-Minded, 1888. Courtesy Archives of Ontario.

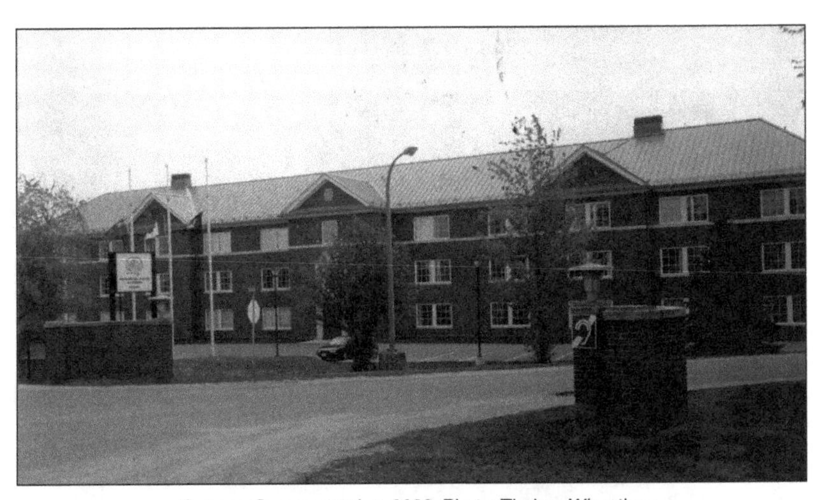

Cottage O, renovated, c. 2009. Photo: Thelma Wheatley.

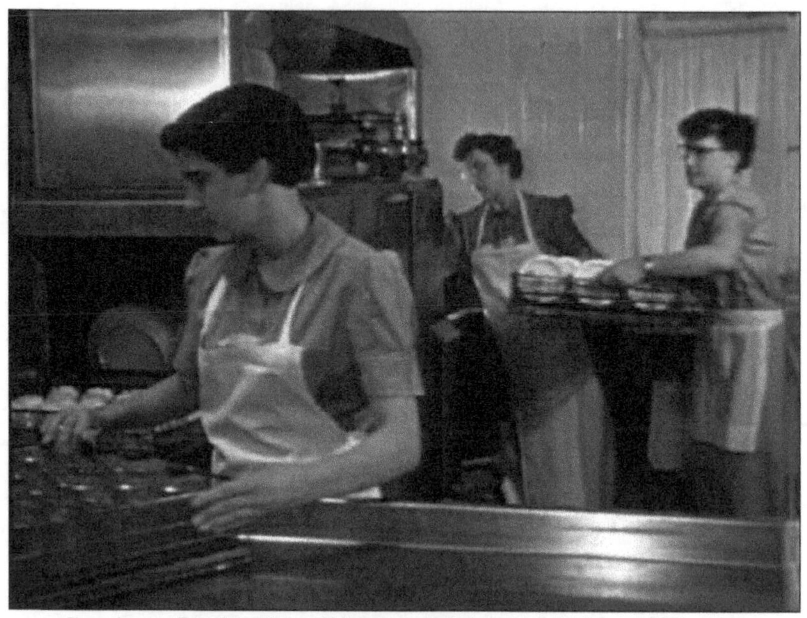

From the top: Female patients at kitchen work, Ontario Hospital School, Orillia, 1960. Courtesy Ontario Archives.

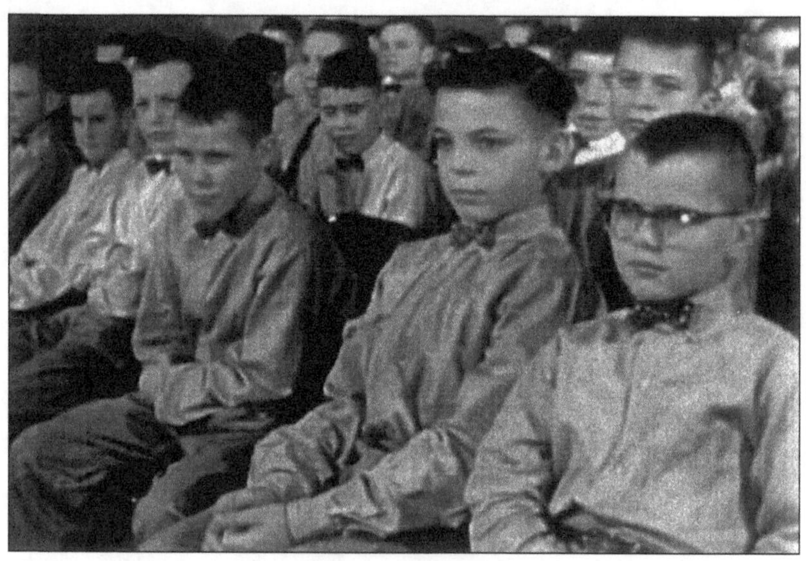

Boys at Sunday service in the gym, Ontario Hospital School, Orillia, 1960. Courtesy Ontario Archives.

To the Parents Key to Grading: B- Very Good
C- Good
D- Fair
E- Poor

Daisy Lumsden
Pupil's Name

HABITS and ATTITUDES	Nov 24	Feb 28	May 15	Remarks
PERSONAL HABITS				1. Timid, but pleasant personality.
1. Sits, stands, and walks correctly.	C+	B-	B	2. Still shy, but is developing well in oral Reading.
2. Keeps neat and clean.	B-	B	B	Keep trying [illegible]
3. Shares responsibility of class.	C+	B-	B	3. Progressing, socially and academically, but hesitant at times.
4. Is courteous.	A	A	A	Keep [illegible]
5. Is honest and trustworthy.	C+	C+	C+	
6. Gets along with others in the yard.	C+	C	C+	
7. Gets along with others in the classroom.	B	B+	B	
WORK HABITS				1. Tries to do neat work, but printing is still difficult.
1. Works steadily.	B-	B	B	2. Neater work, but should keep on the lines (prints 2 lines high).
2. Works neatly.	C+	C+	B-	Passing to new Reader
3. Follows directions.	C	C+	C	3. Finds it hard to follow directions
4. Works willingly.	A	A	A	
5. Finishes work.	C	C	C	
6. Finds new work when done.	D+	C-	C	

HOW PARENTS MAY HELP THE SCHOOL

1. By providing for good sleep habits.
2. By developing habits of regularity and personal cleanliness.
3. By providing practice in dressing, especially street clothes and footwear.
4. By developing health and safety habits.

PARENTS' SIGNATURES

1st Report Mildred Rawlings

2nd Report Mildred Rawlings

3rd Report Mildred Rawlings

PROGRESS IN SCHOOL SUBJECTS	Nov 24	Feb 28	May 15	Remarks
READING				1. Real gain in [illegible] Better understanding of what she reads
1. Is interested in reading.	B-	B	B	2. Difficult, but steadily progressing.
2. Is learning new words.	B	B-	B	3. More effort, Gail
3. Understands what she reads.	C	C	C	
4. Is making progress.	B+	B+	B	
LANGUAGE				1. Still weak in oral expression
1. Expresses himself well.	D	D+	D	2. Keep trying Gail
2. Learns and uses new words.	C+	C+	C+	3. Printing is improving, needs practice
3. Is mastering spelling.	C	C+	C	
4. Printing or writing is improving.	C-	C-	C	
ARITHMETIC				1. Knows facts to 10 – not sure of extensions (15 + 4)
1. Is learning number facts.	C	C+	B	2. Good improvement
2. Is accurate.	C	C+	B-	3. Becoming accurate
SOCIAL STUDIES				1. Greater interest [illegible] now.
1. Shows interest.	C	C+	B-	2. Needs a [illegible]
2. Is progressing.	B	B	B	3. Good [illegible] at home in helping
NATURAL SCIENCE				3. Showing more interest
1. Is interested in world about him.	C	C+	C	
MUSIC				1. Beginning to take whole note [illegible]
1. Enjoys musical activities.	C+	C+	C+	3. Singing with group.
ARTS & CRAFTS				1. Makes a real effort.
1. Is gaining handwork skills.	C-	C	C+	3. Trying hard, needs encouragement.

ATTENDANCE	Sept.	Oct.	Nov.	Dec.	Jan.	Feb.	Mar.	Apr.	May	June
Times Late										
Days Absent		5				4		1		

YEAR'S SUMMARY:
June 27, 1958 – Passed to Gr. 2 in Arithmetic
New Reader "Come Along" Gr. 2

G.A. Brown

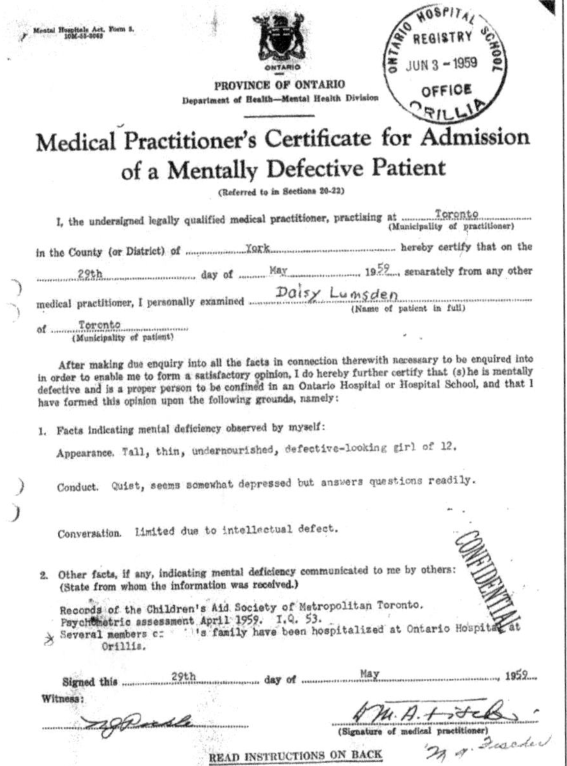

Mental Hospitals Act. Form 3.

ONTARIO

PROVINCE OF ONTARIO
Department of Health—Mental Health Division

ONTARIO HOSPITAL SCHOOL REGISTRY JUN 3 - 1959 OFFICE ORILLIA

Medical Practitioner's Certificate for Admission of a Mentally Defective Patient

(Referred to in Sections 20-22)

I, the undersigned legally qualified medical practitioner, practising at Toronto (Municipality of practitioner) in the County (or District) of York hereby certify that on the 29th day of May 1959, separately from any other medical practitioner, I personally examined Daisy Lumsden (Name of patient in full) of Toronto (Municipality of patient)

After making due enquiry into all the facts in connection therewith necessary to be enquired into in order to enable me to form a satisfactory opinion, I do hereby further certify that (s)he is mentally defective and is a proper person to be confined in an Ontario Hospital or Hospital School, and that I have formed this opinion upon the following grounds, namely:

1. Facts indicating mental deficiency observed by myself:

Appearance. Tall, thin, undernourished, defective-looking girl of 12.

Conduct. Quiet, seems somewhat depressed but answers questions readily.

Conversation. Limited due to intellectual defect.

2. Other facts, if any, indicating mental deficiency communicated to me by others: (State from whom the information was received.)

Records of the Children's Aid Society of Metropolitan Toronto.
Psychometric assessment April 1959. I.Q. 53.
Several members of [illegible]'s family have been hospitalized at Ontario Hospital at Orillia.

CONFIDENTIAL

Signed this 29th day of May 1959.

Witness:

(Signature of medical practitioner)

READ INSTRUCTIONS ON BACK

From the top: Daisy Lumsden's report card, Opportunity Class, William Burgess Public Toronto, 1958. Daisy's Patient File.

Daisy Lumsden's Certificate of Incompetence on admission to Ontario Hospital School, Orillia, 1959.

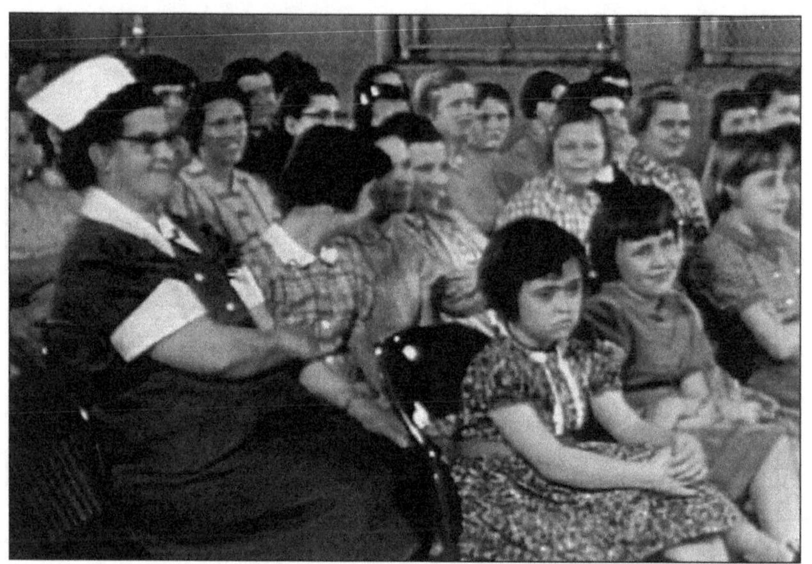

Girls and nurse's aide at Sunday service in gym, Ontario Hospital School, Orillia, 1960. Courtesy of Ontario Archives.

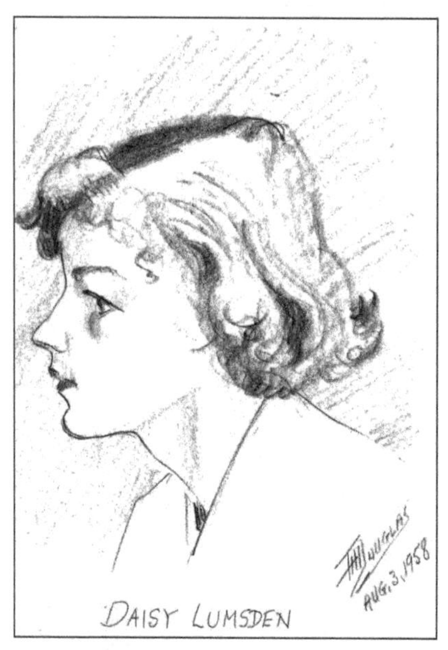

Pencil portrait of Daisy, age 11, by a Lieutenant in the Salvation Army, Danforth Corps, Toronto, 1958. Daisy's Patient File.

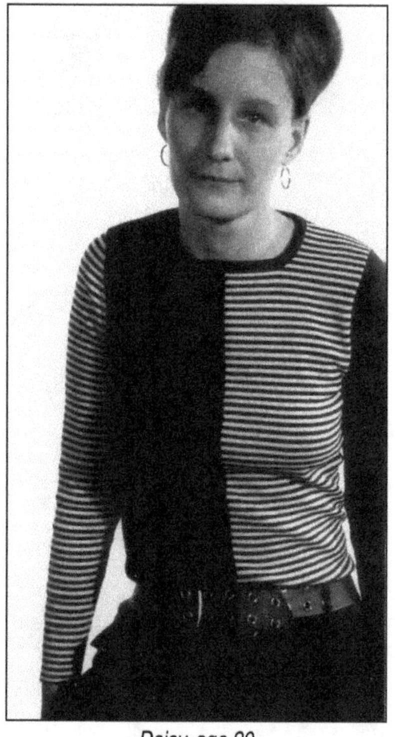

Daisy, age 20, on her release from Orillia, 1966.

PART TWO
THE MENACE OF THE FEEBLE-MINDED

TORONTO, 1900-1932

Who are the feeble-minded? They are people with the mental capacities and abilities of children. In the cities they tend to drift towards the slums. Indeed the slums are largely the product of the segregating of the subnormals.

—Dr. William Hutton, President, Eugenic Society of Canada, 1934

...Criminals and moral lepers are born in the atmosphere of physical and moral rottenness pervading the slums of large cities.

—Dr. Charles Hastings, Medical Officer of Health, Report on Conditions of the Poor in the Municipality of Toronto," 1911

Toronto is roused at last! The terrible menace of the feeble-minded has shocked the community... that 1,445 cases had been examined at the Toronto General Hospital — that of this number a large proportion were feeble-minded; that 285 were habitual thieves; that 120 had attempted to commit murder; that 59 delighted in setting fire to buildings; that 178 were prostitutes of the worst type and for the most part afflicted with venereal disease; that 201 cases were incorrigible in school, and 53 of the latter were found guilty of immorality of the most shocking nature.

—Dr. Clarence Hincks, Psychiatrist, Director of the Canadian National Committee for Mental Hygiene (Canadian Mental Health Association), addressing the Academy of Medicine, Toronto, 1916

19.

SOMETHING HAD TO BE DONE about the feeble-minded, the girls in particular, frowned Dr. Clarke, Charles Kirk Clarke, or "C. K." to friends and colleagues: former Superintendent of the Toronto Hospital for the Insane, first Professor appointed to the new Department of Psychiatry, University of Toronto, in 1908, Dean of Medicine, in 1911. He stood, perturbed, that afternoon in 1913, at the window of his old Clinic on Chestnut Street.

One only had to look about the city to see girls everywhere dressed in the latest fashions, cheap frills and furbelows, silly feathered hats and the rest of it, and skirts above the ankles. They traipsed along the streets, lingering, unchaperoned, outside shop fronts. Though even here there were distinctions; the better educated and employed dressed in conventional white shirtwaists and dark serge skirts.

The five o' clock hooter had gone off for the shift change at the factories that now proliferated Toronto's seedier areas and at the Eaton's store. More young women flooded the sidewalks eager to partake of the pleasures of the city after work: cheap vaudeville shows and burlesque, movie theatres with names like The Eclipse, nickelodeons and dance halls, minstrel shows, gaming palaces, and the so-called "supper clubs" that had sprung up all over the city in the past decade.

While many young ladies still lived at home, helping their families (the decent respectable ones, noted Dr. Clarke, "a good type mentally") thousands were at loose in the city; the government census of 1911 had cited 43,000. Many of the lower paid ones, likely factory girls, lived in dubious, uncertified lodgings south of College Street, mixing with all sorts of strangers — men with whom they reputedly shared the same water closet. The Department of Health, alerted to the problem, were planning to put out Sex Hygiene pamphlets warning young girls of the dangers of "rubbing up against strangers" in public places, about as much use, snorted Dr. Clarke to himself, as trying to dam the St. Lawrence River with a toothpick. Something else had to be done.

The National Council of Women of Canada (NCWC), founded in 1894 by Lady Aberdeen, wife of the Governor-General, was one of the most influential reform groups in the city consisting of many fine ladies and benefactresses from Rosedale and the Annex. Mrs. Willoughby Cummings, secretary, had expressed concern as early as 1890 about "simple" country girls coming into the city and "being taken advantage of." As a medical man, Dr. Clarke had at once understood the inference.

The NCWC had consequently started up a Committee on Feeble-Minded Women that called for the sterilization of girls deemed "not insane, not idiots," in their report — in other words "feeble-minded" — and segregation in institutions such as Orillia. As early as 1897, they had undertaken an enquiry into the number of unmarried women in each province under forty years of age who were either idiotic, semi-imbecilic, weak-minded, or unable to take care of themselves.

The Toronto Local Council of Women (LCW) soon started up a Protection of Women and Girls Committee and, with their own daughters in mind, a White Slavery Committee. This group of women had successfully lobbied in 1912 for the establishment of a Juvenile Court and continued to press for anti-prostitution legislation: "Shoulder to shoulder let us attack this evil, and attack it at a vital point — the law...."

According to Rev. John Shearer, leader of the Presbyterians, 60,000 girls across North America sank into the underworld every year, and 25,000 working girls right then in Toronto lived unprotected away from their families. The Methodists, equally concerned, had warned in 1911 of this "vile and shameless social evil." Dr. Margaret Patterson, first magistrate of the Toronto Women's Court and an expert on prostitution and sex hygiene work (she favoured the sterilization of criminals and the feeble-minded) claimed to have access personally to a shocking list of one hundred traffickers in the White Slave Trade, which she had provided at the Toronto LCW meeting on March 19, 1913. These girls were often lured by false ads in the *Star.* A group of concerned citizens of the Toronto Vigilance Committee had put out pamphlets warning of questions being asked at so-called job interviews such as: "Do you like wine supper clubs?" and: "What are your measurements below the hips?"

The problem lay, of course, with the Morality Department of the police force, frowned Dr. Clarke. It simply was not strict enough in punishing perpetrators, some of whom were Chinese living in the Ward by City Hall, corrupting white girls. The ladies of the Toronto Local Council of Women at least had gotten the government to add a good whipping as penalty for repeat offenders convicted of procuring girls. "The purity of our women is the very foundation of national life" — their admirable motto.

However, as the Toronto Chief of Police had confided to Dr. Clarke, it was not like the old days when girls in the brothels on King Street had been easily identifiable. "We 'ave difficulty, sir, telling a 'good times gal' from a genuine hooker or a working girl." A factory girl dawdling outside a movie palace surely had the right to enjoy herself for a couple of hours after pasting labels on tubes of Colgate toothpaste all day, hour after hour at a conveyor belt, he coughed apologetically.

Dr. Clarke was assured the police force had, however, hired two lady officers to patrol the dance parlours undercover, specifically to apprehend girls dancing hand in hand with men to whom they had not first been formally introduced. The police had been given the authority to devise their own bylaws concerning "vagrants," with added powers to supervise dance halls, saloons, skating rinks, and nickelodeons. Girls could be charged and placed in a reformatory for up to two years under the *Juvenile Delinquents Act* of 1908 or sent to the Jail Farm in Richmond Hill if she were suspected of soliciting. Of course, the Jail Farm was little more than a holding tank at best, bristled Dr. Clarke — one feeble-minded inmate had been in the jail twenty times! An unmarried woman found in bed with a man could also, thanks to the Toronto LCW be arrested under the new *Vagrancy Act*, though the logistics were not clear as to how exactly this would be effected.

Dr. Clarke grimaced, for the truth was many of these girls were incorrigibles and obviously feeble-minded, a threat to the nation's germ plasm. This germ plasm, discovered by German biologist August Weismann, using powerful microscopes, was the physical source of hereditary talents and other mental peculiarities. Sir Francis Galton, cousin of Charles Darwin, and president of the Eugenics Education Society in England, had advocated for the "scientific breeding" of humans — *eugenics* — a term Galton himself had coined in 1883 meaning "good in birth." It seemed the superior classes in society were to be encouraged to produce intelligent, talented offspring, and the "unfit" prevented as such: "Could not the undesirables be got rid of and the desirables multiplied?" Galton had urged. Quite. Degenerates naturally sought out their own kind, threatening to outbreed them all, as Dr. Clarke well knew. One had but to observe the sort of girls coming through his Clinic.

The ladies of the Women's Christian Temperance Union (WCTU), who were against obscene literature, wearing tight corsets, and eating too much meat, had tried to start up a club for them in Toronto, the only requirement being modest dress and deportment. But the ingrates had taken off at first chance for Dottie's Dance Parlour on Yonge Street, and never returned. Clearly, as Dr. Patterson had warned, Toronto was fast becoming a "hotbed of vice."

The mystery was that these girls preferred factory work to being a domestic in a gracious home in Rosedale. The ladies of the Toronto LCW sat concerned one afternoon in Lady Falconer's sun-filled conservatory, as they sipped tea. Elsie, the parlour maid, one of the faithful few in white frilled cap and pinafore, her petticoat slightly bedraggled below her long black skirt, had brought in dainties and *petit foie gras* on a silver tray.

There was an alarming drop in the number of domestics available in upper-class homes, they agreed; the statistics spoke for themselves. Mrs. Emily Willoughby Cummings and Mrs. Florence Huestis, President of Toronto LCW and prominent member of the National Council for the Prevention of Venereal Disease, both well-off philanthropists in the Methodist Alliance, noted that only one quarter of working girls were now in domestic service, even though the female labour force, out of a general population in Toronto of over 96,000, had increased to 42,000 in the province by 1911. The rest were working in factories, shops, and offices. The Ontario Bureau of Industry had investigated the decline in domestic service among working class girls as early as 1887, noting they were turning to factory work and retail jobs even at lower pay. The scarcity of servants "menaced the home life of the country," all agreed. Yet the Protestant Directorate of Female Immigration had reported that in the past ten years, 129,000 domestic servants had entered Canada from overseas.

It was especially exasperating, added Mrs. Huestis, since domestic service offered women room and board and respectable surroundings where they would be safe and cared for. What more could a girl want?

"I had to wear a cap and gown and go out the back door," one former servant had complained to the members of the first Royal Commission on the Relations of Labour and Capital back in 1898, which had been as equally flummoxed by the number of girls choosing low factory work over domestic service. The Commission had been an attempt by the government, as the ladies of Rosedale and the Annex well knew, to quell labour unrest. Over 1,800 witnesses had testified, some employers admitting to paying errand girls as low as $1.50 a week in wages. Nevertheless, the girls still rejected domestic work. "They like to go out in the evenings," Miss Burnett, a milliner on the Committee, had finally surmised, "which I suppose ... is the real reason."

A Mr. Meeks, a Labour journalist from Kingston and representative from the Knights of Labour linked to the Trade Union which supported women workers, had offered the notion that many Masters and Mistresses in big homes expected servant girls to work from dawn to dusk. "And all night too," he had hinted.

Miss Elizabeth Neufeld, Social Worker and Head of Central Neighbourhood House (CNH), a reputable social reform organization in Toronto, had since 1911, along with four Social Work students from the university, investigated the social mores of working girls. At a meeting of the Toronto LCW in April of 1913, she reported on a list she had compiled of thirty-five houses of ill repute and the names of fifteen young prostitutes and the causes of their downfall. Neufeld recommended more healthy outlets for young women and started up a supervised dance hall for working girls on the corner of Elm Street in the Ward. It was agreed that the Toronto LCW, with the help of Mrs. Florence Huestis and Mr. George Warburton of the Young Men's Christian Association (YMCA), would lobby the government to form a Commission to further examine the moral welfare of single working girls. The Toronto LCW also arranged for members to tour Toronto's bookstores and check out the windows for indecent postcards and books.

The Commission, soon known as the Social Service Commission, included four elected politicians, six clergymen, four representatives of social reform organizations, three doctors (Dr. Clarke himself, of course, being consulted), two lawyers, two businessmen and, of course, members of the Toronto LCW, including Elizabeth Neufeld, Florence Huestis, Dr. Margaret Patterson, and Adelaide Plumptre, wife of Bishop Plumptre of

St. James Cathedral of the Anglican Church in Canada, who was engaged in social work at the cathedral. It was to produce a survey of the local vice scene by 1915.

It was soon obvious to the Commission that lower-class women, and factory girls in particular, as Dr. Clarke could have told them, indulged their taste for fun and finery by "supplementing" their wages; how else could they afford trips to Dotty's Hippodrome and Charlie's Minstrel Shows and dancing parlours and the like, reasoned Miss Neufeld and colleagues? Though Shea's Vaudeville on King Street reputedly offered special women's rates for their girlie shows.

Girls, or "good times gals," accepting any favours from a male escort such as a supper, a show, a drink, perfume, jewellery, money, or clothes, were, in effect, practicing a form of prostitution. As a result, they were in need of correction. Though conditions of misery for the poor were reported by Rev. A. Mackenzie of the East Neighbourhood Workers Association — he cited families living on not even half-rations — it was not necessarily true that low wages were the cause for girls going "astray," pointed out Miss Neufeld: there were working girls who managed to remain morally upright and righteous for Christ on as low as $3 a week. On the other hand, one was not certain of the actual security claimed for girls working as domestics. As everyone on the Commission knew, Mr. Christopher St. George Clark, a journalist, had done an extensive survey in 1898 of the city's morals in *Of Toronto the Good, A Social Study: The Queen City of Canada As It Is*. He had cited one boy of sixteen, for instance, who admitted in one interview to having had sexual intercourse with every servant his father had hired. And there was the unfortunate case of Carrie Davies, servant to the wealthy Massey family, reverberating through the upper echelons of Rosedale and the Annex.

On February 9, 1915, Carrie Davies had actually shot to death her Master, wealthy "Bert" Massey, in the driveway of his Walmer Road residence for allegedly being drunken and lewd and trying to rape her the night before, while Mrs. Massey was out of town. Young Bert had pushed Davies, a somewhat plain servant girl of two years' service, onto Mrs. Massey's bed during a wild weekend party, after first tempting young Carrie with gifts of chocolates and a pair of Mrs. Massey's sheer stockings and other personal underwear which he had wanted her to put on. She claimed she had killed him to protect her chastity. There had been sensational coverage in the *Telegram*. The Toronto LCW had appeared at the Police Court hearing in full force, eager to hear the details, the *Daily News* reported excitedly on February 16: "Many of the women were well-dressed and evidently of the 'upper' strata, but they pushed and jostled with the rest."

Of course, she had had to be of unsound mind, Dr. Clarke opined. The Masseys had, in fact, hired an alienist (an early term given to psychiatrists who worked in insane asylums) to test Davies' sanity. After all, she had deliberately shot Bert in public and made no effort to deny her crime. At that, Carrie Davies had become an icon to every low working-class girl in Toronto. Under old English Common Law, a servant was entitled to protection from attack. As immigrant servants from England knew, they had lost that traditional right with no new legislation set in place. Donations had flooded in for her legal support. Operators from the Toronto Hat Factory on Adelaide Street West got up a collection and donated $3. Letters flooded the *Telegram,* many signed anonymously: "British working girl," "Another English Carrie," and, more ominously, "One Who Knows." When Carrie Davies was acquitted, great cheers had arisen from the crowd of spectators.

Of course, it only pointed all the more to how vulnerable the feeble-minded were in the workplace, and that something should be done about them, Dr. Clarke said.

Dr. Helen MacMurchy, Inspector for the Feeble-Minded of the Province of Ontario since 1906, agreed. A colleague of Dr. Clarke and most reliable, she had herself given evidence to the Commission on vice in the city. A sturdy, attractive woman in her forties, Dr. MacMurchy, dressed in a long dark skirt and high-necked jacket, informed the Commission that many low-class working girls were lax morally and were, in fact, feeble-minded, as were most prostitutes: "There is little to distinguish them," she had announced in her decisive way, "being easily led astray."

Which was partly why, indeed, Dr. Clarke had kept the Ward Clinic going for the past four years, since 1909: the first psychiatric clinic in Canada, he liked to boast. It was a dilapidated place, a semi-detached house with a sunken verandah and broken porch on the corner of Chestnut and Christopher Streets, at the edge of the St. John's Ward slum at the foot of City Hall. A notice on the front railing said:

TORONTO GENERAL HOSPITAL
FREE DISPENSARY DAILY 9:00 AM.
GENITO-URINARY CLINIC MEN ONLY.

Above it, nailed to a post, somewhat askew:

FREE DISPENSARY; DISEASES — WOMEN 2:00 PM DAILY.

Similar signs were in Hebrew and Italian: *Dispensario Gratuito*.

This was not exactly what Dr. Clarke had envisaged. His dream had been of a modern Psychiatric Reception Hospital or Clinic, distinct from the Toronto Lunatic Asylum at 999 Queen Street West, which one female inmate, Elaine O. had called in 1910, "*that Prison house of Satan.*"

Dr. Clarke had always prided himself on being a just, modern Superintendent who had fought to maintain a restraints-free approach at the asylum established by former Superintendent, Daniel Clark. Had he not encouraged therapeutic work for the inmates, such as laundry and needlework for females, and wood shop for the men to keep them occupied? He had even founded a nursing school, the first in the country. But this inmate, Elaine O. — insane, of course — had written a spate of letters after her release claiming she had been abused while being transported to the asylum, and all sorts of other uncorroborated sexual abuses: "You needn't think every one insane that gets into that cruel inhospitable uncharitable Asylum get such a claw and paw on me." It was all part of the old erroneous view of asylums linked in the mind of the public with alienists, and inmates bound in manacles and arm muffs, even though Dr. Daniel Clark and Dr. Clarke himself believed in fresh air and exercise for patients.

But that was the past. The new clinic he had envisaged was to be modelled along the lines of Dr. Emil Kraepelin's famous Psychiatric Clinic in Munich, which Dr. Clarke himself had visited in 1907. He had been a member of the Royal Commission appointed to investigate the major psychiatric clinics in Europe and new approaches in the treatment of the insane, the most impressive being Emil Kraepelin's famous Clinic in Germany.

He had soon introduced Kraepelin's classification of psychiatric mental diseases in 1909 for use by alienists in all Ontario Hospitals for the Insane. Psychiatrists at his new hospital would try to *prevent* mental illness by catching it in the early stages.

"Toronto will become a Mecca and lead the world!" he had cried eagerly to colleagues, assured of support from the government and from Sir Robert Falconer, the new President of the University of Toronto. He could hardly wait for construction to begin. Such a psychopathic clinic would be the epitome of good research and teaching, and provide that needed status and prestige for the new "science" of "psychiatry."

Then the government reneged on its promise of $500,000 funding. He had stormed, bitterly disappointed, "Those rogue politicians!" Mr. W. J. Hanna, newly appointed Provincial Secretary responsible for the administration of mental hospitals, including Orillia, had diverted funds promised for Clarke's Psychiatric Clinic to build a new Guelph Reformatory and to rebuild the old Toronto General Hospital on Gerrard Street at a cost of over three million dollars. Dr. Clarke had been outmanoeuvred.

"I love psychiatry, but hate politics!" he had raged. He also suspected jealous colleagues of subterfuge in the Neurological Department. There were rumours of alienists resenting the prospect of Dr. Clarke taking away the curable patients in this new profession of psychiatry and leaving them with the "dregs" of the back wards. Of course, hospital patients from their crammed wards had little idea of all this going on in the government offices and hospital boardrooms around them.

Dr. Clarke had remained undaunted. His was a jolly, exuberant temperament, as he well prided himself, with his high vivid complexion and vigorous reddish moustache. He determined to start a clinic anyway, however small, until the great psychiatric hospital of his dreams was built. He persuaded the board of the Toronto General Hospital to loan him the use of the house on Chestnut Street. He had even invited Dr. Ernest Jones, reputed British neurologist and psychoanalyst, to come to Toronto in 1908 and be the Clinic's first medical director and written personally to Mr. Hanna, the Provincial Secretary, recommending Dr. Jones for the position of Pathologist and Neurologist at the Toronto Insane Asylum (at a salary of $600 per annum). Dr. Jones was one of the best known living authorities on nervous and mental troubles, and colleague of Dr. Sigmund Freud and Dr. Carl Jung, who had worked at the Munich clinic under Dr. Kraepelin, urged Clarke. He was especially strong in the "psychological side of medicine."

One wonders what dapper, sophisticated Ernest Jones, a Welshman destined to be Freud's great famed biographer, and attractive to women, must have thought when confronted with the "Clinic" on Chestnut

Street, teetering at the edge of a slum. He had exulted to Dr. Freud, on his appointment, that he was entering a "new world."

The patients had turned out to be overwhelmingly feeble-minded — a fact not lost on Dr. Clarke. The silly, coquettish girls brought in for their checkups in their lacy camisoles were soon seen in their true light, as they *really* were, once they removed their petticoats and corselettes and lay on the examining table, he frowned, many of them riddled with syphilis and gonorrhea. Not that they felt the slightest shame as they parted their legs. They did not. One such girl of about sixteen — "Suzie" — had given him a saucy knowing wink. "'Aving a good look, Gov?" Dr. Clarke had bristled. For the shocking thing was that she was an *English* girl.

Of course, not a *nice* English girl, agreed the police officers who had brought her in with the others, who also had not had the slightest hesitation in telling their stories. One such girl had exasperatingly chewed gum throughout. The Morality Squad was equally confused by the number of these British girls being apprehended in the dives, brothels and massage parlours on King, Front Street West, Simcoe, Richmond and Seaton Streets, and other such areas of the city. They were obviously the new degenerates of the English Poor Laws being let into Canada lately from the working-class slums of Britain, despite the 1897 *Act to Regulate The Immigration Into Ontario of Certain Classes of Children* – just repealed in 1912. They were a far cry from the noble Anglo-Saxons that Canadians were used to and praised by the Methodist Missionary Society for their "old English strength of character" (still present, of course, in the best families of Toronto). What was needed, frowned Dr. Clarke, was a Eugenics Record Office such as the one founded by their American colleagues in Cold Spring Harbor, New York. This Record Office was, right then, compiling a genealogical registry of dubious American families suspected of carrying defective germplasm.

Dr. Helen MacMurchy concurred. In her Seventh Annual Report as Inspector for the Feeble-Minded, she stressed the *Immigration Act* should be tightened, and the feeble-minded barred from landing. Out of 47 feeble-minded immigrants detained in 1913, she reported indignantly, 24 had been released.

By 1913, the little Ward Clinic on Chestnut Street had begun to peter out with the demise of its director, Dr. Ernest Jones. They had tried to keep it open to the last, Dr Clarke recalled sadly. Dr. Jones had done his best, had been admirable, Dr. Clarke maintained loyally, though there had been little evidence he had ever actually attended any patients — Dr. Clarke himself had attended to 276 patients. Of course, there had been the awkward discovery of Dr. Jones living common law the entire time with a woman, his mistress Loe Kann, whom he had passed off as his wife while living on Brunswick Avenue. When confronted, Dr. Jones had not shown the slightest shame, had even seemed nonchalant: "No, we're not married."

Other rumours had gradually surfaced across the Atlantic of certain sexual improprieties in England. Dr. Jones had apparently been charged with conducting an improper interview with a young female patient in a London hospital, which was against hospital protocol, and consequently forced to resign. And in another incident, he was accused by the London County Council of masturbating in front of two thirteen-year-old mentally deficient girls in a school for the mentally deficient in Deptford — he had apparently been conducting an inquiry into speech mechanisms. Unfortunate. Brilliant man. Dr. Clarke had tried to hush it up, loyal as ever to his protégé. But the Hon. Lieutenant-Governor of Ontario, Dr. Herbert Bruce, incensed, had declared Dr. Jones a pervert and had had him dismissed from the faculty.

Dr. Jones set off across the Atlantic for Europe to study psychoanalysis under Sándor Ferenczi, calling Toronto, on his departure, "Victorian" and biblical in its attitudes.

20.

THE STEAMER HOOTED and a puff of white smoke curled in the air. Florrie, not yet fourteen years old, leaned anxiously over the rail as *The Empress of England* drew into the landing stage at St John's, New Brunswick, in 1913, her first glimpse of her new country.

She was but one of 80,000 British girls and boys brought to Canada between 1868 and 1925 as cheap indentured labour to work as domestics and farm labourers, under the passenger warrant system — words she had heard Mr. Murphy, the agent for the steamship company, Blue Line, say. He had been paid $3.00 Canadian a head for every girl and boy, man and woman he booked for the Dominion.

A long grey wharf topped by an equally long grey building loomed, where immigration officers checked the arrivals. But Florrie, in her long coat and second-hand lace-up boots, had nothing to worry about; she had more clothes in a carrying bag than she had seen in her life, including a petticoat and combinations. All the arrangements had been done in London at the Canadian Government Emigration linking Britain and Canada. Auntie had known all about it though not her actual date of departure. Auntie had been to the Work House School as a child and could read words.

"Canada Wants Domestic Servants!" This notice had been issued by the Canadian Authority of the Minister of the Interior in 1909. "High Wages, Good Homes, Healthy Climate!" Auntie had seen the pamphlets and posters around London's east end, in the fish market even. What more could little Florrie want, it was better than the workhouse, Auntie had said. She could not afford to keep her forever, she had hinted, and no doubt Florrie would meet a nice young Canadian fellow with some dosh in his pocket.

Florrie had lived with old Irish Auntie since the father she could not remember had taken off. Auntie, whose own mother had come over on the boat from Ulster in the time of the Troubles, had come and got little Florrie out of the workhouse. The poorhouses of Manchester and London were familiar to Florrie and Henry, and Daisy's other grandparents, the Lumsdens, all of whom were children of the British Poor Laws and Poor Law Unions. Auntie had her bit of outdoor relief, some cash, from the Poor Law but it was not much. She had lived in a room off Gossport Street, without light. There were rooms upon rooms, stretched out in long galleries. It was subterranean: a place of tunnels and alleys and wretched dens that little Florrie had gotten used to. She was to help Auntie, a washerwoman, with the laundry. At age six she did the scrubbing, her small knuckles worn and bleeding on the rippled steel boards.

What had happened to her mother no one said, only that she had gone to a hard place called the "asylum." "Well where else was a woman to go to what been left dest'ute by 'er 'usband with children?" Auntie had said once, "an' the asylum was better than the work'ouse; *any place* was better than the workhouse."

Florrie had a vague, frightening memory of the workhouse where she and her brothers and sisters had ended up as a cold, dark place of long, hard wards with iron grilles at the window shutting out London; of straw mattresses on wooden platforms each side of a gangway; of people coughing and cold; floors you swept at age five or so; and of big Mr. Beggleby and his bottles of gin, before Auntie come.

At age fourteen, a girl like Florrie "with experience" was in demand, assured Mr. Murphy, as the Canadians in Toronto were all mad for English domestics. At age eleven, Florrie had been a parlour maid — a "dolly mop" they had called her — at the Chisholme-Lloyd's, a grand place outside London, where she had worked from dawn to dusk hewing water jugs up to Master and Mistress's bedroom before dawn for their ablutions. Sometimes, Master had slept in a separate dressing room. She did not know time but Tillie did by the cockerels in the outhouse. She had done the scouring; she had peeled hundreds of taters; she had lugged scuttles of coal for the kitchen fire; and she had slept in a cupboard away from the butler and manservants who were out in the back-house. Tillie, the hall-maid who saw to visitors, had worked for the Duchess of Carlisle up in Scotland (and where was that?) and had said it was better at the Chisholme-Lloyd's than there.

The Duchess had had her head servant make the maids stand in a line and show their pads every month to prove they were not with child. "They'd better bloody well be bleedin'," Tillie had said with a snort, otherwise you were sent packing.

But it would be different in Canada, in Toronto. No front steps to scrub, no brass plates by the doors to polish, and no dark cellars. Amazing. Where did Canadians keep their coal, and Master's wine and the taters? They had basements, she was told. And gas.

Something called the BWEA, or British Women's Emigration Association, saw to the various forms including the medicals, said Mr. Murphy. Canadians wanted the civilizing influence of British women in Canada. Florrie would be absolutely safe, they had assured Auntie. Though had Auntie asked? Young girls like Florrie, travelled in parties with a chaperone or conductresses who accompanied his or her charges on the Great Western Railway, and delivered them safely at the other end to the Women's Welcome Hostel in Toronto.

And so Florrie had set out across the vast ocean that May, 1913, with a ribbon in her hair, unaware that she was passing famous or infamous Dr. Ernest Jones mid-Atlantic, sailing in the other direction. He was returning to Europe, to Budapest, from Dr. Charles Clarke's Psychiatric Clinic in Toronto, the clinic having been finally shut down.

There were hundreds of parties on board: Mr. Bentham's Party, Miss Grisholme's Party, the Home Boys Party, the Catholic Boys Party, the Salvation Army Girls' Party, the Waifs and Strays Party. Florrie had been in Miss Bartlett's Party. Miss Bartlett, a reliable spinster in a dark costume with pleated bodice and a brimmed hat, had already crossed the Atlantic twenty times accompanying her "girls." Miss Bartlett remembered how the ocean had rocked. There were great, great glassy waves and a vast expanse of blue. Large birds swooping about. And many of the girls had been sick.

At night, they all squeezed together into the bunks. There was a smell of hot oil and steam, and the whir of great propellers. Some of the young women in her berth — they had their hair "up" — were being sent as farm domestics somewhere Out West, to a place called Manitoba. The posters at Charing Cross had shown a smiling, rosy-cheeked woman holding a sheaf of corn: "Go West Young Woman!" They likely would end up marrying cattle or pig farmers, they had whispered excitedly, anxious with hope.

Florrie's position, "on one year's probation," had already been arranged: scullery maid in a large home in Rosedale, Toronto, room and board included. The older girls in her berth told Florrie that if the Master "wanted his way," she was to go along with it. She would be "all right" if she kept very still on her back afterwards, and did not move.

21.

YOUNG HENRY HEWITT knew a thing or two about factory girls in Toronto, before the Great War. It was when he had met Florrie. As soon as he saw her in the nickelodeon he knew she was the one: a pretty little thing of about fifteen with golden curls done up fancy on top of her head, and pretty lacy stuff peeking out of her camisole if you wanted to see more. Florrie had skipped lunch for a week to save for it at Woolworth's.

She was with Maudie, a ripping girl, hard as they come. She knew the price of a dollar. You would not have Maude Herrigan up against the factory wall, or your hands up her skirt for naught; a girl had her price, she would say all haughty. But Florrie was different; she was sweet, and all smiles, and had shining eyes; she was soft in his arms.

He had come over as a Union Poorhouse boy on *The Corsican* he told her. He even had new breeches for the voyage.

Florrie had smiled. "Tha's nice, 'Enry."

He had laughed. "You're a funny one."

His name tag had said: "London England: Bound for Toronto." He was bound for a farm in Ontario, with hundreds of other boys going out west, some of them cheering and others crying. They wanted to go home, sobbed the littler boys on the train, changing their minds. "Cheer up, lads, think of 'Is Majesty," Mr. Barnstable had said.

He had been picked up off the east end streets of London with other vagrants, and put into the workhouse where he had learned his lessons in the workhouse school, an echoing desolate place. They had sat in rows on long benches and learned to recite the "Lord's Prayer" and psalms: "I will lift up mine eyes unto the 'ills," longing for the bowls of soup ladled out by the Matron. He had reached Standard 111 (Grade 3 Canadian equivalent) at fourteen — a backward boy, said Mr. Vellicott, who had a bamboo cane that went *crack*! Then they were told they were going to Canada, for their King and Country.

Of course, as soon as he got near sixteen, his bonding over to his Master at the farm as an indentured labourer, he had jumped the train to Toronto and got himself a room off Spadina Avenue, $2 a week with a shared privy. The house was filled with boarders like himself, working men and boys looking for jobs in construction or the new factories.

He earned $6 a week stamping steel plates, he told Florrie eagerly. He could afford to take her to the Minstrel Show at the Gaety next Saturday on her half day; it was 15 cents a matinee.

He had had her one summer night, back in his room on D'Arcy Street. It was a tiny room with a narrow window at the back. A large heavy tree outside swayed, like Florrie beneath him. Ah, she had taken off the dress. Her worn drawers parted in his hands, which trembled. She was a pretty little thing underneath, all pink and swollen, her tight bubs sticking up like pins. She had rolled and gasped again and again. She forgot all about keeping still afterwards.

He had known she had already been taken. She had admitted so at once, had sobbed. It was when she had been at Doctor and Mrs. Rowatt-Gilbertson's doing the scrubbing. She was sorry. "Oh so sorry, 'Enry, want you in me first."

But she had been put in the great big house, in Rosedale called "Rosemere"; houses of the rich had names, like people. It had big trees, and lots of entrance doors that Florrie could not count, and endless windows to clean. You only had to know your door as a servant — the back one by the coal-house. There was a scullery maid, a serving maid (in a nicer skirt and clean white bib), a butler, a man for the heavy work and the horses, and a chauffeur for Dr. Rowatt-Gilbertson's new auto.

The drawing room had lovely deep carpets. She brought in the trays — conversation stopped — laid them on the sideboard and curtseyed as Maudie, the other servant girl, had shown her. Mrs. Rowatt-Gilbertson resumed talking. She was a tall, powerful woman in sweeping skirts. "Do you know to use a dauber, Florrie?" Florrie had whispered, "Didn' know, ma'am." Mrs. Rowatt-Gilbertson had rolled her eyes.

There were vast stairs you got lost on, and hushed landings with closed doors. Which door was she to put the water jug in front of? She had to collect the smelly pee-pots first thing. "Chamber-pot, please," said the cook. "These are gentry." There were endless rooms, and turrets that twirled around until she was dizzy.

She was weary all the time. Her day started at five in her tiny, hot attic room, which was better than the cupboard in England, though the Social Service Commission on Vice did not necessarily record that; for Florrie was a scullery maid at fourteen, not to be trusted yet to wait on tables.

She pulled on her uniform in the early dark: a heavy serviceable apron and bib and mop cap. Underneath, she wore cotton combinations Mrs. Rowatt-Gilbertson had provided, long knickers with a slit for her monthlies (the pads given out and counted by the head servant, Miss Pinsent), a spencer, and a flannel petticoat for winter. She had felt tied in.

At six o'clock, the cook told her to get cold water from the tap for the Misses Emily and Clara, and Master and Mistress' toilette. Then, she had to carry the heavy pails up two flights of stairs via the second back staircase. But which staircase was that? "The one without carpet, silly," said Maudie. She had carried the heavy pots up the staircases and learned to knock carefully on the correct door, to then go inside, fearful, but of what? She was to pour the water into the ewers, and be careful not to look at Master and Mistress in their big feather bed behind the curtains. Oh, the size of that terrifying bed. Once, Master Rowatt-Gilbertson, who was a judge, and snored said Maudie (and she should know), had opened one eye at Florrie and given her a wink. Florrie knew what that meant.

She scoured the kitchen floor, wrung the Rowatt-Gilbertson's sheets through the mangle. There were all sorts of implements: a banister brush, a stove dauber. Confused, Florrie kept mixing up brushes. "Lordie, don't you knows a *dauber*? What they sendin' over from the old country nowadays," cried Miss Pinsent, head servant; she had been in service for twenty-five years and had a different shining uniform and a white straight cap.

Florrie bent down with what she now knew was the hearth duster to tackle the grate. There was the manservant, Charlie, who brought in the silver; she felt a hand press quietly over her buttock. There was the noonday meal of bread and cheese and a glass of beer, then the weekly afternoon chores, would the day never end? No, not until eight o'clock, unless Miss Emily and Miss Clara needed help with their corsets. Mrs. Rowatt-Gilbertson had said in a loud voice down the hall, "What do they always want a half day off for?" Florrie would fall exhausted on her palliasse at night, thinking of Charlie's hand on her buttock.

"Oh, the Austins, now they got a place, Flo, over in Spadina House up on Dav'nport Hill," went Maudie; she had started her service over in their great house. "They has a *pot cocher* in wrote-iron an' glass out front. An' a terrace with bal'strades an' urns." Florrie had little idea what a *porte cochère* was or wrought iron. There were two great houses up there on Davenport Hill — "Ravensbrook" and "Spadina House" — above the oak woods, Maudie went on.

Florrie, worn to a thread from polishing the stairs and fetching and carrying for Miss Emily and Miss Clara, only sighed.

But Miss Emily played and sang beautiful on the pianoforte for visitors, "Oh, for the wings, the wings of a dove," breathed Maudie, who often waited as a maid at these dinners on account of her erect posture and coiled red hair.

The clothes they had given Florrie were so hot, so stifling. And her tiny room at the top of the stairs in the attic was long and narrow and unlit. It had only a thin skylight. The agent had not said Canada was *hot*. In the summer months she often had to open the top buttons of her dress.

Maudie was twenty, she said, to which Billie, the coach-boy, added snidely, "an' the rest." She had been with the Rowatt-Gilbertson's for two years. She knew letters and numbers. More important, she knew a thing or two and more about pleasing the young masters, she hinted, tossing her hair. She gave Florrie a sharp, anxious look. Master Ewan and Master Cecil had come home from boarding school, lads of sixteen and eighteen, and they liked to have their bit of fun, Maudie winked.

But Florrie was too tired to listen. Yet now she feared the nights and the long unlit stairs leading up to the attic, as if she knew it would happen, and of course it did. He was at the top, waiting on the step; was it Master Ewan or Master Cecil? He slid down his bracers that held up his trousers, smiling; his hands reached down and pulled at the rest of her buttons.

"Bleedin' bastards!" Henry clenched his fists, in tears for his own loss as much as Florrie's. "You just a lass."

They had had her first, she had not been able to keep herself for him, he cried bitterly. He'd go there right then to South bleedin' Drive up over the bridge and dig out their balls. Then they wouldn't be able to jump girls no more. He was strong and hard-bodied from his years at the farm. He had hard blue eyes that Florrie liked — the way they glowed.

Maudie said he would swing for it in the Don Jail. Then he quieted down. It was pointless to go to the courts (dangerous places for working girls and men). No cop or magistrate was going to give heed to Florrie over the young Masters' word. "Why 'ad she not resisted?" the judge would say. "She must 'ave encouraged them."

"I loves you anyway, Flo."

Frightened, Florrie had got out of her position, thanks to Maudie. Maudie could read and write a bit, and knew where the Women's Welcome Hostel was downtown. She bet if Florrie threatened to make a fuss about the young masters and what they had done, the Imperial Order of Daughters of the Empire (IODE) would arrange something with the Rowatt-Gilbertons to get her released. Maudie was sharp, she knew a thing or two about toffs, how they would not want a fuss, "And not the Imperial Order of them Bloody Daughters neither, Flo."

The ladies of the Imperial Order of Daughters of the Empire and of the Toronto Local Council of Women had expressed cautious concern at Florrie, standing in the hall of the Women's Welcome Hostel next to Maudie on her half day, in her worn cotton dress and bit of lace, illiterate and no doubt feeble-minded. Should she even have been let into the country?

"What about th' Protection o' Women's Committee?" Maudie had cried, "Warn't no protection fer us."

The Ladies had bristled. These were the Masters, after all, their own husbands in their homes in Rosedale and the Annex. They had initiated the Purity campaign and the White Feather movement, which touted "one standard of morality for all."

"And she needs 'er six months wages, too, how's a girl to survive?'

Maudie had been right. There had been a flurry of consternation. Where this girl really belonged was a House of Refuge or the institution in Orillia, but Florrie had been quietly let go and now was granted wages to cover her for a few weeks, which she kept in a little string bag down her chemise on Maudie's advice.

Maudie gave in her notice too; she'd laughed at Mrs. Rowatt-Gilbertson's reiterations of exasperation about "servants these days." Why would Maudie leave South Drive for a room below College Street and a dingy factory? If Mrs. Rowatt-Gilbertson suspected (and perhaps she had) as she paused in the conservatory, with a slight quiver in her eye, she said nothing. These low-class girls coming over now on the steamers were not the girls of yesteryear.

Dr. Rowatt-Gilbertson had tweaked Ewan's ear affectionately and said simply, "Rascal! Been after the pretty one, eh? Florrie, was it?" Florrie had gone off in a huff; odd, that, he thought, and Maudie given in her notice too. Young Master Ewan returned to boarding school, and Master Cecil was to be articled to his father's old law firm, Maudie had heard when she went to collect her wages. A new little girl had been hired through the BWEA, who had just crossed over on the *Empress of Britain*, fresh from England.

Maudie found them a little room to share in the St. John's Ward near City Hall at $3 a week, "for now," she had said, exulting. She was sick and tired of domestic work; paper box-making was better, or even stamping tubes of toothpaste in the Colgate factory out on King Street was better. They could catch the tram.

"You'll see, Flo," she winked.

They had an iron bedstead to share, a palliasse, one broken chair, a small cracked mirror a former lodger had left on a nail, and a bar of carbolic soap for the fleas. They washed their camisoles and drawers and cotton pads in the chipped sink in the basement and hung them on a piece of string in the window to dry. The house was filled with boarders: a family of ten in the attic, men on construction shift work, and a few clerks who spent a long time in the water closet off the kitchen.

Maudie rapped on the door. "Eh, you gonna wear it down ter nothing in there."

They got work at the Chocolate Factory down on Lakeshore Road where there were rows and rows of low, grey buildings and makeshift hostels for factory girls and men with nowhere to go.

"We're free, Flo. We c'n do as we please!"

That evening, Florrie and Maudie laughed and laughed at the raunchy songs and jokes at the burlesque made popular just then by Marie Lloyd: "Just because I'm a fool don't think I'm Irish" and "She'd never 'ad the ticket punched before!" with a wink from the chanteuse.

And they joined in lustily in the chorus of the minstrel show hits from the 1890s, waving their beers as Daring Dotsie twirled about the stage, her suspenders flashing in the high kicks, her naughty tinsel pasties a-quiver:

I'm not too young, I'm not too old,
Not too timid, not too bold,
Just the kind you'd like to hold...

Oh, the Chocolate Factory! It was hot. Large fans whirred intermittently in the molten air. The girls sat in long lines at the conveyor belt like automatons. Florrie was to drop one dollop of cream — no counting involved — on each chocolate cupcake as it whirred by, hour after hour. She get dizzy over the thrum of the belt, the whirl of chocolate cups. "Goes right through yer," warned the girls.

A bell rang. They all rose and walked in lines to the canteen for break, watched over by Mr. Benedict and Miss Tolston who guarded the water closet. It was shared with the factory boys from Block C who made the Dolly mixtures, and who kept blocking up the pipe with their turds. "Made of fucking concrete they are," complained Clara, the leader of the licorice train, who earned $5 a week. Management had put in a tin with a lid for the girls' pads, by order of the Department of Health — who removed them at night?

Oh, the fun, then, of drinking tea and eating a biscuit. The men sat separately on the other end. Florrie sat with her fellow workers, some of them smoking Black Cats daringly and flicking their ash on the floor. Some had their hair piled up in curls held with glittering combs, or a feather through a hairslide, and wore sparkling bodices with sequins under their pinafores. But there were also girls as young as eleven, their flour-sack dresses tied with string or bits of lace. They had that wan look that Florrie recognized.

"Ooh, he wasn't half a good looker, aye. A real masher! And he come up to me in the Parlour and says ... red sports car..."

"Enough, you girls down there," called Miss Tolston. She was tall, straight as a stick, with a long, severe face, "like she got a poker up 'er arse," said Sophia, and then Maudie said something about stirring a poker in the fire, which Florrie did not understand, but all the girls screamed, "Oh Maudie, you are card!"

Florrie leaned forward in her seat at the trestle table, smiling widely. The things they said! The things she learned!

"You want to get every penny out of them while you can, dearie, the swine," was the general advice about fellers.

She thought of his big red hands that summer. Henry said it was 1914 and that meant the year. It was still hot and sunny when you came out of the factory. You could smell the odour of cocoa for blocks. She felt the excitement at meeting him at the market on Augusta Avenue; she knew it was Augusta because there were live chickens in cages; goats tied to a post; dried pats of manure mixed with dust and peelings; the merry ring of ice cream carts; men in long black coats and beards; a rush of bright signs she could not read; trams rumbling on Spadina, and a horse and cart swaying down the gutters.

He took her out to the island on the ferry that summer evening, the dust of the factory blown away, and streaming skies and birds in its wake, to Hanlan's Point, the merry jetty bright with bunting. You could see the toffs sipping drinks out on the terrace of the Royal Yacht Club, the ladies moving in a haze of long white dresses and straw boater hats. Florrie had a straw boater, too, and a new strip of lace on her camisole. She had skipped lunches for a week to save her pennies for that at the Five and Dime Store — a place she learned about from the girls — "Economics, dearie." There were rides and games and a dance hall. Henry held her hand steady at the shooting gallery. Then, Florrie and Henry whirled round Dotty's Hippodrome. Oh, it exciting to touch of his chest with its hint of curly red hairs she would run through her fingers later.

Later that night it was his fingers that parted her frilly drawers and a layer of petticoat as she lay under him. She felt herself swell under his fingers on the little iron bed under the eaves (there was a tin pee-pot for his piss and turds, which he threw out of the window afterwards in the yard below). Her camisole shone in a new way, her pretty worn stays (the bones sticking through) excited Henry, she knew, as he unfastened them slowly. This was what they had been waiting for all evening, wasn't it? He struggled with each hook, until he had reached the place he wanted and lay pulsing over her, and she felt something open wide that she had never known before.

22.

DR. HELEN MACMURCHY, now in her late forties, was riding down Yonge Street on her trusty old bicycle (later on she used a little electric brougham.) "There she goes!" She was certainly a familiar figure around the city in her sturdy costume and brimmed hat, pedalling furiously that summer day in 1909, on her way to the Ward. She had beef tea in her saddlebag for one of her patients.

Her father, Archibald MacMurchy, had been the first head-master of the Toronto Grammar School, later Jarvis Collegiate, a strict authoritarian, and her mother a "Ramsay," both of Scottish heritage, as if nothing more need be said. Mr. MacMurchy had been, in his time, the President of the Ontario Educational Association, and had written six books on arithmetic. After his retirement at age seventy, he devoted himself to writing a history of English literature. All of which meant, of course, that the three MacMurchy girls, Helen in particular, as the eldest, had had a lot to live up to, as she was well aware, not without a certain pride.

There was a curious photo of Helen MacMurchy that she invariably offered the newspapers for their publicity columns. It was of herself as a young woman, about twenty, in a pretty dress with a low-cut ruched bodice that showed off a strong graceful neck and hint of shoulders. A silly velvet bow in the fashion of the time sat over the breast. Dark, luxurious curls were piled high on top of her head. The expression on her face was earnest and intent; owlish eyes peered through rimless, round glasses giving her a studious air, either off-putting or appealing to a young man in her circle? It goes without saying that the dancing parlours and nickelodeons of Yonge and King Streets were not for the MacMurchy girls. For them, much more appropriate were the occasional socials in the discreet homes of Upper Toronto and Rosedale, and afternoons teas or evening concerts in Lady Falconer's drawing room or Forrester's Hall, the Miss MacMurchys always with their chaperone.

At the turn of the century, in 1901, Helen MacMurchy had sat in her bedroom at her writing desk marking student papers. Being a single woman of nearly forty, she still lived with her father and mother in her parents' home in the old house on Bloor Street East, with her sisters Marjory (a reporter and editor of rising acclaim) and Bessie, also unmarried. The three sisters attended First Presbyterian Church with their parents and, led by their father, said their evening prayers in the family parlour: "Blessed is the man that walketh not in the counsel of the ungodly, nor standeth in the way of sinners..." For the MacMurchys were of the old faith, followers of Reverend John Shearer, General Secretary of the Lord's Day Alliance, which had pushed for the *Lord's Day Act* in 1906 in Toronto, and an end to such ungodly pleasures as skating rinks, Sunday shopping, and fishing in the Don River on the Sabbath. Rev. Shearer also upheld strict punishment, even jail for prostitutes.

There was a sense of loneliness in the quiet *tick* of the clock in the hall below, as Helen lay down her fine quilled pen and paused from marking student work. She took in the sheaves of papers, the sombre desk, the late hour. She was thirty-nine. It was in that still moment that she had known that her child-bearing years had passed in an era when young women were considered spinsters by age twenty-five. Ruefully, perhaps she had wondered, besides, what man had been eligible? Had she ever really wanted him? What she really yearned for was to enter the medical profession.

This is what she had told her father, now retiring, at whose side she had taught for twenty years at Jarvis Collegiate, from the age of nineteen, despite his disapproval of women teachers. She had gone ahead and enrolled at the Ontario Medical College for Women at the University of Toronto, and become a physician at a time when women were rare in the field, part of the challenge, perhaps. She had, of course, done brilliantly: came first in her class; received her degree of M.D. in 1901. Her thesis, "Hospital Appointments: Are They Open To Women?" was published in the *Lancet*. It had at once drawn immense attention to herself. Who was this MacMurchy woman?

After further study at the prestigious Johns Hopkins Hospital in Baltimore, and at the Women's Medical College at the University of Toronto, she had set up practice as a general physician in her parents' home at 133

Bloor Street East, specializing in gynaecology, obstetrics, and paediatrics. She had felt her father's unexpected pride in her. But she also lectured on anatomy and physiology at various women's educational institutions around Toronto, and was appointed Resident Medical Assistant at Toronto General Hospital — another first — with Dr. Clarke himself. She was, in essence, an emerging professional woman of power. But part of her work was also devoted to the poor in St. John's Ward, the slum at the foot of City Hall, stretching between College and Queen Streets, not far from her home, but far enough. Such work was an essential part of her Presbyterian sense of duty to mankind: "Soldiers of Christ arise, and gird thy armour on..."

The "Ward," as it was called, had been somewhat of a shock. Dr. MacMurchy pushed her bicycle between a maze of shacks and sunken houses. There were swarms of flies, mounds of refuse, pieces of stolen firewood, and rats scurrying amidst the warrens of subterraneous rooms added on to houses, broken shacks. She could see Dr. Clarke's Ward Clinic teetering at the edge of Chestnut Street, appreciating what the great doctor was attempting. His brave little venture demonstrated the courage it took to tackle, alone, the problem of the feeble-minded all around them.

The low intelligence of the slum dwellers, Jews from Eastern Europe, the rag-pickers of the city with their strange Hebrew signs over doorways, and Chinese mixed in with the lowest, destitute Anglo-Saxon immigrants, was all too evident. A thousand of the unemployed had actually dared march on City Hall in 1909, demanding work, the first alarming protest of this new underclass, perhaps. Easily put down, of course. They were the doomed ones in the "survival of the fittest" in society, a term coined by the great English philosopher, Herbert Spencer, as Dr. MacMurchy knew from her vast reading. Spencer had made it plain in as early as 1864 that the endowed survived while the impoverished and uneducated died off, as they should: "If they are not sufficiently complete to live, they die, and it is best they should die," wrote the great thinker. Yet, Dr. MacMurchy gripped her bottle of beef tea, in readiness.

Rack-rent landlords rented out these hovels to the poor at exorbitant rates, forcing them to live eighteen to a house, ten people to a room. Municipal reports had recently highlighted the misery of such families huddled together in shacks, as ruthless land speculators, including the Toronto General Hospital, held on to these shifty houses waiting for property values to rise. Dr. Clarke's Clinic in St. John's Ward was itself a piece of dilapidated property, also owned by Toronto General Hospital, a discomforting fact that Dr. MacMurchy and Dr. Clarke did not necessarily acknowledge. Dr. MacMurchy's immediate concern, however, was the state of Toronto's milk: she had written indignant letters to the Department of Health about milk being contaminated from lack of proper pasteurization, as well as the problem of flies and open sewage, which, in turn, led to typhus outbreaks, diarrhea, enteritis, and soaring infant deaths — 180 per 1,000 infants a year — appalling. Well, feces were still being thrown out on the dirt street by the people who lived in these shacks, as if it were the Middle Ages.

Dr. MacMurchy had reached such a foul-smelling shack, swarming with flies. Nellie Gafferty on Elm Street could not afford a physician or even a midwife, nor could the Gaffertys afford anywhere better to live, so she lay on her back on matting on the floor, her legs already parted and her filthy gown pushed back. Six or more children ran barefoot or naked around the room; some were hungry and pulled at Mama for butties. As a gynaecologist, Dr. MacMurchy was exposed to the intimacies of women's bodies, exercising a certain subtle power when examining women. She was intelligent and aware enough to understand that this could be any woman's fate. Perhaps she felt a certain horror at the woman's helplessness; a helplessness that, under other circumstances, she might have experienced herself if married. There was, then, a safety, a certain inviolable physical integrity, to spinsterhood. She would never be vulnerable or helpless or out of control — the horror of it — like this woman lying on the floor in front of her.

There was a sudden gush of water, then long groans before the head appeared: "Push *now!*" she ordered. It was essential to be objective, and in control. She took out her scissors.

A sickly little thing, no doubt feeble-minded like the mother; as a doctor, one could tell at a glance. The new baby trembled in her hands. She put some silver nitrate drops in its eyes. It would not survive. She knelt and offered beef tea to the woman's lips. "Ah, Doc'r MacMurchy, you an angel dear," the woman had murmured. She might not live herself; the fever was soaring. Neighbouring women had been boiling kettles of water, as the little ones swarmed and cried again for butties. The father appeared, shifting awkwardly in the back kitchen, another out-of-work labourer, no doubt. Dr. MacMurchy encountered hundreds of them. There would be no fee.

"The rich baby lives, the poor baby dies," she had once said dryly, not without indignation.

Dr. MacMurchy had been the obvious choice of Mr. Hanna, the Provincial Secretary of Ontario, to represent Canada in New York, at a meeting in 1905 with the British Royal Commission of King Edward VII on the Care and Control of the Feeble-minded. The Commission was touring the British Empire looking into services and facilities for the mentally deficient. The officers included Mr. W. H. Dickinson of the National Association for the Care of the Feeble-Minded and a Mrs. Hume Pinsent, a British Lunacy Commissioner concerned about the rise in mental defectives in Britain, especially workhouse girls who came under the Poor Law authorities of Britain. They had omitted Canada from their itinerary, they had confessed to Mr. Hanna, unaware that the Dominion had any facilities for the feeble-minded. "Oh, but we have Orillia!"

Imperious in her stiff costume, dark stockings, and spectacles, Dr. Helen MacMurchy had soon put the commissioners to rights. The Orillia Asylum for Idiots, established since 1876, was of some repute, she informed them. Before that date, mental defectives whose families could not care for them had ended up in the county jail in wretched conditions, or locked up in a lunatic asylum. This asylum, built especially for the feeble-minded, was a vast improvement. Its massive building alone had a central corridor 550 feet long, with embossed sheet-iron ceilings and hardwood floors. It had its own gas, made on the premises. The ovens could brown 180 loaves of bread at the same time. Dr. Beaton, the Superintendent, a dear man and fellow stalwart Scot, an elder in the Orillia Presbyterian Church (she had once called him a "great man" while he had been known to refer to her as "that certain lady we all admire and esteem") had twice been elected President of the Association of Medical Officers of American Institutions for Idiotic and Feeble-Minded Persons in recognition of his work. He had been the first to start up a little school as early as 1878 (funded by himself) for the forty or so educable inmates with the help of Miss Christie, head teacher, and Miss Jennings, assistant. There had been 75 pupils then, which had quickly increased to 652 residents by 1900. "No child, not even the most severely retarded, need be neglected," had been the great doctor's axiom.

The British Commissioners were impressed. Of course, she did not say that children were sleeping two to a bed, and that the Asylum was grossly underfunded. Orillia was, in fact, the least funded institution per patient, even as compared to those in Europe. "Poor house rates!" Dr. Beaton had cried. Each day in the Orillia Asylum began with the "Lord's Prayer," followed by calisthenics — club swinging by the children in school, dumbbell drill, and ladder walking; the ladder inclined at twenty-five degrees, continued Dr. MacMurchy staunchly of the physical exercise program. By 1905, several low grades could talk, and thirteen could speak intelligibly. The ideal had been to train the higher-grade inmates to be self-sufficient. Dr. John Langmuir, the first Inspector of Asylums, Prisons and Public Charities appointed in June, 1868, had urged the government for a modern training school in Ontario for idiotic and imbecile children, such as those proven successful in Great Britain. The aim was for patients to be returned home as soon as possible to their families after training, making Orillia a sort of boarding school for the feeble-minded. Of course, that ideal would necessarily have to be modified, frowned Dr. MacMurchy, as mentally defective children needed *permanent* care. Inspector O'Reilly, who succeeded Dr. Langmuir as inspector in 1882 had assured that preference would always be given in Orillia to girls at the age of puberty and up, something the British Commissioners themselves were stressing.

For in Britain, Dr. MacMurchy was now perturbed to learn, the problem was out of control. A government census had been taken. Dr. Alfred Tredgold and Dr. W. A. Potts, medical investigators to the Commission, had identified 271,000 mental defectives including lunatics in England and Wales, of whom 149,000 were uncertified. Who knew how many there were in Canada? The medical men wanted certification of defectives under the *British Idiots Act* of 1886. Special classes established by the 1899 *Elementary Education (Defective and Epileptic Children) Act* were being used as "sorting houses" to identify and separate the children of low intelligence.

But the real issue was what to do with them in adulthood, when they were the most danger to society. Every Board of Guardians of Work Houses for the poor and destitute in Britain was familiar with the problem of the mentally defective girl who came to the work house, perhaps five or six times, to bear her illegitimate children. Permanent custodial care was the only solution, as in the United States, where institutionalization was now compulsory in many states, especially for females for obvious reasons.

Another official then cited sixteen feeble-minded women in Liverpool who had given birth to over one hundred illegitimate children.

Dr. MacMurchy had stiffened to attention. Dr. Beaton himself had once received an application to Orillia for a family of seventeen idiots. Three of them, all female, were already in the Asylum. From them, he had been staggered to learn that they had cohabited among themselves, resulting in seventeen defective children and grandchildren. One of them had actually given birth to a child on the road! It was disgraceful that such a state of affairs existed in Ontario, in Canada.

Back in Toronto, Dr. MacMurchy realized exactly what was needed: a province-wide census of the feeble-minded, conducted by herself. Galvanized, she sent out over 3,000 letters in 1906 to social agencies, churches, and police authorities, as well as to the governors of goals, the superintendents of asylums, and the city missionaries and deaconesses, all in an effort to garner information about people who had not been certified insane or idiots, yet were "not able to protect themselves."

The result was the names and addresses of 1,385 persons, 850 of them females, and 411 of them children, 124 males, which confirmed Dr. MacMurchy's predilections: though the parents of some of the children were of the upper classes (a few lawyers, a physician, a church officer, merchants, a clergyman), the "others," who were unable to pay anything at all for the care and education of their defective children, were therefore supported by the "public purse."

In fact, she added, not without compassion, it was only with good care, management, and self-sacrifice that they were able to feed and clothe their normal children. Her second census in 1908 confirmed this. Of the 612 persons enumerated, she reported that only 244 could read and write. Moreover, these 612 persons had given birth to 234 feeble-minded children between them, also supported ultimately by the taxpayer, a burden to "the public purse."

It was essential that the Government of Ontario and the House make provision for these people, and, in particular, the females aged fifteen to forty-five. "We must not permit the feeble-minded to be mothers of the next generation," she urged.

Dr. MacMurchy had soon become part of an elite group of professional women emerging in Toronto, easily identifiable in their dark serge skirts, serious stiff collared shirts, and flowing ties, many of them members of the University Women's Club (UWC) of Toronto, of which she was President in 1905. There were weekly afternoon teas and "delightful talks" in the gracious cosy Club Room, with its potted palms, rows of books, and Indian rugs. Miss Millicent Whitethorn entertained at the piano.

But the UWC women were too excited to discuss the morals of the feeble-minded that February day in 1909. There was the most intriguing guest speaker before tea: twenty-eight year-old Marie Stopes, a palaeobotanist. (She was later to become the champion of Birth Control in Britain.) Absolutely brilliant! Youngest Doctor of Science in Britain. She had apparently obtained her degree in Botany in 1902, at only twenty-three; afterwards, she received a second doctorate at the University of Munich, graduating *magna cum laude* — unprecedented. She had studied under the famous Dr. Goebel at the Botanical Institute. Her thesis subject was "The Reproductive Habits of Cycads," a mystery young Dr. Stopes hoped to solve.

It seemed she had tramped undaunted, a white woman in a topee — short Japanese blue trousers and leggings — through trackless forest and riverbeds in Hokkaido province, Japan, in pursuit of petrified specimens in the coal balls. She was now touring Canada giving talks to women's societies before returning to England.

Dr. Stopes, who scorned corsets, had turned up in a pre-Raphaelite gown of floating silk with masses of jewellery, and a flower at her breast, sensational among the sturdy costumes of the UWC women. Her red-tinged hair was piled softly, loosely, above her head, a few curls escaping; the entire effect was incontestably feminine and sensuous, an effect of which the slim, full-breasted Dr. Stopes seemed quite aware of at the podium.

She spoke on the nature of sex life spores of *cycads,* the origin of angiosperms in plants, as opposed to gymnosperms, in a dramatic, powerful voice — electrifying.

Afterwards, over tea, everyone pressed around Dr. Stopes. Invitations flowed, though Dr. Helen MacMurchy, as president, inevitably took precedence. She accompanied young Marie for the remainder of her stay in Toronto, but a few weeks, the two women visiting the museum, an evening concert of Mozart, *Eine Kleine Nachtmusik* at Forrester's Hall, the botanicals at Allan Gardens (a must!) in between Dr. Stopes's speaking engagements. There were moments under the frozen cold trees of Queen's Park — a sudden exchange of laughter — the fascinating

Marie Stopes calling her "Minky," teasingly, of course: "Minky darling!" Helen MacMurchy, feeling somewhat heady, found herself cancelling appointments, even with the Officer of Health, to be with the lovely and charming Miss Stopes.

And, at last, there was a quiet heart-to-heart talk in the privacy of her study, in the MacMurchy home. For Helen had already divined, from tearful hints and sighs from the young woman over that week, that beneath the brilliant front was an unhappy, restless woman. Marie Stopes was, in fact, a jilted woman.

It all came out. As Dr. MacMurchy — "Dear Helen," murmured Marie, "May I call you that?" — held her comfortingly in her arms, Marie confessed the real reason behind the pursuit of petrified specimens. She had wanted to be with Professor Fujii, Kenjiro Fujii (a married man with a young daughter in Tokyo) whom she had met in Professor Goebel's laboratory. They had fallen deeply in love. His specialty had been the gingko tree and his research paper, "Has the Spermatozoid of Gingko a Tail or None?" was absolutely brilliant. What more could she want in a lover, a husband? But he had rejected her unequivocally in Japan, somewhat shocked at the openness of Miss Stopes' advances and proclamations of love he apparently no longer wanted — here Marie sobbed again — and her sudden appearance in his country. She was broken, she confessed in tears. Yet, she was also often attracted to women; she cried artlessly, "Why do I always fall in love with women?" There was an American she had seen at the Imperial Chrysanthemum Party at the Akasaka Palace, her graceful white neck...

Helen MacMurchy felt giddy. "Darling!" she heard herself say, in a low voice, her breathing coming in unexpected pain, her costume jacket suddenly suffocating her. Marie trembled. Fujii's betrayal, his evasions, blurred. Here was an older woman, Dr. MacMurchy — President of the University Women's Club of Toronto, Inspector of the Feeble-minded for Ontario — in her arms, bending her head, trembling, towards her. There was no mistaking the look on the older woman's face.

A spate of love letters followed. They were impossible to stop. Helen MacMurchy was consumed by desire — felt the danger to her position as Inspector of the Feeble-Minded — yet these strange waves of passion, nor unlike delirium, pulled irrevocably. "My darling!" she wrote, after Marie left for Montreal to board the *Lusitania* for England. "That is what I have been wanting to call you ever since the express took you away from me to Montreal. In that moment I knew I loved you — when I found it in my heart to take you into my arms and kiss you..."

In the quiet of her room in the family home, Dr. MacMurchy paced; light fell from the lamp outside, a low glow. Below, her sister Bessie was practising the hymn for Sunday service at the harmonium: "*Abide with me, fast falls the even'tide, the darkness deepens...*" Helen sat at her desk and took up a quill, an unaccustomed giddiness overcoming her again, of being vulnerable in an unexpected way. At forty-seven she sensed her stodgy face, thickening figure, and increasing vulnerability, which she was powerless to deny. "You have "got me" — dear — ," she wrote, "and what a sweet thing that you had got me and were a little glad about it. I claim you for mine, dear — forever — as you said. You dear genius ... midnight and mail time. It must be goodbye — and was I the only person who kissed you in Canada?"

Snow fell against the upper window of her bedroom against the night. She wrote again and again to her "darling," in the secrecy of her room, after the day's work at the consultation room and clinics and hospitals, and her meetings with Mr. Hanna concerning putting away the feeble-minded, while she kept secret the woman who was superior in gifts and intellect. Dr. MacMurchy was aware all the more of herself now as a spinster at forty-seven, stolid in her long tweeds and spectacles, the forbidden kiss with her darling, recalled over and over, if only she could resist — the fall of Marie's hair loosening from its pins.

"February 24 — Dear, tonight, I wanted to ask you if you meant it all! You see, I know so little about you, dear — and yet so much." Helen MacMurchy was anxious, a hint of her native Scottish caution creeping in; she was vulnerable in a way she had never suspected she could be.

By March the anguish intensified. She lay on her bed one night, her body heavy, bent over after reading a letter from her darling over and over, muffling sudden sobs in the pillow. Old Dr. MacMurchy paused, disquieted, outside her door on the landing, hearing in wonder his eldest daughter's cries. But his was a strict, reserved nature; he passed on slowly to his room.

"...given you your place in my heart and it hurt to let you go.... Then when your letters came and I found you really did care — perhaps I thought very much about you.... It seemed too good to be true that you really cared for me...."

But as "Dr. MacMurchy," she had to be thinking about the problem of those feeble-minded girls, as well as the contaminated milk of Toronto and the hordes of flies everywhere infesting the slums (somehow connected). She wanted a *Milk Act* passed for proper pasteurization, urging the support of Dr. Charles Hastings, Medical Inspector of Health for the city, mundane concerns that a genius like Marie Stopes could not possibly be expected to empathize with.

And there was her report on "Infant Mortality" to write. She had been assigned by Mr. Hanna, the Provincial Secretary, to investigate infant mortality, and was to represent Canada at the British International Conference on Infant Mortality in England in 1909, the first time a woman had been invited to speak There had been no time even for thoughts of Marie — that would come later, at night.

In England, she got in touch with Mary Dendy, founder of the famous Sandlebridge Special Schools for the Feeble-Minded in Manchester. Miss Dendy, daughter of a non-conformist minister and member of the Eugenics Education Society, had testified at the Royal Commission and obviously had the answer to mental defectives. "The feeble-minded," she asserted, were epitomized by a "total lack of moral sense." In particular, feeble-minded women were promiscuous and highly fertile and produced large numbers of defective children that filled the workhouses of Britain (though feeble-minded boys were just "as dangerous").

This, of course, was not unfamiliar to Dr. MacMurchy. Dr. Beaton in Orillia was of the opinion that sending idiots to poorhouses, as had been tried in New York, resulted only in filth and disease and the horror of these vulnerable girls becoming pregnant as a result of illicit intercourse with the very guardians appointed to protect them.

Miss Dendy was not the lovely Marie, of course, but she was an admirable woman, founder of the Lancashire and Cheshire Society for the Permanent Care of the Feeble-Minded in 1898 and in 1902, the Sandlebridge Homes boarding school, supported by the Duchess of Sutherland. There were by now, it seemed, 9,000 children in Special Classes in England, half of them in the London area. But they needed segregation *for life*, stressed Miss Dendy. What was special about her Sandlebridge boarding schools for the feeble-minded was that they provided permanent care. Happy, feeble-minded children worked in the gardens, blacked clogs in the tool-house, and addressed the Matrons as "Mother." Though, since 1902, hundreds had been removed by the Poor Law Guardians to work on Poor Law Union Farms. Dr. MacMurchy lost no time in inviting Miss Dendy to Toronto.

Together, that June, they examined nearly 1,800 children in the Toronto Public Schools, one percent of whom Miss Dendy pronounced, in a matter of days, as feeble-minded (exempting Jewish children; Miss Dendy was of the opinion that the Jewish people had less defective children, perhaps because of stricter marriage customs). Somewhat taken aback, Dr. MacMurchy had estimated the general number of feeble-minded as 0.3%. Miss Dendy addressed the Women's Canadian Club of Toronto as well as the Board of Education, reporting on the problem of feeble-mindedness. Mr. Hanna, impressed, appointed Dr. Helen MacMurchy as Girls' Medical Inspector for the Public Schools in Toronto.

Here was her chance. Inspired by Miss Dendy, she now pushed for Special Classes. In 1911, the *Act Respecting Special Classes for the Mentally Defective* was finally passed which gave legal authority and financial support to the Toronto Board to establish half-day classes in Grace and George Street Schools. The classes would sort out the truly "mentally defective" child from the merely backward for placement in an institution. The first step had been achieved! She had triumphed!

Yet, only a handful of parents turned up for the voluntary registration and medical examination at her office in City Hall, ordered by Dr. MacMurchy in her authoritative way. The parents, fearful perhaps of their children — and themselves — being identified as "feeble-minded" had stayed away. Who wanted to be a "taint" upon the nation? It did not help that Dr. MacMurchy had referred to the "feeble-minded" in her report of 1907 as "degenerates" and "criminals," and feeble-minded children as a "drag" in the classroom. "Typical!" she fumed, exasperated.

What was needed was compulsory registration, legal registers supervised by herself, and Auxiliary Classes, she urged Mr. Hanna. Germany had had special Auxiliary Classes since 1850, the feeble-minded children integrated into the public schools in a most humane fashion, far ahead of the rest of Europe. In 1914, an *Auxiliary Class Act* was passed, and Dr. MacMurchy appointed as Inspector. She was now both Inspector of the Feeble-Minded for Ontario and Inspector of Auxiliary Classes, her youthful photo with a write-up appearing in the Toronto *Daily Star*.

Children and parents were now to submit to examination by order of the school medical officer; the full details were laid out in her treatise,

Organization and Management of Auxiliary Classes, 1915. Personal information about heredity, marital relations, fecundity, conception, gestation, and lactation of the child was now to be garnered by the medical officer. In addition, the medical officer was to provide his "impression of the mother." Of course, Dr. MacMurchy knew such procedures were an intrusion on privacy, and inspectors were urged to "give every consideration to the feelings of parents"; however, parents were also to be "frankly told" the truth about their child's defects.

Once in an Auxiliary Class, pupils would be further sorted out to separate the low grades from the "educable." She urged that the "educable" ones, whom she vaguely termed "backward," should certainly be given the benefit of the doubt, for she was determined to be just. After all, backward ones could simply be suffering from adenoids or poor eyesight (she was, herself, short-sighted). "They should be given every chance!" she averred, catarrh and adenoids notwithstanding. Later she brought out an urgent pamphlet, "Teacher — Save That Backward Child!" The curriculum she recommended was surely impressive for its time - sewing, raffia-work, cookery for girls; shoemaking, farm-work, and carpentry for boys.not forgetting he social graces such as the "proper use of the pocket-handkerchief."

But low-grade children and mental defectives, whose I.Q. was below 50, were destined for permanent segregation and placement, otherwise known as "custodial" care in an institution for life. And what better place than the asylum in Orillia? For no skill, no knowledge, no training — nothing — would ever change a mentally defective child into a normal one, she cried.

Of course, there was still the problem of defective parents (they had absolutely no self-control). One feeble-minded married woman, for example, had a mentally deficient daughter, who, at twenty-eight, was herself the mother of two more illegitimate children. "Three generations of feeble-minded! By this time there may well be four!" she wrote indignantly in 1913.

Soon everyone was reading Dr. MacMurchy's reports. There had never been anything like them in government — they were sensational.As well, influential articles were appearing in the important *Journal for Psycho-Asthenics.* Dr. Walter Fernald, Superintendent of the Massachusetts School for Idiotic and Feeble-minded Youth, founded by Samuel Gridley Howe in 1848, and an authority on feeble-minded girls, had warned of their inevitable promiscuity: "One evil girl can corrupt a whole village." And, more ominously: "The feeble-minded woman who marries is twice as prolific as the normal woman."

Dr. Martin Barr, Chief Physician at the Pennsylvania Training School for the Feeble-Minded, had petitioned in 1905 for the "separation, sequestration, and asexualization" of degenerates to prevent mental defect, urging it as: "The Duty of the Hour." He had personally effected the sterilizations of certain incorrigibles at the school. Indiana State had already, in 1907, enacted legislation for compulsory eugenic sterilization for rapists, epileptics, and idiots. The Americans were far ahead.

Dr. MacMurchy found herself swept along with a fervour approaching a crusade. No less than thirteen mentally defective young boys, all murderers, were even then being tried before the courts in Toronto. Dr. Clarke himself had reportedly seen them passing through his Clinic. Feeble-minded males were, of course, as reprehensible as females, being, Dr. Fernald warned, "frequently violators of women and little girls."

However, the "*real horror*," as she stressed in her report of 1912, was the threat of mentally deficient boys at the Victoria Industrial School in Mimico, Toronto. They were soon to be released, according to the law, at age sixteen when they would be "left to face the fierce passions and temptations of life."

The words seemed to hover in mid-air. Dr. MacMurchy paused, confused. The year before, within a week of the *Special Classes Act*, she had attended the wedding of Marie Stopes, who had returned to Montreal to marry Dr. Reginald Ruggles Gates, a Canadian botanist. Of course, it was a union of superior minds, Reginald Ruggles Gates — "Ruggles" as Marie called him — being a geneticist. They had met, significantly, at a scientific conference. Whatever powerful sense of struggle and loss that Dr. Helen MacMurchy felt that March day on seeing Marie again — she had taken the express train at once through a cold wintry day to Montreal — she kept to herself. It had been a passion, a moment in time. She was now nearly fifty.

The marital union of Marie and Reginald was, of course, in stark contrast to that of the feeble-minded (the horror of such couplings between degenerates still going on in the city and around the province). Concerned citizens, including the Toronto Chapter of the National Council of Women, the Household Economic Association, the Culture Club, and the Salvation Army, who understood the significance of her reports, were demanding something be done. Mrs. Willoughby Cummings of the National Council of Women had pointed out, back in 1903, that feeble-minded girls left to themselves "were the prey of the evil disposed," and the children of such women were of a lower scale of intelligence, which helped to explain the serious increase in lunacy in the province.

In November of 1912, the powerful Canadian Proclamation on Charities and Corrections held its conference in Convocation Hall at the University of Toronto. The Proclamation, an offshoot of the American Proclamation, was the most influential group in Canada, as Dr. MacMurchy well knew, consisting of sociologists, legal and law enforcement officers, psychiatrists, doctors, and public health workers. It was the venue for all important speeches and papers on the topic of the mentally defective. The conference was attended by members of Toronto's social and political elite, noted Dr. MacMurchy, gratified: Mayor Hocken, Mrs. F. H. Torrington (President of the National Council of Women), Mrs. A. M. Huestis (prominent in the Canadian Public Health Association (CPHA) and the National Council for the Prevention of Venereal Disease), educators, and clergymen, all personally welcomed by herself at the door. She also gave the opening address.

The Proclamation wanted action from the Ontario government. They demanded custodial detention for feeble-minded adults as well as idiots, and an amendment of the *Marriage Act* of 1898 to include the "feeble-minded" on the list, and so protect the germplasm of the nation. In 1911, the Ontario Statutes had added to the earlier penalty of $500, a prison sentence of up to twelve months to anyone issuing marriage licenses to "idiotics" and the "insane."

More preventative punishment was needed than this, the men cried (possibly longer jail time). Opposers pointed out the ineffectivenes of the Act, it being impossible to prevent degenerates from having sexual intercourse, for the unfit reproduced their kind regardless of marriage laws. The entire evening had been somewhat of an uproar, and shortly afterwards the Provincial Association for the Care of the Feeble-Minded was formed — with Dr. Helen MacMurchy as its secretary.

The following year, in 1913, the *British Mental Deficiency Act* was at last enacted. Dr. MacMurchy had followed the fiery debates over the Feeble-Minded Persons Control Bill, in the sessions of the British

Parliament. Mr. Winston Churchill, Home Secretary, had urged that everything be done for the feeble-minded in a Christian society, but that they should be segregated under proper conditions so that their "curse" died with them. There had been outbursts and some outcry. A certain Josiah Wedgewood, a Radical MP from Newcastle-under-Lyme alone stood up in the House of Commons and claimed the Bill was the work of "eugenic cranks" criminalizing poor uneducated girls whose only "crime" was being pregnant out of wedlock. Defeated, of course. The Bill was incorporated later into the *Mental Deficiency Act*, "the most important piece of legislation in our time," wrote Dr. MacMurchy. (The British were ever leaders in the world.)

The term "feeble-minded" was at last clearly defined and given statutory status. Until then, there had often been confusion over the British and American usage of the term; the Americans used the word to represent *all* mental defectives, whereas the British and Canadians had tended to use it for those with a higher level of intelligence. Dr. Tredgold, the admirable British authority who had been medical advisor to the Royal Commission, and had written the influential textbook of his time, *Mental Deficiency (Amentia)* in 1908, provided a final definition. Feeble-minded were persons "not amounting to imbecility," yet "unable to care for themselves," and in need of supervision and control for their own protection and for the protection of others. There were four grades of mental deficiency: "Idiots," "Imbeciles," "Feeble-minded," and "Moral Defectives."

She read on eagerly, noting the new criteria for placing mental defectives in institutions. A parent was but required to petition the local authority.

The law also clarified those who had "unlawful and carnal knowledge" of a defective woman. The onus was now on the man to prove he did not know, and had had no cause to suspect that the woman was defective. Dr. MacMurchy tightened. All the more reason to have these simple girls put away.

As the Royal Commission had stressed in 1905 concerning the feeble-minded: "To allow progeny was an evil of the very greatest magnitude."

23.

FLORRIE WAS PREGNANT. She knew because the bloods had stopped. Plaster fell with a thud and a spray of dust floated down from the ceiling of their tiny room on D'Arcy Street. Water would seep in with the rains through every crack, making her cough again.

A little babby of their very own.

"Don't worry, I'll make an honest woman of yer, Flo," Henry cried happily. And he did. He bought her the loveliest little ring in the Five and Dime Store in the market. Now that they were affianced, they could walk together down the promenade past the Palais Royale an' cock their fingers at the Morality Squad, he chuckled. He had filched some bits of wood from the dockyards and started making a cradle for the babby when he comes.

Upstairs, Mrs. Derrick, Esme Derrick, only sighed when she heard. The Derricks lived in two rooms and shared the kitchen stove below with the rest of the tenants. She would help Florrie when 'er time come, she said weakly, for she had just had a babby herself. Mrs. Armagh in the basement had helped. Esme Derrick was a thin, harassed-looking woman, her hair falling out.

"The nurse at the clinic on Dov'court say I gotta 'ave veg'tables an' meats," she told Florrie. She had had her baby on the bedroom floor, as "it come too fast." Little Beatrice, who was ten, had helped with the delivery and boiled up the kettle for Mrs. Armagh to sterilize the scissors to cut the cord. Florrie knew that you put the scissors through the steam to stop infection; she had seen it at the workhouse in London, long ago, with the women on the wards.

"If we 'as one more the lan'lord throw us out," Esme cried. She did not want to go to the House of Refuge, she fretted. What would happen to them all? She had bandages around her belly to keep her womb from wandering. Florrie looked with wonder at the grimy, unravelling strips of cloth. Nevertheless, she sat excitedly at the deal table with Mrs. Derrick, not knowing this might be herself one day, with seven little Derricks running around the kitchen. The children were in rags, and some of the very little ones stood listless, their eyes dull, in the September evening. "They can't go to school; they gots no shoes."

There were a few biscuits and a piece of sausage for their supper. Esme pulled out her breast to feed the baby, who barely sucked, and looked out the kitchen window onto the yard. Eventually she said, in a low voice, "Oh, I so long for a nice cup o' tea an' a piece o' cake, Florrie, a lemon tart say in the bakery window on College." Tears filled her eyes. "Just something ... nice ... for once ... jus' to keep you going."

Her husband Bert was out looking for work. He had been laid off at the docks, as nothing was happening. Esme's face screwed up tight. She was from Manchester, had come over on the steamship as a little girl, as kitchen help, a skivvy. Florrie knew what that meant. That night, in bed, Henry had said things were bad in the job market and he only had a dollar left. People were being laid off left, right, and centre at the steel factory, he grumbled, due to something Florrie now understood to be a "slump." Lots of the girls had been laid off at the Chocolate Factory, too. Now Florrie was working for a Mr. Pearl in the garment district, stringing beads for two cents a chain in a basement off Spadina, squatting on the floor from early morning, until eight at night. "An' bloody lucky you is to have it, too," said Maudie. Maudie had been laid off a week or two, but a gentleman friend, a right toff, had "seen 'er through." Now she was putting spines in women's corsets at the Corset Company, for $6 a a week (it used to be $8 but there was the slump).

"So when's it due, then?" asked Maudie.

She had come to help Florrie and Henry get Florrie's papers from the Women's Welcome House to give the clerk, so she could get married. That's where everything about Florrie would be, filed away when the girls come over on the steamers, she said.

Florrie fluttered; she didn't know.

"Well when did your courses stop?" said Maudie impatiently. "Lordie, Florrie, don't you *know?*"

"A ... long time," Florrie hesitated, confused. "Fireworks for the Queen's Birthday he give it to me."

Maudie rolled her eyes. "Yeah, well," she screwed up her face and computed wonderfully in her head, while Florrie looked on admiringly. "That'll be nex' March or so, 1915, Flo."

Maudie gave a sharp glance at the glass bauble of a ring on Florrie's finger. The she ran her eyes around the small, dank mildewy room with the familiar iron bedstead and broken window and soiled pee-pot in the corner. She saw the swift black fleet of roaches scurrying under the floorboard when you turned on the light. He got her cheap, she thought, and tossed her red hair. "Titian," one lovely bloke had called it, ever such a swanky fellow, a real masher.

But then she turned to Florrie quickly and said, "Say, can yer spare us a crust of bread, Flo?" Maudie was starving.

There was a kerfuffle at the Women's Welcome House. The Imperial Order Daughters of the Empire had instituted an upkeep of all records in Toronto, part of the effort to keep track of the hordes of girls invading the city. Miss Benson behind the desk looked suspiciously at the sturdy yet underweight young man in worn breeches and rough shirt, and the girl at his side whom he claimed to be his "affianced," in a worn dress none too clean. He wanted "'er papers," for the notary, he said. They were getting married.

Miss Benson grudgingly shifted tone, eyeing a breathless Florrie, who was to become joined in matrimony, thus achieving a particular status that automatically conferred on her a certain indisputable position of respect in society she did not yet understand, but which Miss Benson surely did.

"Miss Mallone come over on *The Empress of England* in 1913," said Maudie haughtily. "You got 'er papers here, I believe." Oh, she was a one, was Maudie, in her feathered hat!

"Hmph," went Miss Benson.

"Miss Bartlett's group," whispered Florrie.

The clerk at the notary's office in City Hall swiftly glanced through the papers and then at Florence Mallone and Henry Hewitt standing before him that August day in 1914, and the tall imperious witness, Maude Herrigan. English. Two attractive, fair-haired and blue-eyed young people, fifteen and eighteen years old respectively, with no family, and barely a penny between them, no doubt. He was listed as "labourer"; the original document from the Union said, "farm" labourer, and she was listed as a "domestic." He had been educated to Standard 111 in

England — good enough. She, of course, was illiterate, like so many young girls in service. She made a mark, an "X," scrawled but sufficient. He stamped the certificate.

She was a married woman, albeit pregnant. "Mrs. 'Enry 'Ewitt!" cried Florrie softly. "My 'usbant."

Florrie stood outside the City Hall with Henry, her arm in his. She was allowed to do this now. She was free. With one act she had ended the vague threat of institutions and the workhouse and all the Miss Bartletts. That was in her past now, back in England. There was a rising stench of rot and feces from the Ward slum, as the rickety houses hung together, and the chickens and pigeons pecked at the ground. Thin, worn children ran and shrieked happily with a piece of stick and ball, and the wonderful steamy light of that early August morning before the War had spread wide over the city.

That night, Henry used the last of his money, put away for a wedding treat, and took Florrie and Maudie for dried pork and pickles and a merry glass of ale at the tavern, and then to the vaudeville show, fifteen cents a ticket, half price for the ladies. Oh, how they laughed at Naughty Nancy and her dancing dogs. They joined in lustily and loudly in the pits with the best of them, singing, "*A little of what you fancy does you good*" — nudge, nudge — and other all-time favourites from Broadway: "*I work eight hours a day, I sleep eight hours a day, That leaves eight hours for lovin'...*"

24.

THE LITTLE NEWSBOY ON THE CORNER of College Street was waving the *Globe* with its headline "BRITAIN AT WAR!" It was August 5, 1914, which meant Canada would be too, said Henry, "All stick together, boys."

True enough, the next morning Prime Minister Sir Robert Borden announced on the radio in the factory that the Dominion would be loyal to Britain and the flag. It seemed that far away in Europe, in a town called "Sarajevo," someone called the Archduke Franz Ferdinand of Austria, whom Florrie and Henry had never heard of, had been assassinated that summer on June 28, and Britain now declared war on the enemy: Germany. No one spoke now of the photograph of the former King Edward VII in full regalia, and that he was the cousin of Kaiser Wilhelm II.

Nevertheless, it was exciting in Toronto that fall, with the marches and parades, despite the slump and layoffs, and the long soup lines at the Missions. Parades of volunteers, some already exhausted and undernourished in their broken boots, went up and down Yonge Street waving the Union Jack. Another parade on University Avenue on August 22 with highlander pipes and bugles, tartans and sporrans swishing, had Henry and Florrie standing on the pavements packed with cheering crowds. The boys in the factory, and the thin men leaning against the walls outside, vagrants in worn breeches and broken shoes, cadging for a cigarette or a penny, were signing up at the Armoury. Henry said he had better sign up too, as he did not want a white feather on his chest. Young women were going about sticking feathers of cowardice on any man in the street not in uniform. Posters on billboards and streetcars blared: "Women make your men enlist!" and, "Take up the Sword of Justice!"

He had signed up on October 15, 1915, in one of the battalions, for a soldier's pay of $1.10 a day. "Better 'n' nothin', Flo," he sighed. He had been out of work for months, on the dole, just enough for bread and milk tokens, though things were picking up again now because of the war, due to factory work for uniforms and munitions.

By now the government had promised 250,000 men for the Allied War Effort, and a million bags of flour for the British people. The Order of the Imperial Daughters of the Empire (IODE) and the Women's Patriotic League, aware of the pittance there was for war wives and children left behind, started a Patriotic Fund and made one thousand cups of beef tea. Up in Orillia, the Superintendent of the Hospital for the Feeble-Minded, Mr. Downey, with the aid of the inmates, made 508 pyjama suits for the troops at the Ontario Military Hospital at Orpington in five days, Dr. MacMurchy was proud to document in her Eleventh Annual Report. Thirteen men on staff in Orillia had enlisted and six others, all sons of members of staff, had joined the army "at the call of the King and Country." On their victory, she wrote with fervour, depended not only the fate of the British Empire, but the cause of freedom, of civilization, and of Christianity.

Henry's Attestation Papers of 1915 were still in Daisy's mother's file, the Hewitt file, faded, worn: *I hereby agree to serve in the Canadian Over-Seas Expeditionary Force for the term of one year, or during the war now existing between Great Britain and Germany should that war last longer than one year, provided his Majesty should so long require my services, or until legally discharged,*" followed by his Oath: *I Henry James Hewitt do make Oath that I will be faithful and bear true Allegiance to His Majesty King George the Fifth, His Heirs and Successors ... so help me, God.*

This oath he made on October 15, 1915. He was nineteen. His certificate of Medical Examination was duly stamped with approval by the Toronto Recruiting Medical Officer: "I consider him fit."

He had cleared the Medical. He had felt a certain satisfaction; he was up to par. The officer had ticked off: "speech, without impediment," and "sufficiently intelligent." The criteria had been simple: be anywhere from eighteen to forty-five years of age; be five feet tall; be able to hear a normal voice from fifteen feet in each ear. "Men may be accepted if one or two toes missing as long as great toes are intact."

He had been given his army issue, with a brass tag bearing his name, number, battalion, and religion. He was wearing a heavy wool tunic, breeches, a flannel shirt, cotton underwear, stiff boots that hurt his toes, and a new greatcoat. He had never worn so much clothing in his life and felt weighted down under a staggering thirty kilograms of gear, which including equipment, a water-bottle, and a rifle. The first thing you learned at training camp: how to wind your puttees — a long strip of cloth wound around your socks and legs.

Most vital of all was his little Field Dressing Kit, which was a small package containing a wool pad, a piece of gauze, a bandage, and a pin. Under fire, he learned, he would have to tend his wounds himself first "until help came" out in the field. The *Training Manual* was 250 pages long. Only he did not know that yet.

Florrie was startled. She had no idea where "France" was, but she knew "overseas." The funnel blew and you held on to your hat and there was a cheer and you were for God and Country. Wives and children were allowed free passage (the Women's Patriotic League found out addresses in England). But now she had the babby she was suckling, her darling that she had called "'Enrietta' for 'Enry." You pulled out your teat whenever she cried and put it in her mouth, and out come the milk. That was best, the nurse had said sternly at the Women's Dispensary on Dovercourt Street, and cheaper. Mrs. Hewitt was to drink two glasses of milk a day and eat vegetables and fruit, the nurse had explained, looking sharply at Florrie, who seemed backward. Clearly, a social worker needed to be sent to this house.

This Mrs. Hewitt had not even thought to send someone to fetch a nurse when she went into labour, frowned the nurse, but had apparently had the baby on the floor, though the baby, a girl, seemed none the worse for wear. But that was the poor, they survived. She had indeed given birth in the basement, on sacking. Old Mrs. Armagh, who lived next to the boiler room, had helped, and Esme Derrick had boiled up the kettles, and little Beatrice had wiped Florrie's face with a wet rag as she pushed. She did not know what happened after that. Esme had her hand up there twisting, and after the baby came out little Beatrice wiped the jelly off with a boiled rag. Mrs. Armagh chopped through the cord with the kitchen knife, (plunged through boiling water first ("t' ster'lize it, Flo") and then threw what came out later into the yard for the dogs. It had been a cold and snowy March day in 1915, and the trees creaked outside the cracked panes. In the distance was a rumble of trams.

The babby was in the world and in this tiny room off Spadina Avenue, wrapped in a dirty piece of flannel, but all Florrie cried in a flurry of joy was, "She 'as 'Enry's eyes."

25.

DELINQUENCY WAS INCREASING all over the city, particularly among girls. The editor of *Social Health* was of the opinion it was due to the inevitable lowering of standards in war time. Justice Edward Starr of the Juvenile Court wondered, bewildered, whether it wasn't the girls' youth and foolish innocence that made them so susceptible to unscrupulous, lecherous men.

Dr. MacMurchy, at once concerned, urged Dr. Clarke to reopen his Clinic, only this time linking it to the Juvenile Court. Such a clinic would provide a proper, full, psychiatric study of delinquents. She was, of course, aware of the work of Dr. Charles Goring, the British psychiatrist and medical officer in the English prisons who had written *The English Criminal*, in which he had urged for the supervision of the unfit "in order to regulate procreation." And so, in 1914, the Social Service Clinic — Clarke's preference was "Toronto Psychiatric Clinic" — opened in the basement of the Toronto General Hospital.

It was a resounding success from the start. In the first year alone the Clinic examined over a hundred aments and ten murderers, enthused Dr. Clarke. Dr. Clarence Hincks and Dr. O. C. J. Withrow, young physicians at the Juvenile Court, offered their services without pay one day a week — fine young men. (Dr. Withrow had graduated from the University of Toronto and practised medicine in Thunder Bay. Dr. Hincks' father was a Methodist minister.)

Young Dr. Hincks had himself suffered from a depressive malady that had hit him out of the blue in university, he confided; he had been rendered immobile on his bed for six weeks. An ideal person, then, who could bring to the Clinic a special understanding of those suffering from mental distress.

As well, Dr. William Bott and Dr. E. J. Pratt (later a famed poet) and a Mr. Freeman set up a Psychology Department at the University of Toronto to help from a psychological aspect. Soon Clinic days had to be upped to two, then three times per week.

The very latest scientific methods were adopted. Mr. Alfred Binet, Director of the Sorbonne Laboratory of Experimental Psychology, a dapper Parisian who wore pince-nez on his nose and had a pointed moustache, had published the first "metrical scales of intelligence" in 1905, along with colleague Theodore Simon. This had been at the request of the French Education Department to identify children who were slow learners in school. The Binet-Simon test had been translated into English and revised for North America by Dr. Henry Goddard, a staunch eugenicist and Director of the new research laboratory at the Vineland Training School for Feeble-Minded Boys and Girls in New Jersey. He had just published an important book, *The Menace of Mental Deficiency from the Standpoint of Heredity,* by the Vineland New Jersey Training School, absolutely essential reading. Dr. MacMurchy had gone to New Jersey at once in 1911 to learn how to administer the test under the direction of Dr. Goddard himself and Dr. Walter Cornell, Chief Medical Inspector for Philadelphia's Public Schools. The test included thirty items designed for children aged three to twelve, arranged in order of difficulty; for example, naming objects in pictures, repeating spoken digits, or defining "common words," etc. ("common," that is, in the vocabulary of most nice, educated, middle-class children, something Dr. MacMurchy only sensed rather than gave word to.) But Mr. Binet had also introduced the exciting concept of "mental age," which she understood to mean that if a sixteen-year-old passed the test at a ten-year-old level, he was said to have a corresponding "mental age" of ten and to be deemed "feeble-minded."

There was a flurry of concern at the Clinic. For the purpose of Binet's tests had been to help classify the levels of retarded children in Paris in order to provide them with special classes so as to *keep them* in the school system. Binet asserted that even the intelligence of a feeble-minded child could improve with appropriate teaching, and that one's environment affected performance, openly challenging Galton's claim that intelligence was biologically predetermined for life. He had actually called Sir Francis a "brutal pessimist."

Dr. MacMurchy hesitated. It was one of those moments in time and she knew it. She admitted cautiously that the treatment and training of the feeble-minded indeed "belonged properly under education." But diagnosis had always been the prerogative of medicine. Anthropometry, the identification of stigmata, was primary to any examination of a mental defective, she insisted. Such stigmata as the size of a patient's cranium (phrenology), the shape of the nose and eyes, and any abnormalities of the ears and tongue could only be ascertained only by a trained physician, she averred. Every professional knew that such visible abnormalities were more common in the feeble-minded. The lower the grade of mental defectiveness, the more bodily signs or stigmata were present, and that was the guideline, said Dr. MacMurchy, who believed in calling a spade a spade. German cellular biologist August Weismann had stated that no amount of good environment could offset the germplasm that passed on through heredity from generation to generation. What further proof was needed? She personally favoured a variety of tests, including the measurement of the skull for brain capacity.

Now this Mr. Binet and his "educationalists" were claiming that anthropometry, or anthropomorphy, the skill of detecting stigmata, should take "second place" in the diagnosis of the feeble-minded. He was obviously intent on replacing physicians and psychiatrists with psychologists in the schools. That was the danger.

Dr. MacMurchy decided to throw her energies behind her colleagues, for the very future of psychiatry — a relatively budding profession — was at stake, as well as the importance of institutions like Orillia. And so diagnosis and treatment (including who should go to an asylum) remained the mandate of the medical profession, affecting the outcome for the mentally retarded in Ontario for the next half a century, if she but knew. The "feeble-minded" were to remain firmly under the governance of the Ministry of Health until the 1970s.

But there was no denying the precision of the new tests. There was even an equation. William Stern, a psychologist in Germany, had devised in 1910 a ratio of mental age to chronological age times one hundred, indicating "intelligence quotient," or "I.Q.":

I.Q. = mental age x 100 = chronological age

Here was a powerful tool for classifying delinquents. Under Dr. Beaton, the old classification of 1881 had simply cited "Deaf Mutes," "Congenital Idiots," "Epileptics," "Helpless Cripples," "Dements (lunatics)," and

"Males and Females Capable of Work." Now, Dr. Lewis M. Terman, Professor of Psychology at Stanford University and a eugenicist, did his own revision of the test in 1916, stressing intelligence quotient and adding ninety-two items, including general knowledge questions such as: "Who was Ghengis Khan?" and "What is the boiling point of water?" Terman's *The Measurement of Intelligence* was soon accepted throughout North America and the Stanford-Binet test became standard, acknowledged Dr. MacMurchy. Indeed, Dr. Hincks was the first to apply it in the Toronto public schools, concerned about the "supra-normals." Gifted children needed attention as much, if not more, than the feeble-minded in order to produce adults like Dr. Clarke (a brilliant man, thought Hincks, from fine lineage — Dr. Clarke's father, Charles Clarke of Elora, had been the Honourable Lieutenant-General, member of the Legislature and Speaker of the House in his time).

With the aid of the tests, "Idiots" and "Imbeciles" were now specifically categorized as "below 50 I.Q.," a useful dividing line, noted Dr. MacMurchy. But there was also an important new "borderline" group of defectives, hitherto unsuspected, defined by Dr. Goddard himself at Vineland. These were the "Moron" and "Half-Morons," a term taken from the Greek word *moronia,* meaning "foolish." The problem was they had no recognizable stigmata. They tested as not quite normal, but not feeble-minded, either.

The new classification system left one in little doubt:

TERM	I.Q.
Idiot	below 20 or 25
Imbecile	20-50
Moron	50-70 or 75
Dull Normal	80-90

It was generally agreed that an I.Q. of 70, or a "mental age" of twelve, was the upper limit of feeble-mindedness. The "Moron" females, in particular, presented the greatest problem since they lacked stigmata, the vital physical signs of defect and so often appeared to the unsuspecting public as "normal," even attractive. Canadian law allowed for only Idiots and Imbeciles to be institutionalized, but these ones also needed to be detained in Houses of Refuge or put away permanently in Orillia. Dr. Goddard favoured segregated "farm colonies" for them.

Dr. Martin Barr, Chief Physician at the Pennsylvania Training School for the Feeble-Minded at Elwyn, warned that the "Moral Imbecile" was the most dangerous class of defectives, the male being a sexual pervert "in filthy practices utterly shameless."

The girls also never ceased to shock. They came flouncing through the Clinic from the Juvenile Court dressed in the latest wartime fashions: bobbed hair, shortened skirts, and dropped waists. Of course, they had not a brain in their heads, noted Dr. Clarke.

"Maggie," for instance, was a degenerate from London. She had spent all her wages on Scotch whisky and gin. Dr. Clarke computed that she had already cost the province $350 per annum. Out west, a "Jenny Smith"— touted to be "dangerous as dynamite" — had to be put in an institution at once, where, with the correct supervision, she was happy and under control.

One could go on and on. "Maria P.," eighteen, had not even known the name of Lake Ontario, nor had she even known there *was* a lake at Toronto. Immoral from an early age, she had run away from home. Of course, the fact that she had had "sexual relations" with her father from the age of eleven was but part and parcel of this sort's natural proclivities. She had simply gone on to further immorality, and was a menace to the whole community. She belonged in the Jail Farm in Richmond Hill. And then there was "Betsy," a pretty little butterfly with an undeveloped brain flitting about and sipping at every vice, he wrote. She had left school at thirteen. Like most of her kind, she frequented dance halls, nickelodeons, and Shea's burlesque on King Street: "I was an usher in one of them Vaudevilles." Admittedly, Dr. Hincks himself had been known to enjoy an evening at Shea's in his youth, after a long stint on the wards, no doubt, understandable. "Betsy" had had numerous factory jobs, where she had got "chocolate poisonin'." She had claimed that it got "under the nails." "It goes all through your body," she had confided casually, unaware surely of the implication of her words so lightly given. The point was, "Betsy" had no sense of morality — sex was simply an incident of no importance.

Finally, there was "Peggy," another low-class Irish immigrant from the bogs, only twenty-two. "Her immoralities are many." She'd not stuck at any job, either. After being married at nineteen, and having a baby who had died "mysteriously" (probably of syphilis), she had spent her weekends with what she called a "sporty gentleman," becoming pregnant again. Now she and her new baby both had syphilis. Dr. MacMurchy knew better than most the symptoms of these babies with their horrifying lesions, scarred, depressed noses, and Hutchinson's teeth. But "Peggy" had scored at "age twelve" level on the Stanford-Binet Test and was, therefore, classified as "Normal."

Dr. Clarke hesitated, flummoxed. It was obvious "Peggy," a high-grade moron, must be classified as a "Moral Defective," a category not exactly on any Binet scale but one that it was surely their duty to define so that she could be put away. Dr. MacMurchy was not even sure it was a legal medical category, for "moral" did not have any definitive physical stigmata.

Dr. Withrow, who had been overseas working with venereal diseases at the University of Toronto Overseas Field Hospital No. 4, organized by Dr. Clarke himself during the war, enthused, however, on his return that the Clinic was doing excellent work with these girls. His Third Annual Report of Toronto General Hospital Social Service Department stressed:

> ...Two hundred and seventy cases have passed through our hands in nine months and twenty-nine of these have been placed in institutions where they will be well cared for and trained to a degree, and in some instances taken from a community to which they have been a menace. We are hoping great things from this clinic.

Miss Jane Grant, Head Social Worker at the Toronto General Hospital, who had initially referred to Dr. Clarke's Clinic as a "nut" place, now declared: "Eliminate the feeble-minded and the insane from our communities, and all social work would be a joy!" However, she also cried in a heartfelt way, "How can there be a sight of beauty in the mind of a child whose vision is bounded by bare walls, ash heaps, garbage piles, filth, and grime?" This surely smacked of radicalism, Dr. Clarke frowned. He had arranged for classes two afternoons a week and evening lectures every Thursday at the Clinic for Miss Grant's students and for young nurses-in-training to gain first-hand knowledge of the feeble-minded and realize what the profession was up against.

The fact was, he had come to realize, that well-meaning but deluded social workers like Miss Grant often only exacerbated a situation. They would find a family, dirty and unkept, the children half-naked and uncared for, the house destitute, and, with commendable zeal, proceed to remedy the conditions. Clothes would be bought, fuel supplied, and the family put "on a new footing." Useless, of course. The old situation was doomed to repeat itself due to the feeble-mindedness of the parents.

As Rev. S. W. Dean, noted Methodist preacher in the city put it: "Some may be convinced that the sty makes the pig. There can be no question but that the pig makes the sty."

Dr. Clarke's daughter, Emma de Veber Clarke — Miss E. de V. to colleagues — agreed. She stood erect in a shaft of sunlight in the small basement of the Clinic, stiff in her nurse's uniform, her hair drawn back under its tight little cap. Ever loyal to her father, she never doubted the theory of heredity and the inherent feeble-mindedness of most incorrigibles.

Nevertheless, determined Miss Grant set out with her Social Work students from the university to identify and reform the poor south of Bloor Street. Down Parliament Street and across Shuter Street to that terrible area of Irish slum immigrants (where some were too frightened to walk) and Moss Park, and then west to St. John's Ward, which spread from Eaton's factories down to crowded, innocuous Queen Street and east to Bay Street, another foul slum. In this they were not alone. The deaconesses of the Methodist church — valuable, upright ladies — were conducting surveys of their own to root out degeneracy and moral turpitude.

Young Miss Alice Chown, who had also thrown away her corsets, insisted that church women should model themselves on social workers. Her father, Rev. S. D. Chown, believed the Methodist church could lead Canada in the new Social Science. The Deaconess Training School should no longer simply provide charity for the poor but encourage self-sufficiency in these people. David Archibald, chief of police, complained that outdoor relief money was not going to the deserving poor but to shiftless paupers only encouraging pauperism, while the Ontario Commission on Unemployment noted that vagrants thrived on soup kitchens.

And so, with a certain fascination did the deaconesses and lady volunteers venture into the slum, its overcrowding implicit with sexuality. Rev. S. W. Dean of the Fred Victor Mission had warned that the slum was the haunt of the most "unspeakable crime of incest and degradation." The deaconesses were intent on amassing data in a clinical, objective way, of the "Betsys" and "Marias" and the degraded babies they gave birth to. There were cases right then in the Burnside lying-in ward linked to the Toronto General Hospital; Dr. Clarke made it his business to check regularly on such girls giving birth.

Dr. Charles Hastings, Toronto's own Medical Officer of Health, had identified six main slums in Toronto in his 1911 Report on the conditions of the poor that included "The Ward," which he cited as a "moral contagion," and covered, amongst others, Queen Street from Bathurst to Bellwoods, Parliament Street to the Don River and Eastern Avenue. He further noted the "atmosphere of physical and moral rottenness" that pervaded the slums of all large cities. He was concerned in particular about the number of outdoor privies that still existed reeking with stench, which, of course, also contributed to Toronto's contaminated milk. A *Milk Act* had finally been passed at the fervent urging of Dr. MacMurchy, and, in 1912, inspectors had dumped 900 gallons of unpasteurized milk down the city sewer. Now Dr. Hastings wanted these privies abolished by law. (The social workers and deaconesses plugged their noses as they plodded through.) It certainly was not afternoon tea in the genteel drawing rooms of Rosedale, reciting Charlotte Jarvis' poetry, *Leaves From Rosedale*: "Rosedale the fair and favoured..." Miss Chown insisted that every aspect of the lives of the poor be minutely recorded. "The girl receiving insufficient pay would also be studied," she promised.

There was but one small voice of objection from a certain "Mrs. Morrison," a Methodist out in Saskatchewan who had responded in the *Christian Guardian*: "...Does the girl receiving insufficient pay wish to be studied? Would Alice A. Chown wish to be studied herself? Would you? Would I?"

Enthused nevertheless, the excellent ladies of the Social Work and the National Welfare Bureau organized a National Welfare Exhibit in Toronto in 1916. Citizens and government officials could now view for themselves how slum dwellers lived 365 days a year.

An exact replica of an actual slum house was put together. The Salvation Army Corps provided real furniture taken from slum dwellers' houses. It was not mentioned how they explained to the bewildered families why their furniture was being carried away and it was doubtful if the poor were invited to visit the Exhibit about themselves. What might they have thought of their filthy mattresses with their broken springs, half-chopped sofas, and incestuous iron beds on display before the ladies and gentlemen of Toronto?

As well, there had been a dramatic sketch called "Presenting Some of the Problems of Feeble-mindedness," written by one of the members of the new Advisory Committee on the Care of Mental Defectives in Toronto which included Mrs. Huestis, wealthy philanthropist, and Dr. MacMurchy as secretary. The *Toronto Sunday World* had reported, "A Novel Exhibit to Portray Evils of Feeble-Mindedness — truths thus strikingly presented."

To acknowledge the influence of heredity, there had been a display of the genealogy of the Kallikak family created by Dr. Goddard in Vineland, a potent reminder of what happened when the feeble-minded were left to reproduce their own kind. One but thought of the infamous Jukes family, which had 1,258 descendants from the original five mentally deficient Juke sisters, still living in 1916. The economic damage upon the State of New York by the Jukes sisters' progeny over 75 years, as everyone knew, had been reckoned at more than $1,300,000, to say nothing of the diseases they had helped to spread.

Dr. Clarke glowed. There had been on display samples from the files of nearly one thousand cases that had passed through the Toronto Psychiatric Clinic, by now better known as the "Feeble-Minded Clinic." Citizens of Toronto had read for themselves what was going on in their city. The life stories of "Betsy" and "Peggy" and "Maria" were pinned up for all to see: Peggy's infidelities, Maria's incestuous relations, with nary a thought for patient confidentiality.

The success of the Exhibit was unprecedented. "Toronto is roused at last!" exulted Dr. Hincks. "The terrible menace of the feeble-minded has shocked the community." It was time to press the government.

Of course, the fact that Dr. MacMurchy had once called the conservative government "stupid and absurd" and written in her Tenth Annual Report for 1915: "*Are we doing our best for the feeble-minded? Answer, 'No, certainly not',*" was not exactly guaranteed to endear her to Premier Hearst.

Nevertheless, in her imperious way, her grey hair drawn up in a bun, her monocle glinting, she instigated the petition of the Canadian Conference of Charities and Corrections to Prime Minister Robert Borden and Other Members of the Governments of Canada:

> We the undersigned citizens of Canada realizing the great menace that the feeble-minded are to the moral and social life

> of our communities.... Urge the appointment of a Dominion Commission to study and report upon the provision needed for the country at large to control this menace, and we would even support direct taxation to secure adequate provision for these unfortunates. And your petitioners will ever pray.

First signature on the list: Bishop Plumptre of St. James Anglican Cathedral, Toronto.

The demands had been extensive — laundry colonies, a registry of all mental defectives in the province, a psychopathic hospital, reform of the *Refuge Act*. Dr. Clarke had estimated the number of defectives in the province as 7,000, but added that, "Toronto alone must possess more defectives than that." The Industrial House of Refuge on Belmont Street provided custody for nearly a hundred feeble-minded girls and women, and The Haven for seventy-five, a considerable proportion being unmarried mothers. Dr. MacMurchy wanted these girls detained indefinitely, and the government responsible for morons over sixteen years of age. Like her American colleague, Dr. Goddard, she favoured a special "farm colony" to be built specifically for high grades somewhere on the outskirts of Toronto — here Dr. MacMurchy was vague — at a cost of $200,000, maintenance to be shared between the province and the city. The high-grade feeble-minded, many of whom were almost normal in intelligence though of the lowest morals, would provide much of the labour, making the institution self-sufficient. She envisaged small cottages on the "family plan," fifteen inmates to a "family" with a mother figure in charge. The male and female cottages were to be far apart from each other, on different parts of the grounds, of course.

But Premier Hearst was cautious. It seemed that thousands of so-called feeble-minded individuals who apparently were an even greater menace after age twenty-one, would be turned loose on the city and become the financial responsibility of the province.

He knew already from Mr. Downey, the Superintendent at the Orillia Hospital for the Feeble-Minded, from his Annual Report of 1913, that the institution needed the labour of such high-grade patients to keep down costs. Miss Marion Harvie, head teacher, had noted that many of the girls sent by the Children's Aid Society of Toronto were of normal intelligence; they had just come from poor or bad homes. Indeed, the Orillia Hospital, like the mental asylums, relied extensively on patient labour to remain viable, especially since paying patients were never more than twelve percent of the population. High-grade patients helped with labour, keeping down the cost of hiring help. They even made shoes and clothing, profitable ventures that helped keep Orillia afloat. What was needed, Mr. Downey said artfully, was not the expense of another institution in Toronto, but a farm colony on the grounds of Orillia itself, and so save further and unnecessary costs. He had hinted of Clarke and MacMurchy: "There are certain people who do not appreciate what we are doing here in Orillia."

And so Premier Hearst hedged, promising to "look into the matter" by appointing a one-man Royal Commission under the aegis of the Hon. Frank Egerton Hodgins.

"Picayune!" cried Dr. MacMurchy.

Dr. Clarke, equally incensed, joined the attack — comrades together — accusing the Hearst government of ineptitude, of doing nothing for the feeble-minded. There was only Orillia, he confided to Mr. Newton Rowell, leader of the Liberal Opposition, which was always overcrowded. Mr. Downey was simply incompetent to cope with the special type of high grades they had in mind.

"No one objects particularly to Mr. Downey, but his reign at Orillia has been little better than a joke," Dr. Clarke stormed. Mr. Downey did not offer one thing better than custodial care of a number of idiots and imbeciles. He had no medical degree; the only superintendent of Orillia who was not a physician, Dr. Clarke rounded indignantly; he was a mere former newspaperman and political appointee (friend of Mr. Hanna, the Provincial Secretary, as everyone knew). Motion overturned.

Rumours the government was planning to bring out a Mother's Allowance, as in the province of Manitoba, was even more outrageous. Mothers' allowances only encouraged imbeciles to propagate themselves all the more, promoting the survival of the *un*fittest, snarled Dr. Clarke. "This government lacks grasp, vision, imagination, and common sense!" to the delight of Mr. Rowell.

There was uproar in the Legislature.

It had soon been obvious that the Honourable Frank Egerton Hodgins' Report on the Care and Control of the Feeble-Minded and Mentally Deficient in 1919 was but a ploy to put them off and appear as if the government was doing something. Though the Honourable Hodgins admittedly expressed sympathy for their cause (he had conferred with both Dr. MacMurchy and Dr. Clarke on the recommendations, as well as influential Dr. Fernald of the Massachusetts School for Idiots the Feeble-Minded Youth, agreeing that pregnant unmarried girls and other "dregs" of society should be institutionalized), nothing concrete materialized. No farm colony, no provincial survey or registration of the feeble-minded and lunatics, no Board of Control to manage the financial aspect of the planned Colony and oversee the institutionalization of the morons.

At least the old *Females Refuge Act* of 1913 was finally reformed to include the feeble-minded. The new Act allowed physicians not only to certify a woman as "feeble-minded" and have her detained indefinitely beyond the expiry of her sentence, but *transferred* to a training school, or a reformatory like the Andrew Mercer Reformatory for Females on King Street Toronto, or Orillia, as the physician so deemed. Dr. Hincks, in particular, was delighted. Writing in the *Canadian Journal of Mental Hygiene*, he reminded readers that mental defectives were people afflicted with stunted brain development, urging: "It is necessary to control the sex lives of these classes."

But the battle was far from over. Despite his ongoing cyclothymic attacks of depression and hypomanic frenzy, Dr. Hincks or "Hinksey," as he was known, had founded the Canadian National Committee for Mental Hygiene (CNCMH). It occurred after a miraculous meeting in a home in Rosedale, Toronto, in 1918 with an American, Mr. Clifford Beers, author of *A Mind That Found Itself*. A former mental patient, Mr. Beers had once tried to commit suicide by throwing himself from the window of his three-storey house while in a severe depression, and had subsequently founded the National Committee for Mental Hygiene in Connecticut.

With Beers' support, Hincks resolved to found a similar movement in Canada, the Canadian National Committee for Mental Hygiene (CNCMH). Dr. Hincks' aims for CNCMH included the fight against crime, prostitution, unemployment, juvenile delinquency, moral contamination in primary schools, illegitimacy, military insubordination, pauperism, alcoholism, unfit families, and lax immigration laws that allowed into the country the rag-tags of Eastern Europe and the Mediterranean basin, Jews from the ghettoes of Poland (60,000 alone in Toronto), the Chinese, the Irish, and other undesirables. The CNCMH wanted proper medical inspections at ports of entry to detect lunacy, idiocy, epilepsy, and those carrying contagious diseases such as tuberculosis (and other loathsome diseases).

Excited, Dr. Clarke resigned at once from the Toronto General Hospital to take over as Director of the new venture. Dr. MacMurchy, Dr. Eric Clarke (Dr. Clarke's son, a psychiatrist like his father), Dr. Withrow, Bishop Plumptre at the Anglican Cathedral, Prof. Bott, Judge Mott of the Juvenile Court, Dr. Hastings (Medical Officer of Health), were amongst the members, as well as Inspector Gregory from the police department, and Miss Lucy Brooking, Superintendent of the Alexandra Industrial School for Girls out on Kingston Road. Miss Brooking claimed that most of the girls there were feeble-minded, "otherwise they would not be delinquent," she stressed.

A special committee dealing with mental defectives was struck, consisting of the best minds of the city. The Chairman, Dr. Hastings; the Secretary, Prof. Bott.

The first task of the new committee: to undertake a survey of the mental hospitals across the country, at the request of seven provinces, including Manitoba and Nova Scotia. It was conducted by Dr. Clarke and Dr. Hincks with the aid of capable, kind Miss Marjorie Keyes. Miss Keyes had taken over as head nurse at the Clinic in the absence of Miss E. de V. Clarke during the war. She and Dr. Hincks soon became inseparable (Dr. Clarke did not wish to think how inseparable), touring the provinces together. "Marjorie has been in more asylums than any woman in Canada!" Dr. Hincks liked to quip. In the asylum in St. John's, New Brunswick, they found inmates put to bed in coffin-like boxes with hay at the bottom and slats on top, all boxes except two locked at night. In Edmonton, Alberta, mentally defective children were rolled in long strips of cotton at bedtime, their arms and legs bound, and then piled on a shelf for the night in an asylum. In Nova Scotia, the government had requested a survey of one hundred mentally defective families. The CNCMH study had found that when a father was mentally defective and the mother normal, most of the children were normal in intelligence, but if instead the mother was defective, the children would likely be mentally defective too.

Dr. Hincks' survey of New Westminster Public Hospital for the Insane in December of 1918, and 1919, stressed that the feeble-minded contributed to the province's crime, poverty, and prostitution. Sterilization would be a cheaper, more humane method of restricting procreation. On a visit to Orillia in 1921, Miss Keyes was to report seeing a large room full of commode chairs with helpless inmates of the lowest intelligence tied in them all day. What more was needed to alert the Ontario government?

"Why haven't we got results?" Dr. Hincks stormed at the Social Welfare Congress in January of 1919, not unlike the great Dr. MacMurchy herself. "Because I take it that reforms cost money!"

The new Drury government of the United Farmers Party of Ontario, installed in November of 1919, was suspicious of the CNCMH and "unfeeling," Dr. Hincks complained. "The government says 'Don't knock your province.' Why, we have enough facts to blow up the Parliament buildings!"

Meanwhile, in Orillia, Mr. Downey, the Superintendent, smiled to himself. He was a suave, round-faced, middle-aged man with baby blue eyes, a blond moustache, and wavy hair parted down the middle. He loved the institution and had grown fond of the patients. "The three years I have spent here have been the happiest of my life!" he had written warmly in a little article for the *Bulletin of the Ontario Hospital* called "Among The Children" (which included 60 middle-aged women). "The prevailing opinion among those who have never visited the Hospital for the Feeble-Minded," he observed in an amiable way, "is that it is a very dreary place to live and that work among its population is always disagreeable."

There were annual picnics on the grounds for the patients, with cake and lemonade, he assured his readers, whom of course included Dr. MacMurchy and Dr. Clarke. Once a week a large launch took patients and staff for a boat ride and everyone was accordingly happy. There were moving pictures in the Amusement Hall in winter.

He especially loved the "high-grade" defectives, bright little girls "like little sheafs of sunshine in the ward," he wrote. These same little bright ones had actually put on a cantata, "Fairies of the Season," which had occupied some fifty minutes in the annual Christmas concert and had intricate movements and exacting choral numbers. Premier Hearst himself, a visitor at the event, had remarked that, "the high level of performance of these ones would be a credit to children possessing all their faculties." No one seemed to wonder why such children were in Orillia in the first place.

Indeed, their gifts were useful in other ways, for the brighter ones often acted as "mothers" to the younger children in the wards. They even made clothes for their "children." Miss Hale, one of the teachers at the time, noted they often took better care of them than their own real mothers.

Not all patients were at this level, however. There were certain inmates, the "loathsome ones," who had to be kept separate, confined to special wards. Mr. Downey cut education for these ones (why waste the money?). He knew he was there to cut costs for the government, and he did. These low-grade idiots were seldom seen. Miss Harvie, head teacher, observed privately that she had never seen the inside of the buildings where they were kept, a certain secrecy surrounding them. Even Dr. Beaton had once remarked, sadly, of those "of loathsome visage" who had had to be kept out of sight lest they shock people: "...We have idiocy in all its varied phases, from the semi-bright and confiding child, to the filthy and repulsive adult, without one gleam of intelligence, in whom the soul is indeed locked up, as if in an iron safe."

Of course, there would always be some dissension among patients in an institution, observed Mr. Downey. It was only natural to expect fighting among sixty middle-aged women enclosed in a senior ward. They had their feuds and their scraps. Some were given to violent outbursts that sorely taxed the patience of the nurses, but any group of middle-aged women, he defended, placed together in one ward in an institution, expected to sleep in the same dormitory, dress in the same bathroom, eat in the same dining room, lounge in the same living room, work and play together, would end up, he wrote, in a "real old-fashioned hair-pulling match."

But, on the whole, Orillia was a happy, self-productive place. Mr. Downey recalled Miss Nash's observation of the feeble-minded in Dr. Beaton's time in the Asylum for Idiots that: "their worries are few and fleeting.... All we have to do is keep them safe and happy in their world."

26.

A BABBY CAME, and then another and another, hanging down between her legs. Church ladies had given money for a nurse to come from the clinic but she had arrived too late and little baby Wilfred got born, her fourth in nearly five years noted Mrs. O'Garrity. Old Irish Mrs. O'Garrity from the room next door and Henrietta had done the job. Four year-old Henrietta had held the cooking pan between Mama's legs for the bloods and awkwardly carried dirty strips of cloth dipped in boiling water. It was the best they could do, sighed Mrs. O'Garrity. She had checked Flo's discharge: "What 'ad ter go from red ter brown, even green." Church ladies and someone from the St. Paul's Catholic Church on Power Street had given a layette for baby Wilfred, swaddling and binding cloth for Florrie's belly, that was important said Mrs. O'Garrity, and taken her to the clinic afterwards up Parliament Street. A nurse showed her what to do with her teats (she had not enough milk). She was to get free milk from the depot if she did not have milk coupons for the milkman. The milkman came every morning and you gave him money once a week and he gave you tokens. You put one token in the empty bottle outside the door in the morning and he left a bottle of milk. *You were not to lose them Enry said', or 'Enry'd 'it her over the 'ead.*

They had ended up in lower Cabbagetown after the Great War, the east end of Toronto where they had heard rents were cheaper, unaware they were now living in what was to be known as "the biggest Anglo-Saxon and Irish slum in North America." Parliament, River, Sackville, Oak, Sumach, Power. These were the streets home to generations of poor Catholics like the Hewitts, sprinkled in with refugees, clustered round St. Paul's Catholic Church on Power Street that was to be the Hewitts' world for the rest of their lives, if they but knew.

"There are no poor in Canada!" the Minister of Labour had promised, as semi-skilled workers were guaranteed a wage of $12 a week. Bread was five cents a loaf and coal was four dollars a ton. But that had been before the Great War. The population of Toronto had apparently grown from 96,196 in 1881 to nearly 500,000 by 1919, an increase of over 400 percent. Milk and bread had doubled, strikes were everywhere, and there was no work, reported Henry, glumly. "They says the banks got no money, Flo. 'Can't pay the increase,' they says." He had read the headlines at the corner newsstand. Three thousand metal workers were out on strike in Toronto (the strike collapsed after four days). "And something terrible happenin' called The General Strike in a place called Winnipeg out west, lasted May ter June, 1919, that very year." Florrie, who could not count to three let alone three thousand, only knew the fetid unheated rooms they had rented were full of lice. The further south of College Street you went, the poorer and more broken everything became.

Number 10 on Lower Sumach was the usual small row house — two up, two down — shared with a large noisy drunken Irish catholic family above and other shifty tenants from Macedonia in the basement below. A social worker from St. Vincent de Paul Catholic Children's Aid Society, Miss Dorkins, had written in the Hewitt records quite dispassionately at this time, that she had found them shivering around the stove during the winter, the last chair chopped up for firewood: "*Home conditions of this family poor. Rooms bare and destitute. Bed clothing filthy and entire family almost without clothing.*" She had brought them food, clothes, sanitary pads, and pieces of coal; a used mattress was ordered from the Salvation Army Corps and other basic necessities kindly provided by the Solidarity of the Blessed Virgin Mary at the church.

The baby Wilfred, born the previous year, had woken and begun wailing. Fireworks were exploding down at the bay for Queen Victoria's birthday, May 21,1920, Victoria Day in Canada, which set Henry off again: "*Over th' top!*" he had screamed.

"Oh 'Enry!" Florrie had cringed, wanting to run downstairs for Mrs. O'Garrity. "Oh, what 'appenin?"

"*Over th' top*!" Henry jumped in terror out of the corner, smashing Auntie's piss-pot from England, the china flying about. "AAAGH!"

He had raised his fists and beat her about the head, as she cried, "Oh! Oh 'Enry, na, please 'Enry, is Florrie." There was another explosion inside her ear and she couldn't hear him no more. Was that what war was? Now he was going up on the roof, and she cried out for help. "Over th' top!" he was yelling again, by the chimney pot.

"Ow'd 'e get up there?" The neighbours were coming out. He was going to *jump*.

Dr. Clarke looked cautiously at Henry Hewitt that May day in 1920. He was sitting across from him in the Psychiatric Clinic in the basement of the Toronto General Hospital: a demobilized soldier suffering from the after-effects of so-called "shell shock."

It seemed the fellow had actually tried to swallow a bottle of Lysol before attempting to throw himself off the roof of a house on Sumach Street. He also, by his own admission, had taken to beating his wife at times, perforating her eardrums, and had once turned on the gas and put his head in the oven. That particular episode had taken place during the war, in England — pronounced by doctors at the time as evident shell shock, before he was discharged early in 1915, after which he had stayed on in England until the war was over, before returning to Toronto. A possible psychiatric case. The public ambulance men had rightly brought him days before to the observation ward in the basement next to the Emergency Department, used by the Toronto General Hospital for problems associated with psychotic behaviour, violence, and suicide.

"I didn' know what I was doin', sir. All them firecrackers going off in the sky, an' the babbies screamin' and cryin'."

Was he a malingerer?

"Got half my ass shot off in the war."

Dr. Clarke tensed. "Yes. Quite."

Of course, a certain amount of rot had been said about shell shock. Psychiatrists and neurologists were divided on the issue. One group favoured Freudian theory, delving back into a soldier's childhood to explain away neurotic symptoms of so-called neurasthenia and hysteria in soldiers who had become apparently mute or paralyzed, with no actual physical manifestations. However, His Excellency, Sir Robert Armstrong Jones, a noted psychiatrist, believed such symptoms were due to tainted heredity and that soldiers who had developed psychoses and neuroses during military action would have developed them anyway. In other words, the stress of military service made active latent mental conditions, such as *dementia praecox*. Clarke agreed. He himself knew whereof he spoke: he and Dr. Clarence Farrar, a fine young American psychiatrist attached to the Department of Soldiers' Civil Re-Establishment after the Great War, and Clarke's protégé, had visited and classified one thousand psychiatric cases of soldiers in the Canadian Expeditionary Force (C.E.F.) who had served in France and England and had been discharged from the army due to mental disability, at present receiving treatment in provincial hospitals.

Yet, a great tide of public sentiment had swept the nation for the soldiers, seen as victims of cold-hearted war psychiatrists. The British War Office had initiated a Committee of Enquiry in 1919, still underway, into the supposed torture and abuses by doctors and psychiatrists administering faradic electrical shocks to the soldiers in their care. Dr. Clarke bristled at the mere suggestion. Claims of cruelty had been wantonly misunderstood. Such soldiers were likely malingerers or susceptible to weak hereditary genes, Clarke frowned — mental weaklings.

And this Hewitt fellow was part of that. Dr. Clarke leaned forward to observe him more closely: a small, tough-looking, ill-kept worker from the slums dressed in overalls patched with double seat and double knees. "From England, Hewitt?"

"Yes, sir, I was a Union boy."

Dr. Clarke rolled his eyes. He knew about these feeble-minded paupers of the English Union Poor Laws, 150,000 of them under the parochial system in England in 1900 alone, and all the other riff-raff that had come into the country through Dr. Barnardo's agency — more than eighty thousand — and other such British agencies. He had once had occasion to see a trainload of such immigrant children on their way out west a decade ago, obvious degenerates with dull features, adding to the burden of Canadian taxpayers. He had protested then for reform in immigration laws in 1907, but the profits of the steamship companies bringing them in had counted more.

The fact was, this fellow Hewitt should not have been allowed to enlist in the Army in the first place, being mentally deficient. Who knew how many brave, trusting soldiers on his own side the fellow may have bayonetted to death by mistake in the trenches? His I.Q. showed but 70 in the army's testing: "Moron" level.

Hewitt sat still, his steely eyes looking perplexed. "You was in the war, sir?" He nodded almost shyly at the doctor's missing fingers on his left hand. "There was lots o' doctors behin' the lines in the field horspitals."

Dr. Clarke instinctively withdrew his hand, as he was still self-conscious of the two fingers that had been shot off in a hunting accident as a young boy.

"Some doctors had to stay put and organize the field hospitals, Hewitt."

"Keep the 'ome fires burning, sir?"

Dr. Clarke frowned again. He had personally made himself responsible for organizing and funding University of Toronto Overseas Field Hospital No. 4, consisting of a thousand beds, though Hewitt could scarcely be expected to comprehend his pride in this.

"My daughter signed up for overseas duty as a nurse," he said stiffly.

Dearest Emma. "Goldie" they called her on account of her hair, red like his own. She was the plainer of his two daughters, Margery being the beauty like her mother, Margaret de Veber, who had died on Christmas Day, 1902. The memory suddenly flooded back and the pain of that moment rose again. But Emma was close to his heart. She had done her training at New York Presbyterian Hospital, following his directives, and had devoted herself to his Clinic doing excellent work setting it up. When Emma had left, he had kissed her and put his arms around her, and said, "Dearest one." She was now in charge of mental hygiene work at the Department of Health, Parliament Buildings.

"We used t' call the nurses Our Angels, sir."

"Yes, well, Hewitt."

Henry sat, unblinking. He only knew from other patients on the ward, that Dr. Clarke had been the Superintendent of the terrifying Toronto Lunatic Asylum down on Queen Street. He had little idea that the doctor, a genial-looking man with a kind face, beady eyes and a bushy moustache, was also the first Professor of Psychiatry at the University of Toronto, Dean of Medicine, former Superintendent of Toronto General Hospital, and Director of the CNCMH. But he sensed his greatness, his power, and felt a certain submissive reverence that here was the man who could return him to Florrie and the little ones.

"Look, governor ... please ... don't put me in the asylum," he pleaded in a low voice. "I ain't orff my 'ead, sir, I ain't."

He had only a vague memory of standing on the roof with a saucepan on his head, waving his arms, and of the fire engine roaring down Parliament Street clanging its bells, with Florrie howling below. He hesitated. "All I want is a job, my old job back in th' Ice Company. But they don't want us soldiers no more," he added bitterly.

Dr. Clarke knew that the Winnipeg General Strike of 1919 still reverberated through the nation in a dangerous way, though reporters of the *Star* had sought to maintain objectivity: "There is little or no terrorism." Nevertheless, middle-class citizens of Fort Rouge apparently had had to hide out in churches overnight, terrified of being murdered in their beds. The workers were clearly out of control. And low wages and working conditions had little to do with it. These lower classes were inherently weak, unable to survive in the struggle of life.

"We gort no bread, sir." Hewitt looked anxious.

He knew his name, address, birthplace, the name of his battalion. He knew the war was over and said, in a firm, sincere way, "It was 'ell, sir." He was trustworthy, despite his low mentality. Dr. Clarke hesitated. He wanted to be fair; he prided himself on it. He always made a point of having a mental patient for a servant girl in his Rosedale home. Of course, there was the matter of venereal disease.

"Just that once, sir, I been with a young chippie. You know 'ow it is, away from 'ome. Felt bad about it, about Florrie and the babby. I loves Flo, sir, I do."

"Treatment?"

"We was told soap an' water, sir, on our cocks, and an' ointment they give us, Calomile."

Dr. Clarke snorted. He had personally set up a V.D. Clinic in Toronto offering free treatment with the latest drug, Salvarsan, an arsenic-based drug developed by a German medical student, Paul Ehrlich, in 1909, though difficult to inject, and toxic. In this he had had the support of the Imperial Order of Daughters of the Empire and the National Council of Women, distressed at the immorality of returning troops and the threat to civilians.

Regular checkups for V.D. and chancroid were now mandatory, he pointed out severely, thanks to the *Venereal Diseases Act* of 1919, which carried penalties of up to $500 for non-compliance. Henry and Florrie would have to present themselves at the Toronto General Hospital clinic for a Wassermann test; if infected, they would take a card and submit to treatment 606 for syphilis or irrigation for gonorrhea. He made a mental note to alert Dr. Helen MacMurchy and his son Eric Clarke, now a child psychiatrist, to register the Hewitt children. Eric was making a survey of 38 public schools in poor areas of the city, as medical advisor for the CNCMH.

Hewitt nodded: "Y-yes, yes sir, I understands."

Dr. Clarke glanced sharply at Hewitt. In one sense, here was an example of the success story of psychiatry emerging from the Great War, indicative of the role the profession had played in diagnosing and treating the troops, gaining new respect from the medical profession. He did not seem to be suffering from any real lasting serious effects of war, shell shock or not.

He wrote on Hewitt's form: "No evidence of psychosis," and signed his release.

Mrs. Hewitt was another matter. Florrie, who obviously belonged in Orillia, had just turned up hatless at the Clinic, whispering hoarsely that she had "come ter collect 'Enry," a baby tied to her chest in a wraparound strip of dirty cloth, another on the way, the very sort of degenerate he and Dr. MacMurchy had been protesting about for decades.

27.

THERE WAS NOW Henrietta, Robbie, Edgar, Wilfred, Oswald, Ella, little Georgie "named for 'is Majesty," Florrie told the lady worker, Miss Dorkins, and the new babby, Sophie. It was 1929 and Florrie was not yet thirty, guessed Miss Dorkins, the social worker from the Catholic Children's Aid Society (CCAS). After the baby, Florrie's courses had stopped coming again, "but the castor oil that Mrs. O'Garrity give her did not work," she faltered, and she was "gettin' bigger each day." Miss Dorkins hesitated in the doorway, but how much could Florrie Hewitt, an obvious imbecile, understand of the actions of that awful neighbour Mrs Garrity who thought nothing of sinning against the Holy Father. But Florrie was desp'rite, she said later to Mrs. O'Garrity, after kind Miss Dorkins gone. Mrs. O'Garrity had said "not ter worry," she knew something else that was sure to do it even though Flo was so far advanced: pennyroyal and carbolic. She got it from the chemist on the corner "an' to hell with the Holy Father." She knew who to ask, where to go, she could read: Norforms Zonite, Rendell's "suppositories" what would bring it on. Mrs. O'Garrity understood the implicit messages of Norforms Zonite, supposedly innocuous "suppositories," found everywhere if you knew what windows to look in. But Florrie had to give her some of the milk money Henry had under the mattress.

"Jus' swaller penn'royal first and then we tries the carbolic, Flo." Then Flo was to come to a room at the back place behind the outhouse, last chance, where Mrs. O'Garrity had a mix of carbolic acid and water. Henrietta held the baby who was always poorly, as she had summer diarrhea. Ella stood silently with the boys out back, watching through the doorway, too little to understand. They put a rag in Mama's mouth. There was a long rubber thing that squirted at the end that Mrs. Neale down the street who had been a nurse a long time back had lent. Mrs. O'Garrity pushed it up Mama's inside, high up, as high as it would go, as "I gotta find th' 'ole," she explained.

There were holes up there? Florrie panicked.

"No, jus' one, deary, what he puts 'is cock in every night."

Florrie screamed.

"That's the carbolic, doin' its job," soothed Mrs. O'Garrity.

After a while, maybe that night, maybe sooner, a baby would come out, and it would have fingers and toes, Mrs. O'Garrity warned dourly, because Flo had left it late. If she kept on bleeding she was to send Henrietta or Robbie over for her.

Mrs. O'Garrity pressed down on her belly and out it all came. Henrietta held the pan again between her mother's legs nice and steady, like a good girl. Ella stood by with the rags. A big, bloody thing slipped into the pan.

"Here it be," said Mrs. O'Garrity, huffing and sweating. "Jus' another girl would 'ave bin, Flo." She threw it out in the privy. Later, after dark, the rats came out, feasting well into the night.

Well-meaning Miss Dorkins, social worker, hovered in the doorway of what could only be described as the Hewitts' latest hovel on Oak Street. Behind her was a communal yard pressed in by tottering houses and shifty add-ons (illegal and dangerous). That other awful family, the Lumsdens, also utterly destitute, were on her dossier as well. The Lumsden children, eight or ten of them, ran about in rags like the Hewitts, and were riddled with scabies. Effie Lumsden and her brother, Ernest, both incorrigibles, were slated for Orillia — where else? Ernest Lumsden had stolen a parishioner's bicycle from behind Berkeley Wesleyan Methodist Church on the Sabbath.

Miss Dorkins ducked under a limp line of dirty washing, and stepped into the one room that served as the Hewitts' kitchen and — horrible to consider — bedroom, with its shredded wallpaper and odours one did not want to think of. She had brought more milk tokens, provided for the destitute and unemployed by the Toronto municipality in charge of poor relief, bandages, and underwear for the girls.

Time hung still in the silence of the kitchen. Florrie stood troubled. There was nothing for the baby, as her teats had dried up long ago. Nothing for their teas; the little boy Georgie, in between Ella and the baby, pulled at her skirt and cried, "Butty, Mama!" Ella, the second girl that Florrie said was age four, or was it five?, sat dully by the stove despite the heat. The two older boys were out in the streets scavenging for food and scrap iron with Henrietta. Florrie was not certain how old Henrietta was exactly, perhaps eleven or twelve. All she knew was that she hadn't started 'er courses yet.

"Oh, bless ye, Miz Dork'ns," she gasped, taking the tokens and pushing them under the mattress.

Sunlight played over the dusty yard, the square of dirt they all shared at the back, these families and tenants packed in like rats. Frowzy city trees sheltered the cracked roofs, the tiles tacked together poorly, and now, peeling in the heat. In the kitchen, a sticky flypaper hung from a nail, coated with flies.

Yet, as Florrie stood in the long autumn afternoon after Miss Dorkins had left, she was only thankful for the blood between her legs again. The blood trickled into a dirty cloth held up front and back with two safety pins bought from the old gypsy man from the Ward. He came door to door with his tray full of cottons, needles, and balls of thread; such precious pieces of cloth, and even more precious were the safety pins he had given her for a few pennies. Just the one piece of cloth washed over and over under the spigot, the pins saved.

She lifted the kettle on to the stove to boil water for Henry's tea when he got in; water dripped from the spigot outside and Ella sucked at it.

Florrie was fearful of him now, his tread, his fist, the knot of muscle in his taut arm. He would be back from his shift when the whistle went at the factory. She knew the sound, every woman on the street knew that sound coming from somewhere down Cherry Street. He would come and she would have to ask for money.

The siren went off, along with the ringing in her ears. Then there was the low tramp of feet, of all the workers coming off of their shift. Henry came in breathing heavily from the dust and grime of the factory and sat at once in the chair, his legs apart. "Aaah!" The children ran and hid, and even the baby stiffened. What was going to happen now? She brought him his mug of tea. "No butty left," she faltered, the last crust of bread long gone. He was swilling his tea already.

"On the bleedin' rag agin, I sees," he gave a rough laugh, surveying his wife. "An' jus' when I was fancying a nice bit o' somethin'."

He had read newspapers on the stand on the corner that said Black

Thursday: October 24, 1929. "The 'eadlines says terday there's bin a crash, Florrie. Is Black Thursday." Florrie at once put her hands to her face. "Oh, 'Enry! Who got 'urt?"

"Na, not that kind o' crash. New York stock markit crash!"

Florrie looked bewildered.

"Rich people's money all gorn, Flo. Somethin' bad 'as 'appen' in 'Merica an' we'll git our arses burned too in the end, you'll see."

The baby's face puckered and he lifted up his little fists to protect his face.

That fall, Florrie's stomach was getting big again — another babby — and she was frightened, frightened of his strop. Five-year-old Ella trembled as he stood breathing heavily over Mama on the mattress. He pushed Mama down and rolled her over.

"Na-a,'Enry....."

"Aw Flo, what else a man need after a day at th' bleeding fact'ry?" He was working ten-hour shifts for eight lousy dollars, he grumbled. Grunting, he unleashed his belt. Ella and Robbie crouched in the corner, and the baby lay on his back on sacking. Her belly was too big, and Mama was crying. "Aw, don't make no difference, Flo, come on." The babby would be coming soon, but he wanted up her backside, her belly pushing down on the mattress. Robbie rolled over on to Ella.

"Ma," called Henrietta at the stove. "Robbie's wanking Ella."

Florrie tried to call out, but Henry would not stop.

Ella pushed Robbie off, then stood up tearing her dress. That girl!

"What the bleedin' 'ell now!"

Henry stood over his smallest daughter afterwards, struggling to pull up his pants. "She gone an' torn 'er bloody dress ter pieces! What she do that for?"

Ella lay rolling on the ground beating the floor with her head.

"Hey, she gonna break 'er 'ead an' the floor. Bloody dress in shreds! For Chrissake!"

Ella ran over to the stove. She pulled open the heavy door with both hands where Robbie threw in wood. Flames rose in a sudden heady rush and she screamed with excitement at the roaring red fire.

"Hey! She's gorn an' thrown it in the bleedin' fire!"

Henrietta stood in a haze of flies in the afternoon. Sunlight played over the dusty square of dirt the family shared with other tenants in the other closely packed houses. The houses rose in layers, ever the same, faded and cracked, with shanty rooms tacked on, silent and still. A rat slid lazily out of a pipe.

She hovered in the sun barefoot, her dress tied with string. Wild flowers thrust through the stones: the last of the daisies and goldenrods rising against the sagging fence by the outhouse. You did not go in by yourself, or something would happen for which there was no word, but pretty Henrietta, "a slow girl" Miss Dorkins had once said kindly, stood shyly by, fingering her curls, knowing they would come.

Autumn voices drifted in the air to the slap of a rope, skipping rhymes and songs from long ago that belonged to Mama and Dada, back in the old country of England: "*The water is wide, and I cannot get over. And neither have I wings to fly.*" These were folk songs that had somehow passed into this new world of Toronto. From the place where her parents were born, Henrietta knew from Teacher at Jarvis Vocational School up the road where she learned cooking and other domestic duties.

She pushed back her long, golden curls, smiling at the boys as five-year-old Ella scratched her lice and watched.

The nurse at the clinic said the baby was dead, and noted the year, November, 1929. Miss Dorkins from the CCAS came and took the youngest children to the shelter for a week, as there was a fuss. She had called the public ambulance and Florrie was taken to St. Mike's because someone said she was Catholic. Florrie was carrying a dead baby inside and it had to come out. There were tubes and the cold clear smell of sheets. The Church Ladies paid, but how much? The baby came out dead and was buried and Florrie was not sorry, but poor Henry cried.

Something had to be done about this family.

28.

THEIR APPOINTMENT was on the first Wednesday afternoon in December of 1929, arranged by Miss Dorkins at the Toronto Psychiatric Hospital, Wednesday afternoons having been reserved for the Children's Clinic in the Outpatients Department that had begun in March, 1926. It was run by Dr. Edmund Lewis, a psychiatrist with the Mental Hygiene Service (Toronto Public Health). He was joined in his work by a visiting psychiatrist who came in once a week from the Family Court. General reasons for referral to the clinic, as Miss Dorkins well knew, were behavioural difficulties, social problems such as stealing and truancy, illegitimacy, suspected mental defect, inability to hold a job, vagrancy, backwardness at school, deportation of people suspected of mental retardation or mental illness, and any other number of causes applicable to such as the Hewitts.

Miss Dorkins had explained the day before the necessity for the children to have a bath (and, preferably, Mr. and Mrs. Hewitt). One could hardly expect the nurse and Dr. Charles Meade to touch layers of Hewitt grime and sores. There had been great excitement in the kitchen. It had meant boiling up the kettle and soup cauldron in advance on the stove. Henrietta, with little Ella's help, brought in water from the communal tap out in the yard. Miss Dorkins herself personally provided a bar of carbolic soap, a sponge, and a few (clean) towels. "First time they 'ad a wash since las' Chrismus," said Henry cheerfully. "Better 'n' the dirty ol' Public Baths on Sackville." He brought in an old tin bath from the yard spotted with rust and said he had "cleaned out the spiders an' rat-shit first." Miss Dorkins smiled wanly. The younger children were running half-naked round the kitchen, with Florrie Hewitt laughing, as excited herself at the prospect of dipping herself naked into the water after the others. Fourteen-year-old Henrietta held the soap and sponge as twelve-year-old Robbie stepped in first. Miss Dorkins glanced tactfully away. "Aieee!" he cried. "Oh aye, 'Ettie!" as his sister soaped up his back. Little Oswald — there was something wrong with his legs (but if one looked closely there was something wrong with every Hewitt child) — handed Georgie to Miss Dorkins, a dear child of about twenty months.

"Titties," he lisped. And before horrified Miss Dorkins could protect herself he had pressed his grubby little fingers (who knew where they had been) on her breasts; she had felt them squeezing with childlike need. She had felt an unexpected pleasure at the touch and suddenly, she had wanted to sit down and put her head in her hands and sob.

The Hewitts now had a semblance of cleanliness. Mr. Hewitt lugged the tin bath out the back door and threw the dirty water over the yard. The boys had clean shirts and patched breeches; the girls had second-hand dresses from the Catholic Church ladies at St Paul's. However, no amount of soap and water and new clothes could eliminate a certain odour embedded in this family.

They had got off the tram at College Street and University, Florrie carrying the baby, Sophie, and Miss Dorkins carrying Georgie. Henrietta held five-year-old Ella's hand and Oswald's in the other. The other children of varying ages huddled close. The tram had trundled along Carlton and College Streets past shops, and movie theatres, and Eaton's stores where beautifully clothed women in slender coats with fur around the neck and cloche hats gazed in the windows. The entrance to the new Eaton's store at Yonge Street was lovely, with its tall arched doorway, its fanned windows and clear glass panes glistening as if it were a cathedral. They also caught a glimpse of the dingy Eaton's factories further down the street. The tram conductor called, "Toronto General Hospital," and they got out.

Now they walked, bewildered, by the great sandstone Parliament Buildings in a place called Queen's Park, following Miss Dorkins. Florrie looked in awe at a statue of a man who was looking thoughtfully down the avenue at the city. Miss Dorkins said he was "MacDonald" and that they should be grateful to him. Below him was a boulevard of beautiful oaks that lined University Avenue, then the slums.

They turned the corner up Grosvenor Street along to Surrey Place, and there was the Toronto Psychiatric Hospital (TPH for short, said Miss Dorkins, as if Florrie and Henry understood that). TPH was still new, having opened only four years back in 1925 to great acclaim and excitement in the city. Dr. Clarke's dream realized at last! He himself had been present for the laying of the foundation stone in 1923, before his death on January 20,1924. Dr. Hincks had wept at the funeral, calling him his mentor, a father to him, and "the greatest psychiatrist Canada would ever have." Such were his skills, claimed Dr. Hincks, that he could analyze a man correctly in minutes — a genius. Who else was such a powerful diagnostician, boatbuilder, ornithologist, violin player par excellence (he often played with the Toronto Symphony Orchestra as an amateur), and expert on birds' eggs, all at the same time? Something the Hewitts, Miss Dorkins realized, could hardly be expected to appreciate.

At the opening ceremony, Sir Robert Falconer had called the hospital "a monument to the enlightenment, intelligence, and progressiveness of the efforts now being made to treat mental disease." Rev. Edwin Henry, pastor of Deer Park Presbyterian Church had asked for Divine blessing. The hospital was quite modest, merely eighty beds compared with the Toronto Lunatic Asylum at 999 Queen Street. Dr. Dunlop, Government Inspector, called it a "wart on the landscape." Florrie and Henry saw only a mellow, brick building shaped in a cross, with a small garden to the side, and rows of institutional-type windows with grilles, they noted with alarm.

They sat in Outpatients with their eight children — Henrietta, Robbie, Edgar, Wilfred, Oswald, Ella, little Georgie and baby Sophie who screamed constantly unless she was at the breast — waiting to be called. Florrie was conscious of her ill-fitting skirt. There was a crisp, cool nurse striding around, her stiff white cap on her head like a crown.

Only Henry knew that this place was a loony bin. He had heard about it. The first floor up was for women; some said the wards were sunny and open and some said they were dark with long corridors, and eerie at night with the stink of paraldehyde. Another floor up was for men. There were baths they put you in. You were covered up to your neck in canvas, and then you lay in the water for hours until they took you out. And lastly, the third floor was for the "violent" ones. They were strapped down and locked in, and nobody ever saw what happened to them. There was a curving wooden staircase leading up from the second floor, where you would not want to go.

Dr. Meade appeared in a long white coat, wanting their history. They followed him into the examining room.

What was their history? Florrie fluttered anxiously, shaking her head. Henry was cautious (who knew which floor they might all end up on).

"We's here for the boys, sir. Robbie an' Edgar."

For the first time, Henry and Florrie heard of the process by which they had been directed to TPH, listening as Miss Dorkins explained to Dr. Meade that the school nurse at St. Mary's had reported the boys, aged twelve and ten, to the Medical Officer, part of Dr. MacMurchy's old registry system, for psychological testing. The entire family was to be examined, including the mother and father — perhaps them most of all, something it did not occur to Henry and Florrie to question.

Dr. Meade, the psychiatrist assigned that day, took in the Hewitts at a glance. It was obvious *the entire family* was retarded.

Dr. Meade had, of course, seen the travelling Exhibit on the Feeble-Minded consisting of thirty-one photographs and artifacts organized by Dr. Hincks and the Canadian National Committee for Mental Hygiene (CNCMH) when it came to Toronto in 1924. One useful poster had depicted the "Four Types of Mental Deficiency," featuring faces of real-live imbeciles, idiots, morons and such, to help professionals such as Dr. Meade identify feeble-mindedness and its dullness of expression (dopey eyes, loose mouths, degenerate chins and ears) that he recognized in these Hewitts.

Dr. Hincks, carrying on the vital work of the late great Dr. Clarke, had also circulated a pamphlet, "The Five Thousand Club," put out by the CNCMH, which kept record of this sort of feeble-mindedness, warning it was "deadlier to Canadian citizens than tuberculosis."

Dr. Meade checked out Hewitt's score. Sure enough, Henry Hewitt had an I.Q. of only 70 on the Stanford-Binet test, or "Moron" level — almost "Dull-Normal." The Family History Form, forwarded by Miss Dorkins, noted that on Mr. Hewitt's side his father had actually been a shipwright, which perhaps explained how he had at least reached Junior 111 in school in England. Nothing further back was known of Mr. Hewitt's genealogy — his father was cited as "illegitimate." Enough said.

The oldest girl, Henrietta, fourteen or so (a dangerous age, menarche approaching) had scored an I.Q. 51, which was "Low Moron" level, barely Auxiliary Class level. Her mental age had been pegged at six years.

The older boys were little better, both "Imbeciles" with I.Qs. at 46, and obviously in need of discipline. Robbie was the more serious problem: in the short time at the play box in the corner he had broken every toy and twisted the head off the doll in a shocking way. The younger boy, Oswald, had something wrong with his legs (rickets?) They were now seen punching each other through the open door and being told to "behave" by the nurse, whereupon Mr. Hewitt gave them a clout on the head.

Dr. Eric Clarke, psychiatrist with the Department of Health, and son of the late great Dr. Clarke, had warned of defectives such as these in the Toronto schools in his 1920 Survey: one classroom alone had harboured five imbeciles suitable for institutionalization. Of course, there might be some hope for the younger Hewitts who could possibly benefit from the Dull and Backward Promotional Classes, thanks to Dr. Eric Clarke who had pushed for such classes, along with vocational work.

Dr. Meade turned to the girl, Ella, a dull-looking, expressionless five-year-old child not unlike the "imbecile" in the CNCMH poster, with an obvious squint in her eyes (strabismus). She had uttered barely a word, but perhaps she knew none, as she had undressed behind the screen.

The nurse filled out the particulars on Form 104, headed "Physical Examination":

> Hewitt, Ella: Age given as 5.9 years, height 41 1/2 inches, weight 39 lbs, all standard. Though her vision was stated as normal, the epicanthus of both eyes was enlarged. Tongue, nose, ears, normal. Skin: dirty. Vermin.

On the Psychological Test, Form M, Stanford-Binet Scale, the psychometrist had noted Ella's vocabulary was limited to "dog" and "chair"; she had not recognized "apple" or "hamburger" or any other food items on the picture vocabulary test. As to distinguishing between abstract words, this was a task quite beyond her. On the Mutilated Pictures test she had inexplicably said: "There's rats there."

> Conclusion: high grade Imbecile
> C.A. (Chronological Age): 5.9 years
> M.A. (Mental Age): 2.9.

"'Ow the 'ell can they say she be an imbecile before she even bin ter school to learn 'er letters?" expostulated Mr. Hewitt.

Here Florrie looked anxious, bewildered. She had a vague memory of St. Mary's Catholic School where Robbie and Edgar had attended, the wonderful school with its great stone entrance and shining windows, a wide yard bathed in sunlight, *school* with all its mysterious important knowledge denied her in the workhouse but that her boys would get to experience. She had stood awed and frightened, gripping Robbie in one hand and young Ella in the other with two little ones slung in her Irish shawl. She had heard Miss Dorkins tell the Sister he was already ten years old, late to be starting school. Inside, she had waited in shame, in the office. There was a picture of His Excellency, Pope Pius XI, on the Sister's wall; she had recognized the Holy Father's little white cap and his heavy jewelled cross hanging around his neck from going once to St. Paul's Church on Power Street with Miss Dorkins. Miss Dorkins had handed over the paper called the Registration Form that Florrie had marked with an ugly "X" for what was called the Parent's Signature, which was what she was. Sister St. Clemencia had whispered to Miss Dorkins about head lice, while Robbie and Ella scratched themselves. At age five Ella had not yet attended school, she was barely at toddler level in development, Miss Dorkins had hinted, limited to making mud pies in the yard. And her brother Edgar, who was to follow on after Robbie, along with other numerous Hewitts, was not much better.

"Yes, well, she may improve, Mr. Hewitt."

Dr. Meade was cautious. According to Miss Dorkins' report it seemed Mr. Hewitt had once tried to jump off the roof of a house in a suicide attempt after swallowing — Good God — Lysol. As well, the home environment spoke for itself. The Public Health Nurse had gone to the house last winter to find the family huddled round the stove, the last chair chopped up for firewood. Miss Dorkins had reported, via the Division of Family Welfare Social History, that "numerous agencies have assisted the family, and Mr. Hewitt is on a Department of Soldiers' Civil Re-establishment pension (DSCR) of $14 per month, on which they can barely live. Other agencies involved included the House of Industry, Catholic Welfare Bureau. Neighbourhood House workers which have assisted them for years but squalor and destitution continue."

"Hmph!"

Mrs. Hewitt, being illiterate, was the obvious cause of her children's deficiencies. Florrie had dropped her shift and lay naked, her breasts long and thin, her body undernourished and dark with bruises, as she submitted to the doctor's hands. "The doc'r paintid me insides wiv id'ine affer they fell down," she said, unintelligible, of course. Later, the newly hired stenographer, Miss Griffiths, typed up: "Physical and mental health poor. Reported to be psychologically very nervous, jumpy, and cries out in her sleep according to her husband Henry Hewitt."

Dr. Meade further noted Florrie to be quite deaf, and "easily discouraged, confused and quite childish." Yet she had struggled to do her best on the I.Q. test, the psychometrist had noted, making a gallant effort but to no avail. The woman was illiterate. (How had these people got into Canada?) Nurse Tidwell surmised that over fourteen years of marriage, Mrs. Hewitt must have menstruated but several months. But was not Florrie's life caught, that day, for all time in her list of offspring: Henrietta, b.1915; Robbie, b.1917; Edgar, b.1918; Wilfred, b.1919; Oswald, b.1921, Ella, b.1924; Georgie, b. 1927; and Sophie, b.1928, a sickly baby. She had also had a "miscarriage and stillbirth," and who knew how many more offspring were to follow.

Yet as Florrie stood, thin and worn, dressed again (she had no underwear, the nurse noted), the smallest ones ran and clung to her legs looking up at her familiar face: "Mama!" She was still their mother. Miss Dorkins snapped her briefcase containing copies of the Hewitts' Mental Health Forms for future reference, layers of information explaining exactly what was wrong with the Hewitt family.

Aetiology: *familial.*

Except, of course, for little Georgie, the darling of the family. Dr. Meade had noticed at once his bright intelligence. "The most beautiful of the Hewitt children," Miss Dorkins sighed. Sweet little Georgie, barely twenty months. Dr. Meade judged a normal sized cranium (20 inches), perfectly set ears, big blue eyes, flossy curls, rosy cheeks, and a bright, eager, *intelligent* expression. He walked, he talked, he knew his name, he pointed to things and knew what they were. He had started walking at one year, advanced for his age, Dr. Meade noted, glancing at Mrs. Hewitt who seemed unaware of the baby's forwardness. How could she? She was an imbecile.

Dr. Meade glanced at Miss Dorkins. A subtle message interchanged. Dr. Meade now understood the real reason for this visit. The next step was obvious.

They could not possibly be allowed to keep him. The thought of this lovely little child growing up in the sort of rooms the parents inhabited not far from a brothel known to the Morality Squad, and at least six siblings sleeping at night rolled up together on sacking on the floor, was unconscionable.

Miss Dorkins had an ideal family in mind, an Italian couple looking for a little boy to adopt in a family of girls. They were a good Catholic family, with their own home. She paused. Best Georgie be given up before he got too attached to the Hewitts, to his mother in particular, whom he would eventually realize, to his horror, was mentally deficient.

"But is my babby!" Florrie had sobbed, bewildered. Tears were to be expected. "But you'd want the best for him, Mr. and Mrs. Hewitt. You do have seven mouths to feed." And no bread. Best to be practical. The other young children stood listening, mouths lolling with that dull expression on their faces, a certain stupidity of feature, frowned Miss Dorkins. It was inconceivable to destine Georgie to siblings such as these. The Catholic Children's Aid Society of St. Vincent de Paul would make all the necessary arrangements. Georgie would have a new family and a new name; the Hewitts would never see him again. They would sign an agreement to that, marked "Confidential." Florrie could put an "X."

And so little Georgie became "Giorgio Minelli," and was taken to Hamilton where he would soon forget his family. He would grow up speaking Italian, be a good Catholic boy and son to his parents, the affectionate Mario and Amelia Minelli. He would have his first communion, no doubt, dressed in a white silk shirt and linen knickerbockers.

But Henry was inconsolable. "He was the best 'o' the bunch," he sobbed.

29.

MISS DORKINS HAD BEEN READING *Married Love,* by Marie Stopes, a scandalous book banned by the Catholic church and published in England in 1918, eleven years earlier. The Canadian National Committee for Mental Hygiene, the (CNCMH), directed by Dr. Eric Clarke and Dr. Clarence Hinks, had it cited on their list of "Objectionable Books."

Indeed, there were shocking details on how a husband was to arouse his wife's "passion," for instance, which Miss Stopes referred to as "flower-wreathed love-making" and "transports of joy." Miss Dorkins, who still lived with her elderly mother in plain but respectable lodgings off Bond Street near the cathedral, flushed. Miss Stopes alluded to the sensuality of a woman's breasts, the need to be touched there "once at the crest of the wave of her sex-tide." Miss Dorkins was not exactly sure what this meant, but sensed the passionate intent. There was more about the "mists of tenderness" and "soft touch of his lips," which prompted a feeling of unexpected sorrow at her own innocence.

She felt shock when Marie Stopes switched to the cold facts of contraception: pessary caps, available, apparently, in three sizes, No. 1 and No. 2 being in general use by most women — middle-class women, that is. There followed advice on lubricants and spermicides and actual diagrams of those intimate female parts that Miss Dorkins had not even been aware she had — something called the "os" of the cervix and how to fit a cervical cap over it. There was automatic suction, assured Miss Stopes. No wonder the book was on the Pope's banned list in the Vatican. Marie Stopes had even written incendiary letters urging the use of birth control to Pope Pius XI himself.

Miss Dorkins, who was still a virgin, had been raised on Dr. Mary

Wood-Allen's *What A Young Girl Ought To Know*, published somewhere around 1887. Dr. Wood-Allen had urged girls like Miss Dorkins to think only "beautiful thoughts" and explained that "evil" ones, that is "sexual" thoughts, poisoned the blood.

It was all so disturbing. Miss Stopes — "Dr." Stopes — had dared to open a birth control clinic in 1921 in London, specifically for poor working-class women to offset the fertility differential between the classes. Stopes had also read Galton and understood the threat of overpopulation of the poor and ignorant, and was thus in favour of workers limiting their families, no easy task. She also was a proponent of compulsory sterilization of the insane, the feeble-minded, half-castes and the revolutionaries, excepting herself of course. However, in relation to birth control for the poor, the delicate issue of female hygiene had arisen since the "cap" in question had to be pushed deep into the vagina. One but thought of the unsanitary hands of most working-class women (Florrie Hewitt's fingernails), with no easy access to soap and water, pushing these things inside themselves.

The only birth control technique approved by the Holy Father was the "rhythm method" or celibacy, something that J. S. Woodsworth, a socialist out west in Manitoba, had called "the most abominable doctrine ever taught." Miss Dorkins had heard whispers in young womanhood that a woman's "safe" days occurred in the middle of the menstrual cycle, when ovulation was not supposed to take place. Now it seemed a Dr. Kyusaka Ogino, a gynecologist and obstetrician in Japan, and his colleague, Dr. Herman Knaus, had discovered that it was quite the reverse, claiming ovulation actually did take place in the middle of the cycle.

Dr. Withrow, former colleague of Dr. Clarke at the Social Service Clinic, obviously influenced by this Stopes woman, was now setting up a birth control clinic for the poor right here in Toronto, at 12 Dundonald Street; this, despite the opposition of the Catholic clergy. As head of the Ontario Birth Control League (and also secretary for sex education of the National Council of the YMCA) he was rumoured to have distributed 750,000 flyers, of which many were distributed at Convocation Hall in the University of Toronto: "Birth Control Means Better Babies — Do You Believe That A Sick, Worn Out Mother Cannot Have A Healthy Baby?"

The socialists took up the cause. Birth control information was deliberately denied the poor, they claimed, because under capitalism, the wealthy classes needed a large supply of cheap labour from the working class to run their factories, be their domestics, and fight their wars for them. Another socialist, a woman, Mrs. C. Lorimer, had argued vociferously that doctors and clergymen were only anxious about birth control when the workers wanted it, fearing that workers limiting their families could lead to the emancipation of labour. She actually told Dr. J. J. Heagerty of the Department of Health, to "shut his mouth."

Things came to a crux when Dr. Withrow of Toronto was charged in early 1927 with procuring abortions disguised as "dilatation and curettage" operations. It was disclosed during the trial that he had been banned from the Swiss Cottage Hospital in downtown Toronto due to a number of these suspicious "D and C" operations.

Miss Dorkins felt confused and agitated at heart that Ruth Dembner, a nice, upper-class girl out in High Park, had paid Dr. Withrow $75 for an abortion. Of course, the judge in the case had been careful to distinguish between the licentious slum girls brought before the courts, and the lovely, well-bred Ruth. But Ruth, it seemed, had loved fast cars, late-night parties, and alcohol, her father admitted during the trial: "She went her own way; [she was] headstrong." She had died of peritonitis after getting off the train and collapsing in the snow, haemorrhaging to death.

Dr. Withrow was sentenced to seven years at Kingston Penitentiary, a very shocking thing for someone of his social standing, and for his wife and daughters (one of whom had planned a career in medicine herself, which was now out of the question). Dr. Hincks, Director of the CNCMH, who had once worked with Dr. Withrow in Dr. Charles Clarke's Clinic, was loyally petitioning for his release.

Miss Dorkins moved on to Dr. Stopes' *Mother England*, just published in 1929, which contained many letters written to Dr. Stopes from working-class women over the years, pleas of poverty and sexual ignorance that seemed only too familiar ... one but thought of poor Florrie Hewitt on her back on the floor-boards.

> *I just got to the Door and Callopsed, the Child beining bone almost at once. 13 months after I had a nother girl bone a hour before I could sent for help. 2 year later a boy, and 2 year later a nother boy, this last boy have shutter my nerves....*

> *My husband is so selfish he doesn't care so long as he gets what he wants. What you suffer makes no difference to him in Fack he is a Rotter.*

The letter had lain on the hall table, post-marked 1927, now hidden away in her locked bureau. Dr. Helen MacMurchy had recognized the slant of the handwriting at once, *her* handwriting, after so many years.

She recalled picking up the envelope. Dr. MacMurchy had been appointed Head of the Child Welfare Department in the federal government in Ottawa in 1920, after resigning her post as Inspector for the Feeble-Minded, but came home regularly to the house she now shared with her sister Bessie on South Drive. Old Dr. MacMurchy had died in a tragic accident, run down by a streetcar outside their old home on Bloor Street, years ago. The new Rosedale house was modern and had all the conveniences including an indoor privy and electric lighting. It stood around the corner from Dr. Clarke's family home on Roxborough Drive, and near other social dignitaries of Toronto. Dr. MacMurchy had slit open the letter, in the dim light of her bedroom, trembling.

"Dear Minky," began Marie Stopes, in the old, familiar, outrageous way Helen MacMurchy had once so loved and envied — but that had been in 1909. Marie's nickname for her had struck her at once as startling, shameful even. It had been eighteen years since the last exchange of letters.

Dr. MacMurchy had felt a stab of pain, intense and real at the recognition. Words and phrases had come flooding back: "...the moment that I knew I loved you! ... My darling..."

In the confusion of the moment, Dr. MacMurchy had not yet been able to note that what Marie Stopes wanted was statistical data on birth control in Ontario — information that Dr. MacMurchy, of course, had had no intention of providing this notorious woman. Marie Stopes was now infamous, not just as the author of *Married Love* (scandalous!) but as the British advocate of birth control for the poor and destitute — working-class women. Marie Stopes had once chained a copy of her book on Roman Catholic birth control methods to the door of Westminster Cathedral and had had the gall, in 1920, to send a letter to Queen Mary requesting help to finance her birth control clinics! Ignored by Her Majesty, of course. But most outrageous of all, Stopes had sent out questionnaires to doctors concerning their sexual and contraceptive knowledge, usurping the prerogative of the medical profession — after all, Dr. Stopes was not a *medical* doctor. And there was the unfortunate tragic case nearer home of well-meaning but mislead Dr. Withrow, now still imprisoned in 1929 in the Kingston Penitentiary, influenced no doubt by her to set up birth control clinics. Worse, Marie Stopes had made no effort to conceal intimate details of her annulled marriage to Reginald Gates back in 1914, concerning his inability to penetrate her sexual parts; indeed, there had been certain references to his impotent penis in the notorious public court case, unbehoving any decent Christian woman. If only Marie had stuck to her thesis, the reproductive system of cycads — well, what a brilliant young woman she had been, dear genius!

Helen MacMurchy had been, at sixty-five, at the pinnacle of her career. Her white hair was coiled in a somewhat stylish bun, and her sturdy figure, thickened with the years, held her in good stead. She had a clear vision of herself and her status.

She had sat down, trembling, that day, the gravity of the situation dawning on her. She herself had carefully destroyed all of Marie Stopes's love letters over the years. But she could not be certain that the vain, volatile Marie had done the same: "You see you have 'got me', my dear ... take you in my arms ... kiss. I will love you my dearest for ever and ever." Oh! The things one wrote in the heat of passion, *insane!*

Dr. Helen MacMurchy had sat at her bureau, and with deliberation took up her pen. She had known what was required and had no regrets: a complete break in communication with that woman.

30.

THE HEWITTS HAD SHUFFLED into the examining room of the Outpatients Department for their latest check-up in November of 1932. All had that look of the undernourished. Dr. Meade noted in his report that Mrs. Hewitt, a thin, shrivelled woman now in her thirties, with fading hair drawn back in a haphazard knot, the pins falling out, was advanced in yet another pregnancy. Or, as her husband put it, "She got one insides 'er agin." Not only that. Seventeen-year-old Henrietta, the oldest daughter, was also very pregnant; he judged her to be in her seventh month.

Mother and daughter, pregnant at the same time. Miss Dorkins, social worker for this family and familiar to Dr. Meade, nodded, looking sombre. Dr. Meade did a swift computation in his head. This girl, starting at age seventeen, could possibly produce another fifteen or twenty children before menopause, like her mother, which made at least thirty-five even forty children between them, all likely mentally defective. Dr. Meade's mouth pursed.

"I told 'er to keep 'orf of them boys," Mr. Hewitt had protested to Miss Dorkins.

"But they likes it," said Henrietta.

The father of the child was purported to be a delivery boy, Ronnie Phelps, though Henrietta was not quite certain (she had been flustered at the question). The girl had not even reported her missed monthly flow to her mother as she had not understood what it meant. And Florrie Hewitt had not noticed the drop in the number of rags they shared each month. Well, of course, Florrie could not count; Miss Dorkins hesitated.

"'Twarn't 'er fault, sir!" Mr. Hewitt insisted. "'E bin got at 'er when nobody lookin', an' caught 'er bendin'. She's a good girl, can read 'er letters an' write, an' bake a tart, and boil taters."

Florrie Hewitt, unbelievably, looked proudly at her daughter, at this. Henrietta, her first-born, could read. She could write. She had access to the mysterious power of language all around her denied to Florrie. Henrietta attended the wonderful Jarvis Vocational School up on Jarvis Street, established, unknown to Florrie, for children developing delinquency. Henrietta went with all the other smart boys and girls from all sorts of streets that Florrie only suspected lay beyond the confines of seedy Sumach Street. Of course, Henrietta's school days were now over.

The girl smiled vaguely, and twirled her long fair curls in her finger. She was wearing a tent-like dress over her swelling belly, about which she seemed to feel no shame.

Her mother had been equally vague during the physical examination. "Undress and lie down on the table please, legs apart, Mrs. Hewitt." When asked by the nurse when her last courses had been — they wanted to assess the due date — Florrie had looked around, bewildered, and murmured something about flowers.

"Flowers?" Nurse Henley had echoed. Did she mean *spring*? Nurse Henley tried to keep patient as taught in Toronto Nursing School, but it was hard dealing with these women all day.

Dr. Meade tried to grasp the implications of the Hewitts and their multiple offspring, all presenting that certain facial look that he now knew marked the feeble-minded, all backward in school in terms of development and speech. There were the two older boys, followed by Wilfred, Oswald, Ella (Georgie had been adopted and none too soon), the baby Sophie who had apparently died of chorea (or was it "summer diarrhea" since the last session with this family was in 1929?), but soon replaced by Cedric, now aged about two, and an infant-at-arms called Violet born in 1931 — the fecundity of these feeble-minded women! Oswald, whose stunted legs seemed to have straightened out over the past two years, talked in the same garbled way, unintelligible except to his mother. Clearly, another candidate for Orillia. (*All* the Hewitts belonged in Orillia.)

"Maternal grandmother committed to Rainhill, an asylum in Liverpool, England," read Dr. Meade in the Hewitts' Family History Form provided by the Welfare Agency. Rainhill was an infamous pauper asylum, as far as he knew, to which Florrie Hewitt's mother, Rose Mallone, nee Murphy, had been committed as insane after being deserted by her husband. Well, that answered the question of aetiology: "*Familial*" — "hereditary."

He moved on to the girl Ella, now eight. Apparently, she was a potential arsonist; it appeared she regularly threw her clothes in the flames. She had heavy features and a squint. She would need watching so as not to go the way of her sister. Once again, she had done poorly on the tests (Revised Stanford-Binet), stringing only two beads in 50 seconds in the Stringing Beads test. In her Picture Response, there had been no reaction to "Grandmother's Story" nor to "Birthday Party," but she had recognized "Wash Day."

"Wan' sucky!" little Cedric, suddenly cried. Whereupon, there in the waiting area, in front of rows of patients waiting their turn, some insane, Mrs. Hewitt casually pulled out her other breast and shoved the nipple into the two-year-old's mouth. She now sat with one at each breast, the infant suckling lazily, and the older boy standing on his toes to get at it. "Hung'y," she smiled, a flash of a grin with two teeth missing, at startled Nurse Henley. These women!

Dr. Meade made some ticks on a chart. Essential to stay focused. Henrietta, of course, would be dealt with. Affable Henrietta, reclothed, emerging from her examination smiling, unaware. But of equal concern were the two older boys, Robbie and Edgar, now age fourteen and twelve respectively, slated for Orillia, and none too soon. According to Miss Dorkins, they were running wild and half-naked in the neighbourhood, getting into trouble stealing from vendors or wringing the necks of the neighbour's pigeons, which Florrie promptly threw in the stewing pot. "We needs meats," she had explained.

Robbie, the older boy, tall for his age, with a faint line of hair on his upper lip, was the more attractive of the two with a thin but ruddy face, and thick brown curly hair. Both boys had attended St. Mary's Catholic School, Robbie for two years, and Edgar for a few months, both having been "excluded" as incapable of learning. Robbie had spent his time in his seat in Jr. 1 poking other boys. Neither had attended auxiliary classes, nor had the little girl, Ella.

Mr. Hewitt was of the opinion that "Cath'lic School's better with the Sisters an' th' Soldar'ty of the Blessit Virgin." As well, he countered, "I 'eard auxil'ary class you ends up in Orillia." But Robbie and Edgar had tested at the Imbecile range, with I.Qs. of 45.

Dr. Meade proceeded. The two boys could dress and feed themselves — Miss Dorkins had ticked "Yes" under sub-section: "Habits" on the Family History Form. They did not use tobacco, nor were they cruel to children or animals. They did not masturbate, although the neighbours had complained otherwise.

Being Imbeciles, Dr. Meade now explained to the Hewitts, the boys had not been eligible for regular school. "There is a difference, Mr. Hewitt, between chronological age and the boys' 'real' age inside their heads. Mentally, they are children." They were, in fact, years below their chronological age and properly belonged in Orillia, he urged to a crestfallen Henry.

"They will be well looked after in Orillia," assured Miss Dorkins. The Ontario Hospital, often still alluded to as the Hospital for the Feeble-Minded and before that the Orillia Asylum for Idiots and Feeble-Minded, was a fine place that would provide academics at the boys' intellectual level in the school, and vocational training, possibly carpentry, tailoring, or farm work. Here Miss Dorkins became vague.

Henry nodded, considering the Depression. Over 100,000 unemployed as a result of the crash, mostly in the city, reported the newspaper headlines. Desperate men, protesting on University Avenue, waved placards: "WE NEED BREAD." Everyone seemed to fear a repeat of the Winnipeg General Strike of 1919 out west. He saw for himself daily the hundreds of canvas beds that had been set up in Queen's Park and the St. Lawrence Market for homeless men — many sleeping on old newspapers. He himself had been laid off from Anderson's Paper Company himself, and had to make do on the dole and the food coupons that the Ministry in charge of relief handed out. He hesitated. At Orillia, the boys would have three meals a day, room and board — they were getting big and needed more food — and discipline. They would be locked in firmly in Orillia, assured Miss Dorkins (perhaps forever). The meeting concluded on a practical note; the amount to be paid per week by Mr. Hewitt was nothing.

Miss Dorkins would mail the necessary documents for their committal to Miss E. de V. Clarke at the Department of Health for approval, whence the Applications accompanied by the two Certificates of Incompetence signed by doctors at the hospital would then be forwarded to Orillia.

As to Henrietta, arrangements were underway for her confinement at The Haven, a refuge for fallen girls run by the Salvation Army Mission. Those curls would have to come off, of course. And, afterwards, she would have to be institutionalized. Thanks to the reform of the old *Houses of Refuge Act* in 1919, she could be detained indefinitely and transferred at the will of a physician to Orillia or a similar such place, and perhaps even sterilized, thought Dr. Meade. There was talk of a Bill urging the sterilization of women who had had an illegitimate child to enable their release from the women's institution at Cobourg, where many such immoral morons were confined at the cost of the taxpayers.

When would Ontario follow the example of the other provinces, and of America, and initiate a sterilization act? Dr. Charles Hastings, Toronto's admirable Medical Officer of Health, had done his best, organizing a meeting of the Eugenics Education Society in Toronto in July of 1924, after being in touch by letter with the Eugenics Society in England. That same year, Dr. Meade recalled, a host of concerned groups across the nation, including the Social Service Council of Canada and the Church of England Social Service Department, had banded together in support of eugenic policies (one had to be realistic, witness these Hewitts). Finally, there had been the first meeting of the Eugenic Society of Canada (ESC) on November 6, 1930, under the leadership of Dr. William Hutton, Medical Officer of Health for Brantford. Members included Dr. Hincks; Dr. Herbert Bruce (the Lieutenant-Governor); Dr. Clarence Farrar, (Head of the Toronto Psychiatric Hospital and protégé of the great Dr. Clarke); and, Professor Madge Macklin, leading geneticist at Western, who felt that only the fittest germplasm should be allowed in reproduction. But so far, no legislation had been passed in Ontario.

At least British Columbia had approved an *Act Respecting Sexual Sterilization* in 1933, following Alberta's example in 1928, thanks, in part, to the excellent surveys conducted by Dr. Hincks and Dr. Clarke in both provinces a decade earlier on the incidence of feeble-mindedness.

The Act in British Columbia was being ardently supported by the Imperial Order Daughters of the Empire, the National Women's Council, the Women's Christian Temperance Union, with their little white bows of purity, and the United Farm Women.

"But what 'ave I done bad, Miss Dork'ns? I just 'ad a babby." Henrietta began to sob, clutching the baby. "He mine! "

"Now, now," said Matron Gilmour sharply. "You should have thought of that before you gorn with young lads having your fun."

Henrietta was being difficult. There were rules. A girl like her giving birth out of wedlock was allowed to live at The Haven for six months following the birth of her baby, in order to breastfeed it and provide it with immunities. The Haven, run by the Salvation Army since 1891, had experience over the decades in aiding the feeble-minded and had been willing to admit Henrietta (the Catholic St. Mary House being full). Otherwise, Henrietta would undoubtedly have ended up having it on the kitchen floor like her mother.

The baby was to be handed over to the Catholic Children's Aid Society of Toronto and be made a ward of court, something Henrietta had been told from the outset, reminded Miss Dorkins. "You must be sensible, girl."

But Henrietta cuddled baby Cuthbert closer, and put her little finger between his darling lips, which were pursed like a rosebud. He cooed and pulled at his mother's breast with chubby little fingers, then blew little bubbles of contentment. "Oh, ain't 'e lovely, Miss Dork'ns!"

Miss Dorkins sighed. The baby was obviously feeble-minded. At six months his level of development was more like two months; he had poor muscle tone, he was slow at turning his head, and he was slow at sitting up (all of which, of course, negated any chance for adoption). But Henrietta did not care. She did not want to give up Cuthbert, or breastfeeding. She liked him at her titties, she fretted over him, and cuddled him close.

Henrietta had a good record at The Haven for doing laundry and domestic work, as well as participating in daily Bible classes and prayers, all part of The Haven's reformatory process. The very act of scrubbing and mangling hundreds of sheets was conducive to cleansing the soul, to overcoming evil tendencies and sexual passion, explained the Matron to the Hewitts, as well as productive to the Home. This meant that Henrietta was a good candidate for Cobourg, explained Miss Dorkins.

Henrietta had had her hair cut short according to regulations. "What the 'ell 'ave they done to 'er curls?" cried Henry, as they was ushered into the visitors' parlour. "It were 'er one beauty." He turned to the Matron accusingly.

Matron Gilmour refrained from saying beauty was not needed where Henrietta was going. "Out of the way, for domestic work, Mr. Hewitt," she said briskly. She knew how to handle people like the Hewitts, in their threadbare clothing and cracked shoes. On the other hand, parents seldom turned up to support their daughters. These ones were exceptions, though lost to Christ.

Henrietta was being transferred to the Ontario Hospital School in Cobourg, while she was still seventeen, and still under the wardship of the CCAS of Toronto. This was her chance to be saved, and, it was where Miss Dorkins knew she could be detained indefinitely. The CCAS of Toronto had "powers of Child Protection," as Miss Dorkins well knew, sometimes extended to age twenty-one where circumstances saw fit. The Medical Officer of Health had already gone to the Hewitts' rooming house to verify the need for placing the girl under government supervision. Henrietta would be placed where they deemed fit.

Cobourg, a small institution compared with Orillia, had originally been the Victoria College for Ladies, part of the University of Toronto, in the late nineteenth century; then, it was a provincial asylum in 1921 with 530 women patients; and, finally, briefly, a military hospital. It still confined feeble-minded females and specialized in training girls like Henrietta for domestic service, explained the Matron. There was no room at present in Orillia. Dr. Horne, Superintendent, had informed Miss Dorkins that they had more than enough females on the wards, some with two or three children.

"But she was a good student in Domestic Science, cooking taters," objected Mr. Hewitt. "She was at Jarvis Vocash'nal."

Henrietta was a pleasing girl, agreed the Matron. She could eventually be put out to work in one of the big houses in town.

At this, Florrie Hewitt let out a hoarse cry — the only time Miss Dorkins had seen Florrie Hewitt express an opinion. "Na. Na, na servant girl, Miss Dork'ns!" Florrie rocked back and forth on the chair, shaking her head violently and slapping herself. "Na-a!"

Ignored, of course. Mrs. Hewitt, an imbecile, obviously did not comprehend the situation, frowned Matron. She was to calm down.

"But little Cuthie is our gran'son," cried Mr. Hewitt. "Where is 'e?" Mr. Hewitt looked about as if the baby were hidden in the cupboard.

Henrietta started to sob, "Cuthie ... Cuthie."

What did one do with such logic? Such people?

And so Henrietta was sent to Cobourg, a three-storey institution, about thirty miles from Toronto, which held over 300 so-called feeble-minded women of dubious morals. The white building with its Greek columns, porticoes, and cupola, stood back from the centre of town on a slight incline. Below was the superintendent's house on a tree-lined avenue. A quiet Ontario lakeside town, Cobourg sported a curving beach, a pretty lighthouse, and sleepy houses with verandahs and roses round the doors, pink in the summer sun. Henrietta would be locked in with the hundreds of women, many of them of normal intelligence, who had transgressed the law or had had illegitimate children. She was to live on a ward crammed with beds, rise at five-thirty in the morning to scrub, scour, wash sheets, learn to cook, and be a domestic for her mistress, a Mrs. Dunn on College Street.

The institution, assured the Matron, had an excellent system of probation, and the girls were let out into service to the women in town at good cheap rates. Henrietta would be allowed to keep half her wages.

31.

June 13,1932.
School, Orillia

Attention: Miss E. de V. Clarke
Department of Health.

Re: Robbie and Edgar Hewitt
Enclosed you will find two sets of Physicians' Certificates which I would be glad if you would have completed in the cases of the above boys. Upon receipt of these we will advise you as to when admission can be awarded. I regret that there is nothing we can do to assist you at this time concerning the girl Ella, as we have absolutely no accommodation for females at this time.
Yours truly,
S. J. W. Horne, M.D.
Medical Superintendent

Overleaf, the usual government stamp:

N.B. No person will be admitted to any Ontario Hospital without the approval of the Superintendent or the Deputy Provincial Secretary, and the person should not be forwarded to such Hospital until notice has been received from the Superintendent or Deputy Provincial Secretary that admission has been awarded.

A ROUTINE VISIT to the Outpatient's Department at the Toronto Psychiatric Hospital on June 20, 1932, was in order for the Hewitt boys, for their certificates. Miss E. de V. Clarke contacted Miss Dorkins of the CCAS of Toronto, at once concerning these Certificates of Incompetence, necessary documents for admission to Orillia. Dr. Smith and Dr. Hodge were two physicians on duty that day to provide statements, a matter of protocol.

Mr. Hewitt sat uncomfortably in the now familiar waiting area with the two boys. Robbie sat on the chair next to his brother, Edgar, swinging his legs. Mr. Hewitt, the father, an obviously low-grade labourer in dungarees quite worn through with a certain unpleasant odour (it reminded Dr. Smith of birds) sat tensed, perplexed, unable to grasp the proceedings. They were soon called into an office where the doctors interviewed the boys.

"No physical stigmata," said Dr. Smith.

Dr. Smith and Dr. Hodge corroborated that Robbie Hewitt was, indeed, "insane" and an "idiot." As the certificate stated, "If the insane person is an idiot, add 'and that the said (Robbie Hewitt) is an idiot.'"

Dr. Smith, examining physician, wrote on Robbie's Certificate of Incompetence the facts indicating Robbie Hewitt's insanity: "Childish, restless, swinging about on his chair; talks with his hand to his mouth, indistinctly. Cannot read or write."

> I, the undersigned (a) Harold Smith, M.D., a legal qualified medical practitioner, residing and practicing at (b) Toronto in the County of York hereby certify that I, on 29 day of June A.D. 1932, at Toronto separately from any other medical practitioner, personally examined (c) Robbie Hewitt of (d) Toronto (e) schoolboy and after making due enquiry into all facts in connection with the case of the said Robbie Hewitt necessary to be enquired into in order to enable me to form a satisfactory opinion, I certify that the said Robbie Hewitt is insane, and a proper person to be confined in the hospital for the insane.

Other corroborating facts, noted Dr. Smith on the Certificate: "At school this boy was almost considered uneducable.... Played childish games." The certificate was duly signed by Dr. Smith, and Mr. Hewitt, and witnessed by Miss Dorkins and a Miss Mildred Blossom, followed by the same for Edgar. The documents were to be forwarded that summer's day to the Ontario Hospital Orillia (formerly the Hospital for the Feeble-Minded but still often referred to as such) via Miss E. de V. Clarke, daughter of the eminent, late, Dr. Clarke.

Later, Henry walked the boys along Carlton Street to Parliament and down the various streets to the house on Sumach, unaware of the full significance of the forms on their way to the Department of Health. Yet, he felt a vague sense of alarm and confusion at losing them for he loved the boys, especially Robbie, his first-born son.

That summer morning the city trees were in full foliage and mauve shadows fell over the worn pavement. But something was wrong. Shop fronts were boarded up. They passed a shabby pawnshop and grimy pubs. A horse clip-clopped slowly drawing a van, the driver wearily holding his whip. There had been more demonstrations in the streets, and police officers on horseback charged at the crowds. Men shouted and waved placards that read "WORK NOT BREAD." He had heard the police officers call them, "Bolshies" and "Reds!"

"WHEN DO WE EAT?" said other big placards carried by protesters marching regularly now through the streets. "WE WANT TO BE CITIZENS NOT TRANSIENTS." There were more clashes with police, until you got beaten and thrown into the cells in City Hall, he had heard. He tried to keep the boys away from the protests, and, especially, away from the taverns.

They passed a mission where the soup lines were already forming down Parliament Street, which Henry himself and the boys joined daily. Turning the corner, he saw there was a bit of a commotion near Sackville Street. Another evicted family was out on the pavement, with their pathetically few belongings: a broken table, a few chairs, a shredded sofa, some pots and pans. "EVICTED" said a sign some neighbour had drawn so everyone would know. The woman held a suckling baby to her breast. The man stood dejected, holding on to the littlest ones. They had about nine children.

Henry knew what would happen. Slowly, the men on pogey themselves would appear as if one by one to help with the sticks of furniture, to do what they could. Some would come from the tavern on Queen Street. Then, miraculously, women of the neighbourhood would emerge from their houses. Slowly they would offer to take bits of furniture to mind for the family. Some of the women would take in the older children. The missus, a Mrs. Mathews would weep silently. All must help before the bailiff come, Henry said to the boys, when he would board up the doors and windows. And there was Florrie, his own missus, now coming up the street with a kettle of tea. "'S all I gots," she said, breathlessly.

A wave of sunlight passed over the scene. Henry anxiously recalled his time at the Clinic that morning, and the Statement he had signed about each of his sons: "*Is Insane and an Idiot. To the best of my knowledge the history as given by informant is correct. Henry Hewitt. June 20, 1932.*"

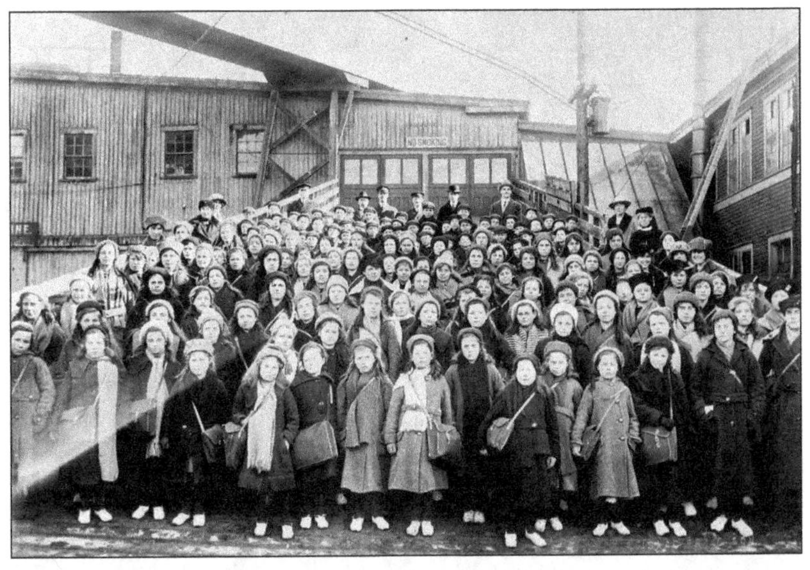

Home Children at landing stage, St John's, New Brunswick, early 1900s.
Courtesy of Library and Archives Canada.

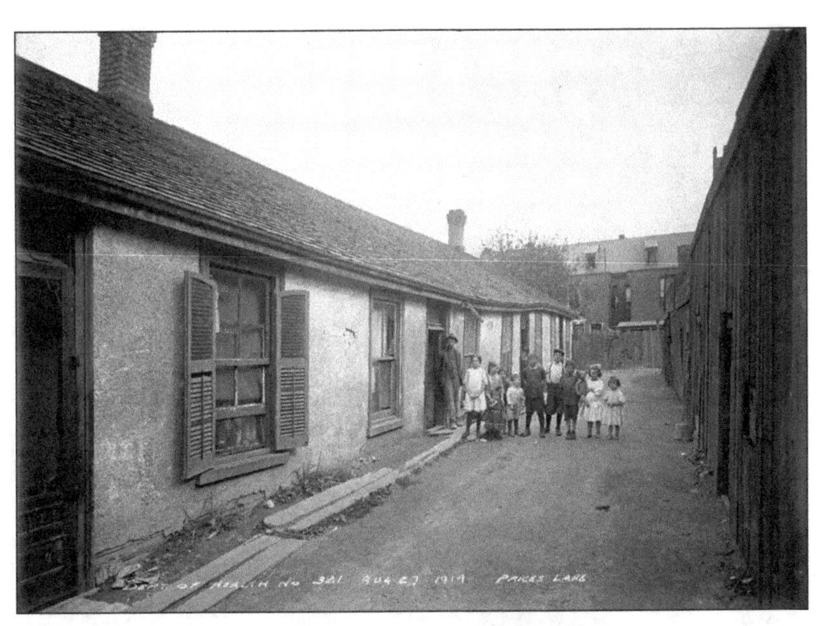

Prices Lane, slums of Toronto, August 27,1914.
Courtesy Toronto Archives.

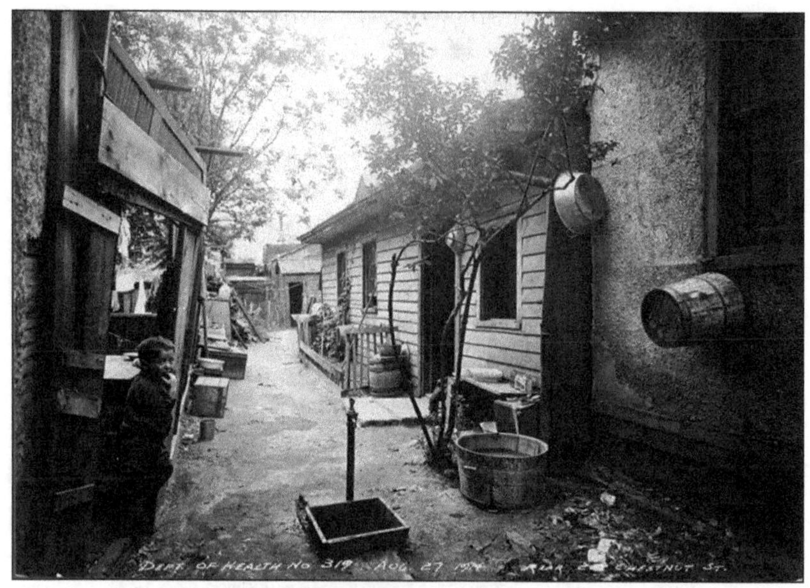

Rear of Chestnut St., "The Ward" slums of Toronto, August 27, 1914. Courtesy Toronto Archives.

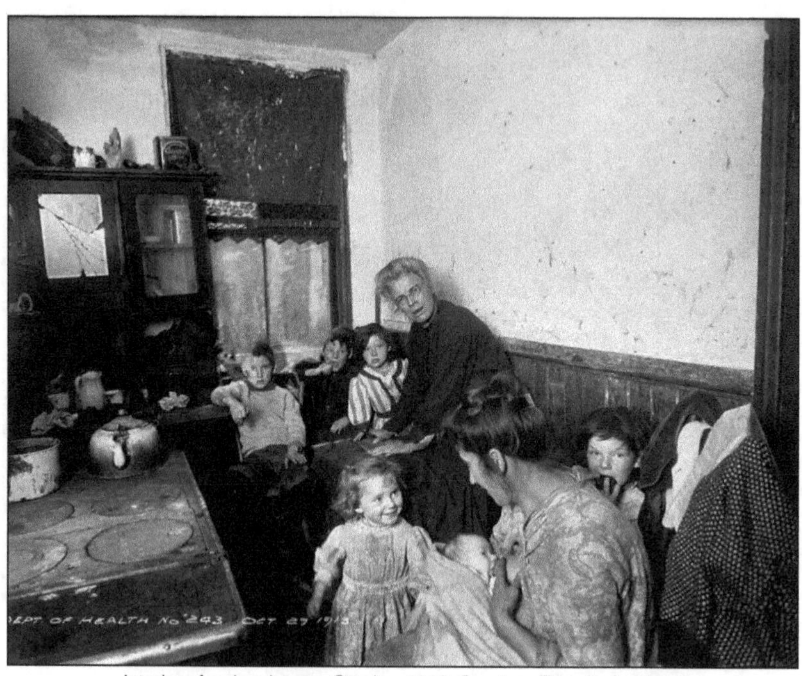

Interior of a slum house, October 1913. Courtesy Toronto Archives.

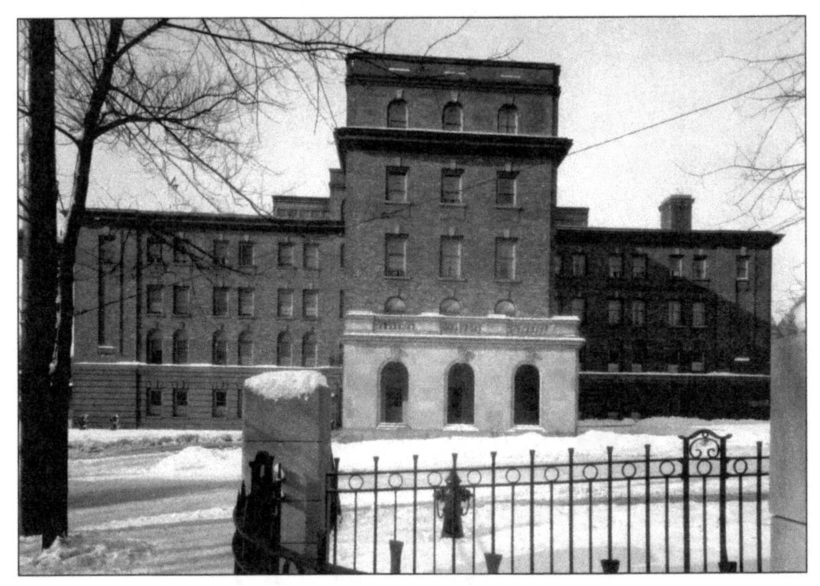

Toronto Psychiatric Hospital. Courtesy CAMH Archives

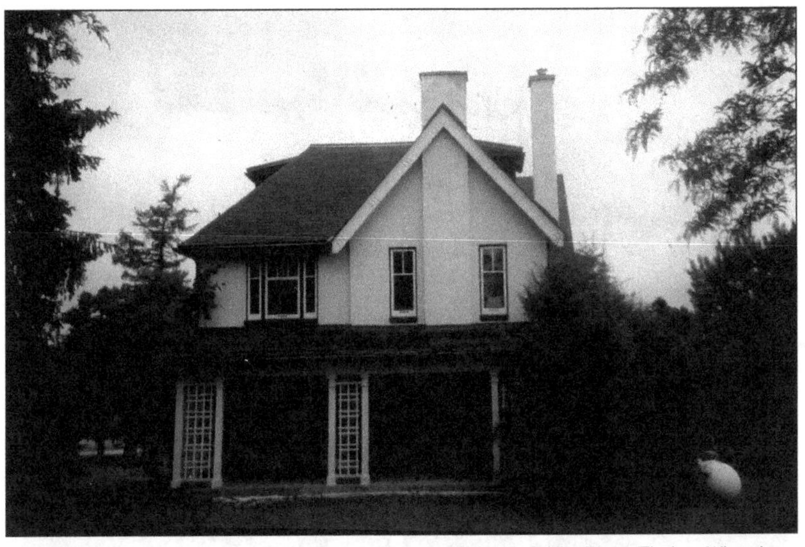

Superintendent's house, grounds, Ontario Hospital School, Orillia. Photo Thelma Wheatley.

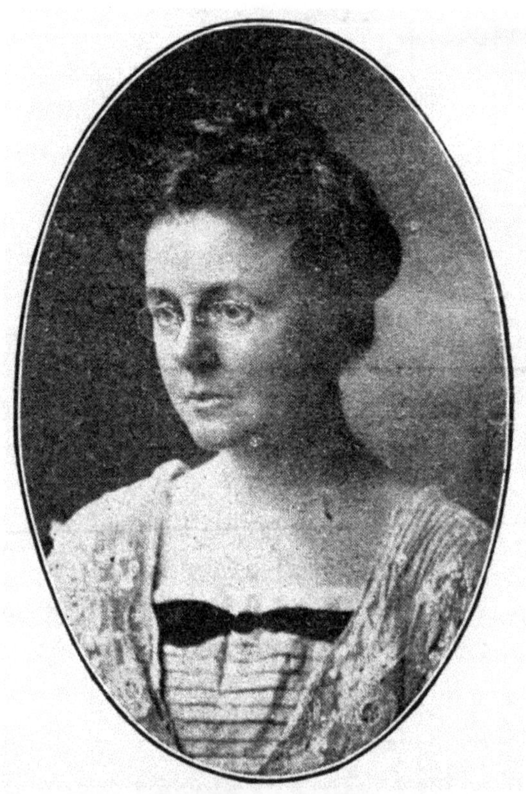

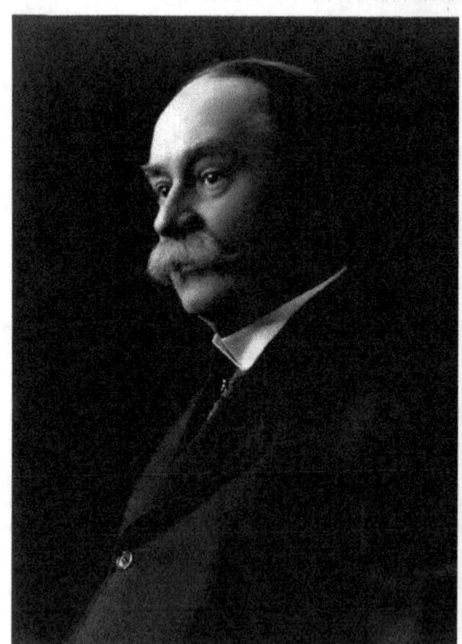

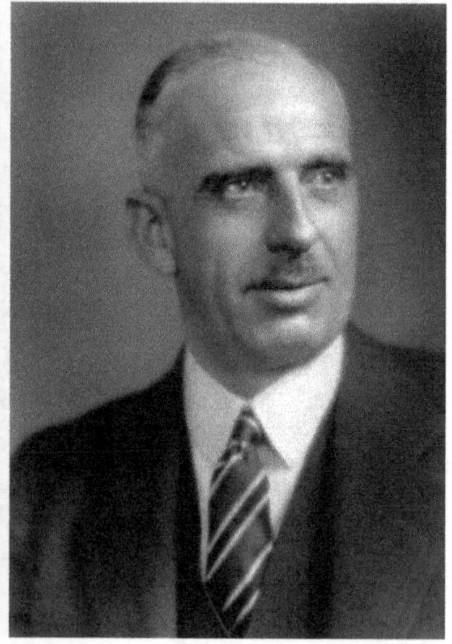

Top: Dr. Helen MacMurchy as a young woman. Courtesy of University of Toronto archives.
From left to right: Dr. Charles Clarke, Dr. Clarence Hincks. Courtesy CAMH archives.

PART THREE
Hospital for the Feeble-Minded

ORILLIA, 1932-1939

...I believe, too, that this Asylum will tend largely to decrease the number of idiots in this Province—for this reason, every female Idiot, if young, when sent here, will be placed beyond the chance of giving birth to her kind, and thereby a prolific source will be cut off, as it were, at the fountain head.

—Dr. Alexander Beaton, Superintendent of the Asylum for Idiots and Feeble-Minded, Orillia, Annual Report, February 25, 1889

We have here the flotsam and jetsam of the human sea....

—Mr. J. Downey, Superintendent of the Hospital for the Feeble-Minded, Orillia, 1919

32.

THE TRAIN HAD STOPPED at a wooden station within the Hospital grounds. "Orillia!" shouted the station-master. A man on the platform had raised a semaphore flag. Robbie and Edgar scrambled out dressed in their only suits of clothes: rough woollen knickerbockers, ill-fitting jackets, and peaked caps. They stood with strange Miss Nesbitt from the Department of Health. The boys had said goodbye to their parents at Union Station in Toronto. They were young men now, Dada had said. They were to learn their letters and be good and he had given each of them a quarter, and Robbie a penknife as he was the eldest. Now they huddled together. A path led up a steep slope to a huge building. Behind the boys was a hedge, and through gaps in the hedge, a glimpse of water.

"Ah, Lake Simcoe!" breathed Miss Nesbitt.

A young man wearing a black uniform, white shirt, and a knotted black tie as if he were going to church greeted them. "Mr. Hansbro, ma'am, attendant. Your charges from Toronto..." He had a list in hand: "Anderson, Forbes, two Hewitts..."

They walked up the slope. The grass was dazzling and Robbie felt dizzy. He held on to Edgar whose chest was wheezing. Figures of children and adults in the distance bent over gardens, hoes in hand, stood out in the distance. Silence. Soon they reached a pretty terrace filled with flowers at the top of the hill. The immense red-brick building was close now; it had rows and rows of windows, the lower ones meshed and grilled. "The Administration Building," someone said. There were steps leading up to the main entrance. It was much bigger than St. Mary's School, as big as the Don Jail with its high grim walls.

"Lovely lawns," trilled Miss Nesbitt to the attendant.

"Oh, aye," said Mr. Hansbro. "And an 'ealthy breeze from the lake.

Gateway to cottage country," he said in a pleased way.

All seemed silent in Orillia. Around the big Administration Building were other red-brick buildings called Cottages, said Miss Nesbitt. Robbie and Edgar would be placed in one, but which one? The Cottages looked like long oblongs in the hot sun. A group of old men, their mouths drooling and moving constantly, shuffled into view, their hands pulling at their trousers. Some of the children around Robbie and Edgar, who were also being admitted that day, began to cry. They were to go through the double glass doors at the top of the short flight of steps into the Administration Building, and wait in the hall for the receiving officer, while Miss Nesbitt saw to their papers.

Edgar slipped his hand inside Robbie's. "Wanna go 'ome," he whispered.

"No talking, there!" said a woman's voice with a sharp tone.

Robbie felt for his knife through his breeches' pocket. Miss Nesbitt had disappeared, perhaps for a cup of tea with the Matron and a bite to eat before catching the train back to Toronto. Their own train had gone. The Canadian National Railway (CNR) track that ran along the edge of the lake on the Orillia property had disappeared forever into the trees and bushes on its way up north or west. No point looking back.

"Git into line," said Mr. Hansbro. "An' keep tergether."

They were to go to something called the "Infirmary." They followed Mr. Hansbro through a heavy door that banged shut behind them, then down a steep flight of stone steps to another door. Mr. Hansbro got out a wad of keys and opened it up, and they found themselves in a low underground tunnel, the "tramway," he said. It was suddenly cool because of the cement floors. The Infirmary was a distance from the Administration Building, said a voice to Mr. Hansbro. They were to be taken to the Admission Ward, said another.

Edgar clutched Robbie's hand, and Robbie felt for his knife again. Who knew what was down here? There, on a door, a notice they could not read warned: "This door is to be kept locked at all times."

They had reached the Infirmary. They went up another flight of stairs to another door that was unlocked by Mr. Hansbro, and opened to a bright sunny central hall with large windows. Two wings stretched out, one on each side. "Females to G," said a nurse dressed in a white uniform with grey sleeves. "Males to B."

The boys' Ward was damp and hot. Mosquitoes whined at the mesh windows. They were in a basement. "Fans on the blink," said an attendant to the Matron, disgusted. "Ventilation gone again."

Miss Nesbitt had forsaken them, gone, back to Toronto. Edgar had tried to cling to her at the last moment in the entrance hall as she gathered up her case. "None of that, a big boy of fourteen like you! You'll be well taken care of. And you've got Robbie."

The new boys had brought no nightshirts (perhaps they had none), frowned the Matron, Supervisor of Nursing at the Infirmary. Mr. and Mrs. Hewitt had been sent the requisite Clothing List: two felt suits of strong outer clothing (had Florrie known what "felt" was?), three coloured shirts, one pair of braces or belt, one pair of leather bedroom slippers, one toothbrush. On the list it indicated that, "[l]ittle boys who wear short trousers will need three cotton jerseys, and two pairs of rubber pants." The list added, for incontinent boys like the Hewitts: "Untidy children who soil and wet frequently need large amounts of washable, cotton clothing." The two boys would have to make do with Institutional wear.

There were rooms called the Examining Room, the Operating Room, a Treatment Room, the Laboratory, the Dental Room, the X-ray Room, and, on the other side of the walls, forbidden rooms you were not to enter without an attendant. "Understand that, you morons." New patients were to be checked over the next day.

More wards beyond these walls were filled with patients who were not sick; the overflow from overcrowded Cottages on the grounds, said the nurse to Mr. Hansbro. One could hear the voices of boys and the deeper voices of men, yelling and moaning as mattresses dropped to the floor in a series of thuds. "Packed in there like flies."

The boys of Ward B were hungry and tired, and something else. They were tense from the journey, and frightened, all this strangeness. What was going to happen?

There was a long dining room.

"Atten'*shun*!" shouted a monitor at the head of the table. "Bow yer 'eads."

The older, retarded boy of about twenty, perhaps, said "Grace": "May the Lord makes yuh truly thanksful."

Dinner was bread, gruel, potatoes, and stew with bits of meat floating around. And something called "tapioca pudding."

Robbie ate hungrily, slopping down his gruel as fast as he could; he had not seen so much food at one meal in his life. In the soup line at the mission all they'd ever had was soup and a piece of butty dried up and stale without butter. Edgar would not eat, he felt sick; he did not like this place, he whimpered. He wanted to go home at once and be with Mama.

Afterwards, they had to line up to go back to the dorm to pee. The boys urinated in the tin lavatories with no doors. They had to wait, as there were crowds of boys pushing in. "An' no wanking!" said Mr. Bayliss, the Night Attendant, with a smirk.

There was a cracked, scummy mirror and a row of basins with taps. The new boys were to get in a line, said Mr. Bayliss. They knew at once he was to be obeyed, as he had a leather strop in his hand. "And out!" And they were to hold out your right hand for talking. Which was right? What did that mean? *Bam!* Robbie's head burned from the blow. "Stupid moron, don't you know yer right 'and from yer left?"

"Lights out," Mr. Bayliss shouted.

They were in a long ward with rows of iron cots, packed in tightly together. Each bed had a grey sheet, a blanket, and a hard lump called a pillow. Rows of frightened boys lay on their beds in rough nightshirts given them by the attendants that they did not know were dirty. Their dicks stuck out through the flannel — perhaps because of the exciting disturbance of the other boys naked together. The boys had dropped their clothes to the floor in piles. Night began to fall beyond the grilles. Where were the street lamps? It was darker than Toronto; a thick, deep blackness like a cloak. Strange bird calls coming from somewhere outside where the sky had seemed to lower.

Robbie and Edgar, who had never slept apart, were alarmed. Edgar crept into Robbie's bed. Far down the ward was a small station where the Night Attendant kept watch, and further down a screen and an overnight bed for the monitor, if there was one. Robbie and Edgar lay in the dark, their arms intertwined. They were in Orillia. The hot room was heavy with the breathing and sobs of the smaller boys. There was a tread of feet between the beds. It was Mr. Bayliss with the keys. There was a heavy clunk, and the grate of a lock at the end of the room. For the first time Robbie understood, with a cry, that they were locked in.

33.

"NEXT." A NERVOUS CHILD, Mellors, stepped forward. The Night Attendant, Mr. Bayliss, had tweaked him playfully that morning at something called "Roll Call" before directing him with the others to the examining room. The attendant accompanying the doctor held a list in his hand. The boys had to line up for their physicals, which were done first, though they did not know that.

The Examination Room was dim; a greenish light filtered through the grimy window mesh above their heads.

"Hewitt, Robbie."

The attendant checked his clothes. "He's got a *knife* on 'im, Sir."

"A knife?" Dr. Stroud turned to look at the attendant, his eyebrows raised.

"'S mine, you codger! Dada give it me!" Robbie tried to grab it.

"Hey, watch yer language to the doctor. Don't need no knives here." The attendant put it in a bag and marked it with Robbie's name, as well as the date.

"But it —"

He cuffed the back of Robbie's neck. "Who asked you ter speak? Git yer clothes off, moron."

There was a big metal weigh scale Robbie had to stand on for the attendant to note his height. Robbie shivered, naked. His penis wobbled as he stepped up. He put his hand over it. "None of that!" admonished the attendant.

He slid a brass rod over Robbie's head and wrote something down on a form, calling out to Dr. Stroud: "Hewitt, Robbie: 62 inches, Sir. Head measurement: 17.75 centimetres length, 13.5 centimetres width. Circumference (this was important): 53 centimetres."

Nose normal. Mouth negative, frowned Dr. Stroud. Ears, large. "Note that," he said to the attendant. Dr. A. F. Tredgold, the expert on mental deficiency in Great Britain, had had a lot to say about the ears of the feeble-minded most notably concerning twisted lobules.

"Both testicles descended," wrote Dr. Stroud on the form, under "genitourinary." His hand had slipped between Robbie's legs and cupped his testicles with an expert grasp.

Robbie's knees had buckled as Dr. Stroud bent, the huff of his breath expelling over Robbie's thighs.

"Family history of syphilis," he wrote, "Unknown."

The attendant motioned to Robbie to get back in line.

Regarding the Hewitt boys, Dr. Stroud already knew their background from the important Family History Form 120 forwarded from the Toronto Psychiatric Hospital. These personal history forms, to be used throughout the province and often pages in length, had been stressed by former Superintendent Dr. Bernard McGhie as vital for the correct placement of a new patient in the hospital. One of the main considerations to be verified was whether a child was to be a "permanent resident" (custodial), and what were his or her educative potentialities. Observations noted on the form were based on a ten-point scale developed by Dr. W. Fernald himself of the Massachusetts School for the Feeble-Minded in the United States, which included the physical exam that Dr. Stroud had just performed (cranial and other developmental defects to be noted) as well as a chronological and personal history of the patient: his mentality, his social habits, his motor capacity, his court record, etc.

Most important was the "family history" concerning legitimacy and whether the family's "social conditions" made immediate admission "imperative." The Hewitt boys, noted Dr. Stroud, were of a familiar type: working-class Toronto slum children. Half of the inmates at the hospital were from the slums of Toronto.

He glanced through the family's history. It documented the usual litany of feeble-mindedness completed by workers at CAS and by professionals at the Toronto Psychiatric Hospital which would, of course, now remain for all time in the Hewitt records — unbeknownst to them — to be passed along to any subsequent social workers and psychiatrists concerning this family. The father, Henry Hewitt, shell-shocked in the Great War, had attempted suicide (good God — had put his head in a gas oven). The mother, Florrie Hewitt, was classified as an "Imbecile" who cried out in her sleep. They had eight living children so far: Henrietta, Robbie, Edgar, Wilfred, Oswald, Ella, Cedric and Violet. Mrs. Hewitt had had a "miscarriage," one still-birth; one child, Georgie, given up for adoption, while another, Sophie, had died as an infant from summer diarrhea. "Parents not blood relations," the psychologist had noted. The boys' grandmother had been put in an asylum in England — an important piece of information, of course, that needed to be passed on indefinitely in the professional network, demonstrating as it did the heredity obviously at work here. He glanced sharply at Robbie: second generation feeble-minded. His younger sister, Ella, had an application at Orillia pending. Dr. Stroud had soon got the drift of the entire family.

Robbie had sensed rather than understood the importance of the strange tests that Mr. Finkle, the psychometrist, had called "Stanford-Binet." Mr. Finkle had a little blue case that snapped open containing the wooden shapes and pegs and pictures that decided everything: which school division you were placed in (if any), and which Cottage.

He had caught a glimpse of a Cottage in the distance while walking up from the train yesterday, a large red-brick building with glassed in verandahs. He knew he was here to learn to be a carpenter, Dada said. He had looked anxiously at the puzzles that Mr. Finkle had put before him from his blue box. He wanted to do his best, to please Dada and Mama, to believe Dada's words: "My boy smart."

"The size of Lake Ontario?" Mr. Finkle asked. What did that mean? He had scrawled his name with difficulty — though he had done his best — in the large shaming block letters Sister St. Clemencia had taught him in St. Mary's School in Grade 2 in Toronto.

"Cannot read or write," noted the psychologist briskly in his report, under " Mental Age." The Hewitt boy had scored poorly; for instance, on Definitions (Year IV) he had known "bed" — to which he had answered "ter sleep in" — but he had not known "wash-day" or "birthday party."

For the Materials section, he had known a house was made of bricks, a window of glass, but when given the word "book" he had said, inexplicably, "father." He could not thread a bead chain or repeat three digits in reverse.

Edgar, the younger Hewitt boy, had done only a little better. It was obvious which Cottage both boys belonged in: Cottage D, for the low-grade ones.

Assigned to Cottage D.
Some academics recommended: Lower Academic School, Group 15.
Vocational Training group: Coal Pile.

Clinical Record: Hewitt, Robbie. Case #7834
Admission Note: August 18, 1932.
Patient is well-developed, clean adolescent.
Ears are large, tonsils atrophied. No stigmata.
Numerous small haemorrhagic nodules on legs and arms, probably insect bites.
Otherwise examination negative.
Dr. Stroud.

Psychological Examination:
Subject was a dull, apathetic-appearing lad. He co-operated quite willingly.
Attention easy to gain but the span was poor. Showed no nervous symptoms.
Test: Binet. CA: 14.0. MA: 6.6. I.Q.: 46. Imbecile.
Examiner: Mr. Finkle

34.

COTTAGE D was a long, solid red-brick building adjacent to a road called Memorial Avenue, and a row of wrought iron railings. Robbie learned from kindly Mr. Atherton, an attendant, when he asked him, "Where is we, sir?" that it was the newest Cottage, built that year in 1932 for 200 boys along with Cottage O for girls, which was identical but not yet finished. Both faced the main road at the front of the grounds and stood side by side at a suitable distance. Mr. Downey, a former Superintendent, had set his heart on the road being planted with a boulevard of elms in memory of the young boys who had lost their lives in the Great War, something that had been dear to his heart, said young Mr. Atherton in his quiet but firm voice. The landscape gardener, with the help of the patients, had put in rows of saplings down the boulevard, fine young elms. But the trees had long since wilted, and the boulevard became forgotten with the passing of time. "After Mr. Downey's death, it just went to pot."

The dormitory windows on the other side faced the grounds and several more large, red-brick, oblong buildings also housed 200 or more patients. Robbie and Edgar, who kept close together, soon learned that the next big building over on the other side was the Nurses' Residence, a long, dark block similar to their own. You saw the nurses coming and going in their cloaks and headbands, hurrying to the different Cottages or the Infirmary. Then there was Cottage C for the older, smarter boys, some of whom came and went to Dunn Farm a half a mile down the road. They looked like men in their dungarees and boots, coming back from a day's work at the farm for their shower in the basement of C, and then their suppers. Others shuffled off to the coal piles or the swamps, and did not attend Academic School. Further along from C was Cottage

L for old women, many of them senile; and Cottage M, for older girls and young women who were allowed to go to the Socials where they danced with boys from Cottage C, said Fletcher, a tall lanky boy who was helping Robbie orient himself and was looking out for him. Robbie at once wanted to get into C.

An attendant yelled and the boys rolled out of bed for morning Roll Call. He heard Mr. Bayliss say to the monitor, "Eighty-five all told, one sick." Then they pulled on their clothes from under their bed, or their school clothes were picked out from an open cupboard by the monitor and tossed to the school group — any shirt, any breeches, and any shoes that looked as if they might fit, it did not matter. The Ward boys going out to labour in the yards put on different clothes, rough-looking loose shirts and coarse trousers made of sackcloth. Robbie pulled on dark breeches and a shirt too tight for him.

Where were the clothes he had worn from home? Who knew? They lined up to go down to breakfast in the dining room on the second floor, a long line of untidy, sleepy boys, some trembling or whining or coughing. A monitor slapped the heads of the slow ones and pushed them on.

Breakfast was porridge, bread and butter, and a cup of tea. Some of the boys had strange, squished-in faces with funny eyes. They were frightening. "Mongols," explained Fletcher. "They don't harm no one." Others seemed flabby and shapeless, waving their big heads, strings of spittle drooling down their chins. A boy banged his head against the wall.

"Settle darn there," called the senior monitor, "or you'll git it."

They lined up again to go down to the underground tunnels called tramways, a vast network of tunnels underneath the institution interconnecting the different Cottages and Infirmary, Robbie learned, frightened. It was lit up by lighting in the ceiling, and felt dank yet cool. Arrows on signposts on the walls at intersections pointed the way for the attendant: "To School," "To Cottage C." There was a flight of steps and a fire door at the top that the attendant unlocked with the monitor bringing up the rear, and they came out upstairs in the Administrative Building.

The schoolrooms were at the back. It was different from St. Mary's, which was a proper school with its own yard, classrooms, and the head-teacher's office where Sister St. Gabriel lived. Here they were in a large airy room with large grimy windows and a lead fireplace. Different groups sat together: Lower Academic at one end, and Upper Academic at the other end. Smaller groups for little children, imbeciles, and idiots, were in the basement doing bead work and tin foil sorting and such, said Fletcher. They sang songs from *Song Echoes From Child Land* like "Pit-a-Pat" and "The Bumble Bee," their tuneless voices drifting up. There was a boys' band that had triangles, clappers, castanets, whistles, and sticks as instruments. Fletcher once played the "kazoo," he said, a strange word to Robbie.

Edgar wanted to go back to St. Mary's, he whimpered to Robbie, "to Sista."

"Forgit Sista Sin Clement," whispered Robbie. "Forgit Sin Mary."

A voice said, "Group 15," and then Robbie's name and Edgar's were called. A woman teacher, Miss Hale, in a dark skirt and white shirt and a loosely knotted tie, said, "Hewitt boys?" She was in charge. She looked at the new patients and thought them sleepy and dull. But she would try to do something with them, she sighed. She pointed to two empty desks for today. There was a blackboard and rows of desks. And girls. Robbie glanced around. The girls sat together in the front, and the boys sat together in the back. A big girl in another group at the other end of the room turned and winked at him and he grinned back, excited. She had books on her desk and a pen and inkwell. She could read and write! The girls all had short haircuts and wore black school tunics and white open shirts and heavy shoes. But girls!

"Do you know your letters, Robbie?" said Miss Potter, the teacher's aide, not unkindly.

Robbie nodded cautiously. It had been a long time since Sister St. Clemencia said to Dada that he had reached his limit.

"What letter is this?"

"A."

"And this?"

Robbie was silent. Was it "S" or "Z?" His head already ached.

He was to write his name and the alphabet, to show what he could do. Robbie could not hold the pencil properly in his clumsy fingers. He did not know where on the paper to put the "R," which Miss Potter said was a capital at the head of his name. Robbie sweated and bent his head, ashamed he could not remember. The "R" was to come round at the top and then down at an angle, she said.

"R for 'robin,'" she said patiently. "You know what that is, Robbie?"

Robbie thought. "Is a bird what Mama put in th' stew wiv pigeon bits, ma'am." For some reason Miss Potter looked stricken.

"Sit still, there, I say! Don't swing yer fuckin' legs." The attendant slapped a belt across the offender's head. The child whined then fell silent, a wheal rising on his cheek. Robbie tensed, keeping his face still. "Too many kids and not enough staff," he heard a voice say.

They were benched. For how long? Forever. You had to sit still, your back against the back of the long wooden bench, until the attendant said "at ease." Rain fell against the Day Room windows mottled with damp dust and old flies. The long wooden benches were like church pews against the wall. "Bench!" an attendant yelled and you were to run and sit still, and be silent, your arms wedged tight against the boy sitting next to you, all to give the attendants a break. A boy somewhere hit his head with his fists and sobbed for mama. "Quit that snivelling!" yelled the attendant, "or we'll give ya' something to cry about."

Hundreds of boys filled the Day Room in Ward D-2 after morning school. Robbie and Edgar had never seen so many boys. Robbie recognized a few from the streets where he lived in Toronto. There was Bertie Lumsden from Oak Street where Robbie remembered they had lived for a time in a run-down sort of place, the houses huddled in shambles one on top of the other. Bertie's mother, Violet, was a worn-out woman like Florrie. He had a sister, Effie, who was somewhere in the hospital. Bertie glanced at Robbie and said, "Yew from Sumach Strit?" Then he ran off shyly. There were other boys he recognized from around Bleeker and Shuter Streets: Alfie Evans, and Paddy O'Reilly, and Arnold Grady from Moss Park, another low-down place.

In their free time, the boys would tussle and wrestle on the floor — what else was there to do? They fought and rolled around the floor while the attendants stood laconically by until they had had enough. Then, they would tackle a boy "for lip" and push him headfirst into a bucket of cold water. The small boy, Mellors, rocked in the corner, his hands over his ears. He had peed the bed again in the night and been punished by the attendant by having his head shoved down the toilet. Boys in straightjackets stumbled about, their arms pinned backwards at a funny angle. Robbie watched them, terrified; he had never seen such a thing. There were laces at the back tied tightly that pulled their arms back in place. The boys stumbled across the floor, their bodies swaying until they lost their balance and fell hard. No one took notice. You could spit in their face and there was nothing they could do about it, said Fletcher. Robbie had given him a piece of his bread at breakfast. "I c'n tell you 'bout this place, kid, what you needs to know."

There was a small room to the side of the Day Room called the Punishment Room, said Fletcher. "That's where you go you give trouble, boy, you give lip." Presently, the door opened and an attendant came out with a slop pail. "Here!" he said to a monitor, Jones, who got extra bread at table. Jones took the pail to the lavatory as it was overflowing with bilge. A boy suddenly fell with a thud to the floor; he was jerking and frothing at the mouth. "Davey's 'aving a fit, sir!" called someone.

Mr. Atherton and old Mr. Snow, the aide, pushed through the wrangling boys. "Okay, okay, boys, let's get back, give him air." Mr. Atherton rolled Davey Wilkinson over on his side and held Davey's flailing arms. Davey's head swung side to side as he let out gurgling noises. His eyes were rolling, noted Robbie, frightened again. There was so much to frighten you in this place, yet the boys continued play wrestling, unconcerned, as Mr. Atherton held down Davey. "Watch his tongue he don't swallow it. Go ring emergency, Snow."

"It's fits," explained Fletcher. Fletcher was proving useful; he knew everything, Robbie was coming to understand. "You aint seen ep'leptics?" Mr. Atherton and the aide stood over the boy guarding him until a nurse came. "He'll pass out an' be quiet soon," said Fletcher.

A nurse had come and the monitor helped Mr. Atherton lift up a now lifeless-looking Davey and carried him to a bed in the dorm.

The ceilings were high and strange, and so far away. Robbie wanted the small room at home that he shared with his brothers and sisters. He wanted to be home to see the baby at Mama's teat, his tiny sister, who had not yet been given a name. The attendants in their black suits and thin black ties stood with their backs against the wall, with a good view of everything around them. Old Mr. Snow wore a dicky bow. Presently, he brought out a bag. "Watch this!" He winked at Mr. Atherton. "Okay boys, git to it."

He tossed down candies and the boys whooped like birds — ugly, pecking birds digging out each other's eyes for those precious treats — pushing and shoving, the boy Mellors at the back crying. Robbie pushed his way in and grabbed some Dolly mixtures, fisting the next boy away to get at them. The boy fell and groaned, but Robbie did not care because he wanted the sweets. The lucky, the strong, and the rough crammed them into their mouths. The Day Room reeked. There were mattresses against the walls stained with urine from the extra boys who slept in the room at night, part of the overflow.

Beyond the window, Robbie glimpsed other Cottages through the mist. Cottage C with its white lattice verandahs seemed ghostly and pale, its patients locked-in like himself. He thought he saw faces at the windows looking out at the mournful landscape at Cottage M and R, and further down to old Cottage L. An old woman had come out in the rain, holding out her skirts with her hands, swaying in the wind, yelling; a lunatic. Presently, a nurse's aide came out and led her inside. There was a scuffle and another aide came and together they seized her by the arms and dragged her inside. And beyond them, the back of the Administration Building, heavy and solid, reared through the mist. It contained, Robbie now knew, Cottages A and K, where there were more rooms full of penned-in boys and girls and old men. Then there were the strange, vast, empty slopes down to the lake. "Lake Simcoe," Miss Nesbitt had said on Robbie's first day, long ago now.

Robbie missed crowded Parliament Street, the pawn shop, and the rattling wooden trams. He tried to remember where he lived; was it Shuter or River Street? Where were the shoppers, and the factory girls, and the women in their short dresses and bobbed hair coming off of a work shift? Where were the factory whistles, the lovely thick smoke? Here the air was fresh and cold and comfortless. Here, in the country, there was only grass and an endless, lonely lake. There was no amusement park like the one at Sunnyside where Dada took them sometimes in the summer when he had pennies in his pockets. Here there was no Ferris wheel, no merry-go-round, no hurdy-gurdy, no noisy bands, no shooting galleries, and no cotton candy for half a penny.

He longed for Levi, the rag-and-bone man and his old horse named Ned; and he longed for old Mrs. O'Garrity in the room behind the kitchen with her sweets and comics. He longed for home.

Clinical Record: Hewitt, Robbie. Case #7834
Sept. 3. 1932
Transferred from Infirmary: August 20, 1932
Settling in well. Cottage D.
Says he's been here 2 months, but really it is 2 weeks.
D. F.

35.

"YOU C'N SIT WITH ME," said Fletcher at lunch, which was bologna with shreds of another kind of meat, turnips, bread and butter, and date pie. Fletcher, a tall lanky boy of nearly sixteen, had been on the ward a long time, four years he thought, after coming up from the Children's Dorm.

"Watch out fer Bayliss at night, Robbie," Fletcher had warned him that first day, "he likes new ones, but he likes 'em little, too. An' watch your arse in the showers."

"Showers?" What were they he had wondered.

"Ugh, you'll fin' out."

Now he knew: a row of iron shower heads in a stall that you ran under; sometimes the attendant shot a hose pipe over you, icy water if no water came out of the heads that day, and yelled "Git on with yer!" The attendants whacked wet towel sheets over your backside if you weren't sharp enough.

Fletcher had looked Robbie over — a handsome boy, he thought, with curly brown hair, merry eyes, and rosy-red cheeks. "They'll be on to you, boy. Good with yer 'ands?" he grinned. He jerked his hand up and down, fast, over his crotch.

Robbie had flushed. "Don't nobuddy jumps me, Fletcher." But he had been anxious and had run fast through the water spray before they got him, the older boys pushing and guffawing.

Then, that first night, Ellcott, a big boy on the Ward, had pushed into his bed and put a hand over his mouth. "Cry an' you're dead, kid." He shoved his cock in Robbie's hand. Soundlessly, Robbie had wanked him good and hard and he had come all over the blanket; his bed smelled of piss and spunk. But that was not enough. Ellcott wanted more. "Go right down, boy," he hissed. Then he turned Robbie around and pulled him up on his haunches, and Robbie knew. "Na," he had pleaded in a whisper. But Ellcott shoved his head down and thrust himself inside his bum. "Agh!" Robbie gurgled into the blanket. "Agh!"

The attendant had called out, "Wha's that gorn on darn there?"

"Jus' goin' ter th' can, sir," said Ellcott, "I gotta." The next morning Robbie pushed the bloody nightshirt under the mattress, frightened. He would get a knife, he thought.

Now at the dining table he nodded at Fletcher. Fletcher knew his way around Orillia. He was smart, in Group 25 of the Upper Academic School. He could read and write well and do figures. In the afternoon he did shoemaking in the Trade Shop. Fletcher boasted: "I c'n turn six pair o' shoes a day."

"They took my knife!" said Robbie fiercely.

"You 'ad a knife?"

"Doct'r got it. Dada give it me when me 'n' Edgar come here."

"I bet by arf!"

"Yes 'e did! Got it in a pawnshop on Parl'mint."

Fletcher was silent. "Well, I got a dad, comin' any time now ter git me. He'll be taking me away now I'm turnin' sixteen. I'll be on probashun."

"Wassat?"

"You git a job outside. You c'n leave th' grounds an' go inter town by yerself, cuz you 'as a pass, an' so they c'n trust you not ter run orff."

Fletcher knew *everything*. Robbie leaned forward eagerly. He gave him a slice of his bread, his butty ration.

"Take me with yer?"

Fletcher hesitated, confused. He would be a man at sixteen soon, and not a ward of the Children's Aid any more, he thought. He should rightly be put on probation for six months, earn wages of his own. But would he be released? A feeble-minded patient like him could be kept in the hospital indefinitely, he knew, perhaps turning out shoes forever for the institution. He was a smart fellow, who made good money for the hospital. He was needed. He trembled at the thought that they might not let him go.

Robbie understood little of this. "I getting outa this place!" Robbie vowed.

"You ain't goin' nowheres, boy, but to coal," grinned Fletcher.

"Coal?"

"Is better 'n' carting sludge from the cesspit, by 'alf."

"I be in carp'ntry," Robbie faltered. Dada had said so, proudly.

"You ain't goin' to no carpenter shop, you ain't smart enough. You in Group 15, so you's an imbecile. You's coal."

Fletcher was right. Robbie's name was called after lunch for Coal Group by the attendant: "Coal Pile."

Edgar was gone to Ward Work, scrubbing out Cottage D, helping with the garbage, and emptying out the shit buckets. He was too weak-chested for the Coal Pile. Boys who were in morning classes at school were to return to the dorm, change out of their school clothes and put on work clothes and follow the attendant. The freight train had come into the station below the Administration Building, with its load of coal. Coal came in by rail or by barge. Robbie joined the big boys from Cottage C and men from G and walked down to the train, shovels in hand. They were to unload the coal into the waiting wagons to be drawn to the coalhouse near the lake, a half a mile down from the Administration Building. Orillia produced its own coal gas.

"You knows your job, boys. Git to it."

"Aye, aye, sir." Others grunted and wheezed.

The boys and young men tackled the coal, shovelling it down and heaving it into the wagon. Robbie was soon sweating, which made him tremble. Soon his hands and face and clothes were layered with sooty dust and grime; he even tasted it on his tongue. His back and arms ached from the unaccustomed labour; he had never worked so hard. He longed to throw off his scratchy rough clothes and take a dip in the lake that lay between the trees. A gang of boys were picking up wood with great difficulty among the trees, very onerously, their arms and legs out of coordination, their heads wobbling. Others in the distance were shambling about trying to rake leaves across the grounds. An attendant lit a fire and the odour of wood smoke rose over the scene — a sweet, sharp, sad scent. Robbie laboured, breathing in huffs.

Soon the wagon drew away and the boys and men took their shovels up and trailed slowly up the hill past the Administration Building where the Superintendent gazed out of the front window of his office approvingly. Robbie saw in the distance to his right, between trees, a pretty white-and-brown house with a deep verandah trailing with vines: the Superintendent's house.

More gangs of boys and older men from other Cottages were already working with shovels to transfer the coal into the coalhouse. At last it was tea time. They lined up and followed the monitor down the tunnel to a door that led into a wash-up area that had showers and sinks and soap. There were dirty towels on the floor.

"Bloody water's off again, so no showers," grumbled the attendant, Mr. Hawkins. "Just wipe over 'ands and faces, boys."

They moved along the tramway again to a door that the attendant seemed to know led to Cottage O. He unlocked it with the keys that were clicked to his belt, and they filed up noisily and hungrily to the dorm to change back into ordinary clothes. Robbie grabbed any shirt or breeches, yearning for that cup of tea in the dining hall, for a piece of bread and butter with jam. There was also a slice of pound cake each because they were working men, said Mr. Atherton. The boys grinned and jostled.

"So 'ow was yer day on coal?" Fletcher grinned.

"When your dad comes, Fletcha, c'n 'e take me?"

"We-ell, it'll cost yer. You got pin money?"

"Dada give me a quarter. Mister Ath'ton got it an' gives me pennies for tuck." This was at the canteen at break.

"Gimme two penny down, an' a nickel when my father comes ter take us away."

Toronto, November 30, 1932
Dr. S. J. W. Horne,
Medical Superintendent
Ontario Hospital, Orillia

Re: Robbie and Edgar Hewitt, Case #7834 and Case #7835

Dear Dr. Horne,
We wish to thank you for your conference reports of November 20, 1932, on the above-mentioned boys.
Yours sincerely,
E. P. Lewis, M.D.
Director, Outpatient Clinic,
Toronto Psychiatric Hospital

Mr. Walker, Administrative Assistant to the Superintendent, filed the correspondence into the Hewitt records, after it was checked over by Superintendent Dr. Horne; a matter of protocol for the Minute Book.

Hundreds of boys and men moved in lines up and down the stairs, and hundreds more moved in the central wide corridors of Cottage D after Roll Call in the dorm. The buzzer went off and then came a voice — Mr. Atherton's? Mr. Fowler's? — they changed shifts every few days. "Okay boys, git to it."

Boys rolled and grunted, tossing back their blankets. Those who had slept on the floor, rolled up their mattresses, soiled with urine and feces, and pushed them against the walls. Dim, early dawn light filtered through the windows. There was a long line of boys at the sinks. More lining up for breakfast in the dining room hall — porridge, bread and butter, a cup of tea — before Academic School and the Training Yards. Robbie was shovelling and picking in the Coal Pile again, and Edgar was on Ward Duty.

A glimpse of leafless trees beyond the grilles. The boys moved in unison. Mr. Bayliss was on duty.

At night, Edgar shared a bed with a smaller boy at the other end of the dorm, two by two. Robbie was with the older boys. He lay in bed squished against Samson, a bigger fellow than himself, who was now sharing his bed due to overcrowding, said Mr. Bayliss. He could feel Samson against him as they curled up against one another, back to front. Then they reversed and it was Robbie's turn. The next bed on either side was inches away. Lights out was when the sobbing and the shuffling began. Mr. Bayliss slept behind a screen at the end of the dorm. Samson half rose on his knees and it would begin. Robbie tensed and lifted his nightshirt. The grim pulsing in Samson's hand, pushing against Robbie's buttocks. There was a sudden pool of wet against his back. Around him, others moved furtively, shuffling under blankets fast, intense, moaning; they all did it.

When Mr. Bayliss was on duty, he let them do it in the showers, or over the open cans, always standing by, always watching. But Mr. Atherton said good-naturedly, "Come along, you young bucks." How they loved Mr. Atherton. Sometimes he brought comics from his home in town.

Then there was silence, a fitful silence down the ward of slumbering boys. And only then Robbie knew the other thing that happened behind the curtain that Fletcher had warned him of. Oh, where was Mama, Dada?

Mr. Bayliss moved stealthily between the mattresses of sleeping boys in his grey nightshirt. He paused by one, and carefully lifted the boy into his arms. Robbie heard a faint squeak like a little rabbit caught by a hunter.

He caught a glimpse in the moonlight of Mellor's small face, his eyes squeezed in pain as Mr. Bayliss's huge shadow rose and fell rhythmically against the partition. Robbie shut his own eyes, and then waited. And he felt the darkness, like a cloak, descend. Night falls swiftly in Orillia.

Clinical Record: Hewitt, Robbie. Case #7834
Nov. 30, 1932.
Ward 4, Cottage D.
Fairly obedient. Careless in appearance. Occasional enuresis.
A rough and tumble lad. Attends School, Group 15.
Good and willing worker in Training Yards.
Has a brother Edgar also in Cottage D.

36.

"WHAT DO YOU WANT TO SAY to Mother and Father?"

Robbie was silent. He and Edgar sat with Miss Potter who was to write a letter home on their behalf. She said it was time.

Wants to go 'ome," said Edgar softly. He had a cough. He always had a cough in this place.

Miss Potter frowned. "Come along, now, Edgar. You can do better than that. You don't want to worry them. What do you *like* here at the Hospital, boys?" Miss Potter smiled brightly.

There were, after all, gym classes, silent movies on Saturday night, skating on the outdoor rink in winter, the Thanksgiving Dinner and party, she urged. The Women's Auxiliary Club from town had brought in presents of toffee apples and cookies for the inmates. There were occasional moving pictures at the Orillia Opera House. As one inspector had declared, these patients had more amusements than they ever experienced in their own homes.

Robbie looked bewildered.

"Sweets from Mister Ath'tan...."

"What about new friends? And your training work?" she urged again, though it was obvious from the ingrained grime and soot in the boys' nails and faces in which group Robbie and Edgar belonged.

"Coal," proffered Robbie, understanding at last that the Coal Pile was classified as "training." "Shov'lin' coal, ma'am."

Miss Potter sighed and wrote that the boys were enjoying their stay in Orillia and were happy. They were doing poorly in their academics, she knew, and would soon be demitted from the school program altogether. Robbie, the elder boy, now looking big and strong after three regular meals a day, though grubby and smelling of certain odours, would be more useful in the Training Yards where they were short of hands.

"You c'n smoke darnnstairs," whispered the girl, sliding up to him at break. You weren't allowed to talk to the girls unless given permission. Her name was Elvina Thomas, she said quickly. "Wha's yours?"

"Robbie."

"Robbie what? What Cottage? "

"'Ewitt. Cottage D."

"'Ow old is you? Where you's from?"

"Sixteen," he lied. "Sumach Street."

"A'm seventeen."

Elvina had red hair and brown eyes. He loved her.

"Loves ya, 'Vina," he said at once, thickly.

"Talk in basement — canteen," she hissed and then ran into the Girls' lavatory.

The female attendant had come by. She had a big hard face and big red hands. "Enough there, Thomas."

Robbie was excited. He had seen her the previous afternoon on her way to Laundry. She had turned in the line and waved to him, covered as he had been with soot, sticking out her tongue saucily, before disappearing into a long, low building called Trades. Another day she had tossed him a note in class that he pretended he could read as she walked by to her group at the back. He knew, now, that rows of "x's" at the bottom of the page stood for kisses.

The little canteen was downstairs in the basement, underneath the Administration Building, where the patients could buy "tuck": candy, chocolate bars, and fizzy drinks, if they had any pin money. There was a wooden counter, and a small seating area with benches. It was already crowded with patients — boys and girls, men and women. Attendants and nurses' aides kept watch from the hallway. They were allowed to talk, but they could not sit together too closely (though who was really paying attention?). The attendants and pretty nurses were having a break, too. The men lit up smokes. "What the 'ell, they gotta have some fun — it's 'armless."

There was a worn sofa, a barred window, a steep flight of stone steps leading to a door that, in turn, led to outside. The older male patients, the ones who could work, could smoke after Training Yards — the Smoking Room was further along the tunnels from the canteen.

"Let's go to th' Smokin' Room." Elvina stood in the tunnel waiting by the canteen door, "Nobody will notice."

Oh, she was a smart one, thought Robbie. They could see men inside a small room near the Boiler Room, smoking. They had their own tobacco tins, said Elvina, and papers to roll their own cigarettes. Sometimes a patient gave her a ciggy if she was nice to him, she winked. She pulled out a battered cigarette from her apron pocket. "Say, yah gotta light for a poor lonesome gal?" she called through the doorway. Soon she was drawing on the ciggy, waving it around. Robbie had a puff, and blew out a smoke ring. She touched his mouth with hers, quickly, sticking her tongue inside his mouth and wriggling it; he felt like swooning.

"Elvina! Elvina!" he whispered over and over that night as he throbbed.

He needed a knife. He had got used to Samson, who was the biggest on the ward and had rights. But Fletcher's words echoed over and over: "And ain't nothin' you can do about it."

At dinner — stew, bread, and tapioca pudding — Robbie slipped a knife up his sleeve while the boys stood scraping back their chairs.

"You ain't no imbecile. I seen," whispered Fletcher.

At bedtime he quickly slid it under the mattress as he bent down to pull off his shoes. He had been given no socks that day. Boys were milling around undressing and others were pushing forward at the basins to brush their teeth, the monitor busy handing out tooth powder. Everyone had to pee last thing. Mellors trembled at the can, sobbing again. "Hurry on, boy," bawled the monitor, giving him a cuff. Robbie pushed in. When he got back from peeing and brushing his teeth, he felt for the knife; it was gone. He wheeled around. He felt under the next boy's bed, and then the next, and then Fletcher's. "Saw ya!" sniggered Fletcher. He pushed Robbie's hand away.

"'S mine!" cried Robbie. "Give it. 'S ma knife!"

"Three pennies."

"Bleedin' bullocks!" Robbie butted his head at Fletcher's chest.

"Hey, hey! Wha's the hell goin' on darn there?"

"He got ma knife!"

"Knife? You got a *knife,* boy?" Robbie struggled with Fletcher, clutching at his throat the way Dada did when he got a pigeon; he remembered to squeeze tight. Fletcher flailed about, gurgling across the bed. The knife had gone flying. "Bleedin' bastid!"

Mr. Bayliss came bearing down. "Call for 'elp." That meant press the red buzzer. The monitor ran to the station. Soon Robbie's arms were pinned back and pushed into canvas sleeves that pulled them backward. He lurched his face and bit into Mr. Bayliss's arm. "The devil! 'E drawn blood! Tie 'im up tight," heaved Mr. Bayliss, out of breath.

"Na-a-a. Oh na-a! Dada! Dada!" Robbie sobbed. "Won' do nothin' ever agin, Mister Bayliss, oh please!"

"What they doon to Wobbie?" sobbed Edgar, pulling at the monitor.

Mr. Bayliss dragged a trussed-up Robbie into the Punishment Room. The laces were pulled up tightly and then knotted. Robbie toppled over backwards and landed with a thud. Mr. Bayliss slammed the door and turned the key. Boys were overexcited now that there was pandemonium in the dorm. The more feeble-minded ones ran about screaming and banging their heads on the walls; others jumped gleefully on the beds. Little Mellors was rocking in the corner, his hands over his head, weeping.

"Enough!" snarled Mr. Bayliss. "Christ!"

Mr. Bayliss duly recorded in the Ward Report: "Robbie Hewitt foun' with knife under bed at bedtime, 8:00 p.m. Got vilent, had to be restrane." He passed it on to Dr. Horne's office at nine p.m. to be recorded in the Superintendent's Minute Book.

"Well, now, you didn't ought to have had a knife, Robbie," said Mr. Atherton.

Robbie was silent. He'd had a whipping from Bayliss, the lashes had cut deeply into his buttocks as he had straddled the bench. Now he sat painfully on a stool in the Punishment Room, struggling for words.

"Was Ellcott. Come on me, in bed, wanting jizz," he said finally.

"That is why you stole the knife?"

Mr. Atherton's face tightened. He knew this sort of thing happened on the wards, of course; he had done night shift on the older wards in his time in Cottage B. But there was an unspoken code about telling on a fellow worker (half of whom were related in some form or another to half the townsfolk in Orillia. Entire families often worked in the institution. There was pride in this, a bond). He feared for his job if he spoke out. And who would believe an imbecile?

"Boys'll be boys," said Mr. Bayliss later when Mr. Atherton ventured to hint tentatively about older boys troubling younger ones at night. Mr. Atherton was not certain about Mr. Bayliss himself, as there had been rumours out at Cottage F on the Dunn Farm when Mr. Bayliss had been night staff there.

"What d'you expec, hun'reds of boys locked up in they teens, full of spunks sleepin' two to a bed?" cried Mr. Bayliss. "What' re we suppose ter do ev'ry time it happen? Gotta git it outa their system some'ow, tha's what I says."

True, perhaps, yes. Yes, Mr. Atherton did see that. He also knew that little would come from reporting Bayliss, except a great deal of animosity for himself from other attendants, bound as he was by an unspoken code of loyalty amongst staff. Yet was not his loyalty also towards these defenceless ones? He hesitated unhappily; he was but one person working one isolated shift, like Bayliss, to whom he was distantly related on his mother's side in town. "Well, well don't do it again, Robbie," he said lamely. He had brought, as usual, comics and comic stips from the newspapers for the boys in the Day Room, the adventures of Buck Rogers and Dick Tracy he knew the boys loved, trying to put out of mind Robbie's disturbing confidence.

Yet, as he crossed the grounds later by moonlight, Mr. Atherton paused fearfully outside Cottage B. There was always a shortage of attendants, the male imbeciles inside unsupervised at night except for a high grade monitor, one of their own, on duty. Mr. Atherton could only imagine the horrors enacted under cover of darkness, but he hurried on, blocking out the night.

Sometimes during the day Robbie saw the freight train rolling along the track at the bottom of the slope — long trains with transport boxes. At night he heard the long distant echo of its wheels along the lake. Men clung to its roofs, men who looked familiar. They were the hobos of the city, their ghastly faces covered in dust from the tunnels. They were anxious men in their broken dungarees and collarless shirts. "Goin' out west," said Mr. Fowler peremptorily, pausing at the shrubbery. "Lookin' for work that ain't there, poor buggers." These trains did not stop at the Orillia Station. They flew sadly, mysteriously by with their cargo, and were gone. Up north and westward along the Great Northern Railway, said Mr. Atherton as if it were important. But what did it mean?

Gradually, over the past year Robbie had become aware of buses, too, on the move, in and out of the hospital each day. He was working in Landscape now, in the mornings, under the charge of Mr. Atherton and

Mr. Fowler, who was an older patient from F helping out. Robbie had been taken out of Lower Academics in 1933. "Has reached his limits," he had heard Miss Hale tell Mr. Atherto, and Mr. Atherton had looked saddened and said something like, "Damn shame."

Robbie had grown tall, and was big in the shoulders now like Dada. Mr. Atherton had looked for bigger sized clothing for him in the dorm. "What they feeding you, boy? Soon you'll be moving over to Cottage C to do farm work." Something about the sound of this Robbie had not been sure of. Was he not ever going home? he had thought, suddenly anxious.

He swung the pick into the air, a heavy implement made of iron, with a curved blade. "Swing it up, boy, over yer shoulder. Mind it!" Mr. Fowler would yell. They were doing fall clean-up on the terrace, readying the beds for winter, pruning the roses, cutting them back to the stump, and turning the beds. He also had a wooden fork to break up the clay soil after he had sundered the ground into pieces for the Superintendent's beds. Dr. Horne was watching approvingly, again, from his office window.

Robbie paused, watching the bus curve around the drive from Entrance A, while Mr. Atherton decided which flower beds they were to tackle next, and how to divide up the labour. Robbie knew by now that the bus came in the morning and stopped at the Administration Building by the terrace, dropping off incoming attendants and staff for the morning shift — he knew shift work from Dada. The bus then picked up the doctors' children who were standing in a happy, jostling group with their attendant, to take them to school in town. They were the children of Dr. Horne, and other important staff members like Mr. Zarfas, the Steward, a kindly man who lived with his family in the apartment above the main entrance. The children wore smart clothes that fit. The boys sported corduroy breeches and fresh white shirts with high stiff collars. And Robbie had never seen such lovely boots. The girls had long, curled hair under their bonnets, and carried books and lunch baskets. One girl was leaning against the lamppost actually reading to herself.

Robbie felt his shabbiness; he was conscious of his ugly canvas apron, peaked cap and big split work boots. He was aware of something about himself that was so different from these shining children who seemed to come and go at will, and who, most of all, had mothers and fathers there on the grounds.

Sometimes these children joined in the activities of the hospital, coming to the concert at Christmas, to the annual dance and picnic. The Horne boys (both kind children) and Mr. Zarfas' sons sometimes came skating on the rink in winter playing hockey, joining in with the higher grade boys from Cottage C, said Mr. Atherton approvingly. They had been told by the grown-ups never to make fun of the patients, nor stare at them, and always to treat them with respect. "There but for the grace of God..." was the dictum set by Dr. Horne, who had been a Captain in the Great War and was also an Arch Mason at the Masonic Lodge in town, a secret fraternity. At this Mr. Atherton lowered his voice — there were certain handshakes only they understood, and oaths about following the "light."

Mr. Atherton knew all this because Mrs. Atherton played something called "bridge" with the doctor and his wife and the Hamiltons once a week, Robbie understood. They had treats and after-dinner drinks, and Mr. Atherton even called him "Sid" at these parties. Mr. Fowler nodded. "Oh aye, he's a good man, the doctor, he don't put on side."

Robbie, as he listened, had a sense of another world going on all the while around him, a world that was not for him, a world far from Sumach Street and Dada, Mama, and Mrs. O'Garrity who saved comics for him. A world from which he was forever separated. For the first time, he understood he would never read or write as Dada expected. That what the doctor had said of him long ago in some hospital was true: he was an imbecile.

Mr. Atherton was chuckling, for they had come to his favourite part of the story: Dr. Horne's first Annual Picnic the year before, a story that Dr. Horne himself loved to recount at bridge. Sidney Horne had been standing up on the slope, watching the games of leapfrog and British bulldog below, when an old feeble-minded man, probably from Cottage B, had come up to him and asked him who he was. "I'm the new superintendent," Dr. Horne had said proudly. "Oh yeah?" said the old man. "And I was Napoleon when I first come here."

For some reason, Mr. Atherton and Mr. Fowler would roar with laughter at this, so all the boys laughed too, everyone happy to take a break from the digging.

"Oh aye, he treats us fair," said Mr. Fowler.

The bus had long gone with the children, who would not return until afternoon. The sun rose over the Cottages and the Infirmary far down the slope by the trees, the great Administration Building nearby. Groups of boys and girls were moving in separate lines around the grounds with their nurses and attendants.

"Watch them roots, boys," said Mr. Fowler. "Blend in the manure."

It was cow manure from the hospital's own pasture on Dunn Farm.

The boys got points for not peeing the bed, and points for lining up pronto when told. They stood naked in the centre of the dorm if they had peed the bed, and if their cock went up, Mr. Bayliss tweaked it and said, "Cock-a-doodle-doo," and all the boys were supposed to laugh, and they did.

Mr. Atherton took the boys who had earned their points into town to skate and listen to the band in Couchiching Park where the institution used to be years before, years and years back, under Dr. Beaton. The town had been full of people Robbie seemed to recognize from another life, ordinary men and women from Sumach, Shuter, and River Streets, like Dada and Mama, going about their business, pushing prams and holding toddlers' hands, telling them to stay close. He had felt tears prick his eyes, but why? There were girls, too, in pretty skirts and coats to their knees and cloche hats; girls who walked the promenade and looked away when the institution boys passed with the attendants. Some children pointed.

"They're from the idiot asylum — keep away!" a mother said sharply to her little one.

There was a letter in the Orillia mailroom from Mr. Hewitt of Toronto, stamped 1933, and addressed to the Hewitt boys, Robbie and Edgar, Cottage D. The boys would not be able to read it, of course, Mr. Walker, administrative assistant to Dr. Horne, decided. One of the attendants, possibly Mr. Atherton, could relay the contents to them in the Day Room, though not the references to "going home." That was absolutely out of the question.

Mr. Henry Hewitt
22 River Street
Toronto

Dec 7

Dear Robbie and Edgar

Received your letter yesterday and was very glad to hear from you both. Also glad to hear you are well Mother and I also Henrietta, Ella Oswald, Cedric and Vi'let and baby Agnes, the new little 'un, are all well but Ella and Oswald had the chicken pox so you had no chance to tease them but it is all over now.

I am going to try and get you home for xmas or New Years but I have no work yet and no money so I wont be able to pay for your fare. So you might do me a favor for me try to see your Master for me and find out if they could arrange for your transportation, and let me know as soon as possible don't delay. How are you making out with your learning you never told anything in any of your letters. I hope you are good boys and doing your best to learn because you know dad and Mother wants to see you grow up smart boys. So you know I'm expecting You both to do your very best. Mrs. O'Garrity has been keeping all the comic for you and I am going to send them on to you they were asking about you.

Well I have very little more to say only do your best to let me know if you can get home for xmas or New Year So bye bye till We see You with lots of love from
Mother and Dad
XXXXXXXXXXX

The letter still lay in the records, written in Mr. Hewitt's forward slope, a surprisingly mature handwriting he had, no doubt, learned in Junior III in school in England. Yet there was no comment of surprise expressed by Mr. Walker at Henry's skills. He frowned at Mr. Hewitt's overly effusive "bye, bye till We see You..." and childish X's. The Hewitt home situation was less than satisfactory, as he knew: "Home absolutely destitute of furniture, the beds filthy, mattresses soaking in urine," a social worker had written in one report. The older sister, Henrietta, had been pregnant out of wedlock; the father had been suicidal and, at one point, had tried to swallow Lysol; the mother was an Imbecile; indeed, the *entire* family was Imbecilic and likely Idiotic.

He couched his reply in no uncertain terms:

Orillia, Ontario

December 19, 1932

Mr. Henry Hewitt
22 River Street
Toronto, Ontario

Dear Sir:
Re – Robbie and Edgar Hewitt

In reply to your letter of recent date regarding your boys, I may state that that they are enjoying very good health and appear to be quite contented in their present surroundings. As regards arranging transportation for your boys to be home with you over the Christmas season, I may state that this would be inadvisable and almost impossible as we have no means of carrying out your desire. I may state that both Robbie and Edgar are conducting themselves quite well and are getting along very nicely in the hospital.
Yours truly,
N. L. Walker, M.D.
(For Medical Superintendent, Dr. Horne)

37.

DR. HORNE had glanced out of his window that January day in 1933, pen poised. It was time to write his Annual Report to the Minister of Health: "I beg to present the Annual report of the Ontario Hospital Orillia, for the year ending 1932..." As the new Superintendent, he was anxious to prove himself. The position of superintendent of a big provincial hospital like Orillia was a coveted one, held in high esteem by colleagues and political patrons, as he well knew. He wanted to improve the Hospital and make his mark. In this he was inspired by his predecessor, Dr. Bernard T. McGhie. Though Dr. McGhie had been superintendent for but a few years, 1927-1930, he had initiated a number of reforms and changes that Dr. Horne had certainly admired, not least a complete overhaul of the educational and training system with the help of the Psychology Department at the University of Toronto, no mean feat.

Dr. Horne was a big-shouldered man, with a balding head, an affable face, and large, kindly eyes. He prided himself on the high moral tone he demanded of staff and colleagues as well as himself, keeping his personal motto as a mason ever before him, "to be good men and true."

His Annual Report was, in part, a response to the report of Dr. D. R. Fletcher, Inspector of Hospitals, for the previous year ending October 31. Inspectors came up to Orillia from Queen's Park three times a year to examine and review the hospital, the plant, the operations, the buildings (no one ever minced words there), the staff, and the school. Dr. Horne, as former senior physician in residence at the Orillia institution for a number of years was already familiar with the protocols and procedures of these inspections that could last anywhere from two days to a week.

Dr. Fletcher, a breezy man, had been up at the crack of dawn the previous February of 1932 to go out and inspect the ice-cutting down on the lake at eight-thirty a.m. Dr. Horne had a vision of him shivering in below-zero temperatures observing the work-gang harvesting the ice. It was heavy, tiring work. Steam rose from the lake, and the horses pawed at the ground. As the cold wind whipped up from the lake, the huge blocks of ice were drawn by teams on flat sleighs up to the icehouse, to be stored in sawdust for summer use. Dr. Fletcher had written approvingly of the patients: "They were properly clad and seemed happy although it was zero weather." Following this, the energetic inspector had gone on to visit Dunn Farm after which he had brought up the need to pay older patients something for their labour.

Admirable though this might be, the whole purpose of patient labour was surely to cut costs for the hospital, frowned Dr. Horne. Dr. Fletcher had written:

> Payment of Patients: I believe those patients who are considered fit for probational discharge should be paid a sum sufficient to buy their clothing. This would not cost the Government very much and would teach the patients to be careful of their money.

And had that happened? snorted Dr. Horne. Like Dr. Beaton before him, Dr. Horne held a certain irritation for government inspectors. It was all very well that they came up from Queen's Park to make recommendations, but when had funding ever been forthcoming? Orillia had always had the unfortunate distinction of being the most underfunded asylum in North America, and even compared with the whole of Europe. It cost $134.68 per annum per patient in Ontario compared with $227.75 spent on patients at the Pennsylvania State Asylum in the United States, for example. Attendants were also always paid less than their American colleagues: $29.32 a month compared with $73.82 in American institutions. This meant, of course, that American asylums attracted a better class of worker. This extended also to superintendents' salaries, noted Dr. Horne dourly: a medical superintendent in America received above $4,000 compared with the $2,000 the superintendent of Orillia received.

The asylum was also overcrowded, to say the least. Over the fifty or so years since its founding in 1876, Dr. Horne reflected that Orillia had increased in population from 40 patients in Dr. Beaton's day to 654 residents by 1902 to well over 1,000 residents in 1932. More land and buildings had been acquired along the way, of course. Under Mr. Downey, two more residences as well as a 200-bed infirmary had been erected in 1926. Now, two more cottages were under construction again, along with the Nurses' Residence — all of which meant a massive institution packed to the brim, with a waiting list of a thousand.

Wages and overcrowding aside, Dr. Fletcher's report had followed the usual protocol. He had written approvingly of the construction of the two new cottages for high-grade boys and girls nearing completion: D and O. Cottages B, L, and M, the oldest, stood in the large central area behind the Administration Building, facing each other in a rectangle. A distance from these, down by the lake, was the Infirmary. It was a good walk around the grounds, which was why the underground tramways were so useful in inclement weather, Dr. Fletcher had noted, to convey trolleys of food and lines of patients hither and thither.

Here Dr. Fletcher had moved on to the question of staffing, noting that there were 1,427 patients (732 males and 695 females) to 140 nurses and attendants. Also on staff were six officers, nine Department Heads, eighteen teachers, and teaching aides, as well as six laundry workers, ten farm workers, thirteen engineers, five kitchen helpers, and fifteen domestics. High grade patients assisted in Ward Work.

Dr. Fletcher had gone on to inspect the Nurses Training School, which he had pronounced "large enough as it stands at present." He had examined the nurses' Sitting Room, the Canteen, the attendants' Sitting Room, and the Medical Library. In the Infirmary, he had noted that the dentist worked five mornings a week, and that he apparently gave his own anesthetics and that the dispensing was done by the doctor. Dr. Forrester had done two tonsillectomies that morning, the Operating Room in full swing. He had queried of Dr. Forrester. Essential to keep up the records. Dr. Fletcher took pains to record every detail, including the patients' and staff's evening meals. That day, for dinner, patients had been served: stew, mashed potatoes, tapioca pudding. Staff: soup, roast mutton, potatoes, carrots, raisin pie.

But it had been Dr. Fletcher's inspection of the Wards and Cottages that had caused Dr. Horne the most concern. His report had been nothing if not scathing. Of Cottage B (Low-Grade Adults — Male), Dr. Fletcher had reported:

> 206 patients, 12 attendants — 1 to 17 patients. This building is in bad repair.... The guarded side rooms for two patients each are bad. The toilets

> and lavatories are very dirty. No toilet paper and no privacy ... patients take exercise walking about the Day Room, do not go out except occasionally in fine weather.... Four patients were in straightjackets. Some patients had no beds. No fireproof inside staircase.

He had noted, severely, of another cottage: "On the top flat one patient dressed in short skirt only." The following day, on February 11, his observations of Cottage K (Males) had been similar in tone:

> Dormitories crowded with beds.... I found in one ward six cases of scabies locked in with no attendant. In another room I found fourteen unfortunates locked in with no attendant — no ventilation and little attempt at cleanliness. I note that in these cottages there are patients on night duty with no apparent opportunity to sleep in daytime. I think this is a dangerous practice.

No one would deny the truth of Dr. Fletcher's accusations, but, again, where was the funding from Premier Henry of the conservative government for extra staff? thought Dr. Horne testily. Dr. Fletcher had moved on to Cottage M (Higher-Grade Females):

> Even here we have girls with almost normal intelligence. The toilets were absolutely without any privacy. The case of Charlotte Jones was brought to my attention as one who can make a good living, but who is liable to sexual indiscretions.... Cockroaches in considerable numbers principally in the sculleries.

The next morning, February 12, breakfast had been recorded as: "Porridge with bread and butter, marmalade. Some had sausages from the day before. One patient took two epileptic seizures. There was no disturbance."

Concerning Cottage A (241 beds, eight male, three female attendants, two night attendants), it had been duly noted that:

> Here as elsewhere in the Hospital, the helpless patients are on the top floor. The toilets face the ... basins and here as elsewhere, there is no attempt at privacy. I had nearly said decency.

"Hmph!" went Dr. Horne, leafing through Dr. Fletcher's report once again before starting on his own. Of course, Cottage L (Low-Grade Elderly Females), one of the oldest Cottages in the hospital, was in a state of dilapidation (superintendents had drawn attention to it for years). Dr. Fletcher had found several patients in straightjackets. One patient had apparently been washing in a toilet.

Dr. Fletcher had continued, much in the same vein:

> I noticed that the water had been cut off and was informed it was off for hours. Low-grade patients locked in without care. Verandahs should be heated. I saw cockroaches in the daytime in the Dietetic Room....

He had concluded: "Washroom toilets are a disgrace to this province."

Dr. Fletcher had also made comment re: Jamie D:

> Case of Jamie D.
> No report from doctor. Patient found to have syphilis. No discussion as to whether he should continue as a barber.

And so the complaints and praise went on.

> SHOEMAKING — 25 boys part time — an excellent trade school. The shoes now being turned out are much better than formerly.
> SEWING ROOM — 35 girls. An excellent vocational center.
> LAUNDRY — 2 male, 5 female employees, 30 women and a variable number of boys. The upstairs is constantly dripping water. The floor is wet and the ironing tables are wet.... The laundry after a few washings — that is, the ward laundry — is of a dirty grey colour. The laundry man says it is due to it coming in so dirty.
> HAIR PICKING — a group of low grade patients — good vocational.
> THE AMUSEMENT HALL. Large — poorly ventilated. Are the moving pictures to be discontinued?

Dr. Fletcher continued, and here is where Dr. Horne flushed with anxiety: "Mortuary — found dried blood on table from last autopsy, and rusty instruments."

Nevertheless, Dr. Fletcher had concluded: "I believe we have here what may be an excellent institution."

That had been the previous year's inspection, but Dr. Horne was determined to be optimistic. The fact was Dr. Horne was fond of Orillia. He had been born on Wolfe Island in 1896, and his mother still lived there (he was not a city man, he prided himself). His wife and children were also happy in Orillia; the two boys had their schooling in town with Dr. Hamilton's boys and Mr. Zarfas' son, Donald, a bright boy. Dr. Hamilton and his little family were also happily ensconced in a separate house on the grounds, while Dr. James lived in the apartment above the Infirmary.

Thin wintry sunlight fell over the desk at which the great Dr. Alexander Beaton himself had once sat at the beginning of the century, no doubt as irritated by government inspectors as himself. Old Beaton, a feisty Scot, had not been one to suffer fools gladly. Dr. Horne considered his response to Dr. Fletcher again. He was annoyed by the reference to *grey* laundry — the inspector just did not realize those women and girls did over *28,000* pieces of ward sheets and clothing items per week.

As to the inspector's complaint concerning the use of restraints, Dr. McGhie before him had put in a request to Dr. Edward Ryan, Director of Medical Services down in Toronto, for the installation of four continuous baths in the hospital for Hydrotherapy, two on the female side, and two on the male side of the hospital. Dr. McGhie had even recommended a company, the Powers Company, who manufactured continuous bath mixtures. This had not materialized for the moment. Nurses had to rely on basic techniques: cold wet packs, Scotch douche (Dr. Horne was not quite sure of them), irrigation, and full hot blanket pack — all of which were vital in getting control of overexcited or violent patients.

He took up his pen again, determined to stress the achievements of staff and patients alike, after being careful first to congratulate Dr. McGhie on his promotion to Director of Hospital Services on Nov. 1, 1930. He enumerated the successes of Orillia: the first class of Nurses had graduated from the School of Nursing in the hospital on May 28, 1931. The Physical Instructor had given 1,495 gymnasium classes and 180 special corrective classes as a result of which two spastic paraplegics had been taught to walk.

He continued proudly, concerning the Mongolian patients:

> During the past year a complete survey of our Mongolian patients was made by J. G. Dewan. On January 16, 1932, Dr. J. H. Forrester did a Wassermann series on all our patients with a view to promoting special work with those suffering from congenital syphilis, the tests sent down to the Connaught laboratories in Toronto.

Under Mr. Downey, the laboratories had proved useful on several occasions testing new toxins on the inmates. The Connaught Laboratories in Toronto, where vaccines, serums and antitoxins were manufactured, were saving the lives of hundreds of thousands of people in Canada and across the world. When a scarlet fever epidemic had broken out in the institution in 1925, under Mr. Downey's superintendency, over one thousand "Dick" tests were carried out, with 297 positive reactions to which experimental immunization had then been given. Mr. Downey had regarded it as a service to the public as well as to themselves — epidemics spread quickly within the crowded wards. "The subsequent observation of this work proved a factor in the standardization of the protective dose of scarlet fever antitoxin, a matter of inestimable public importance." There had been consequently no deaths from scarlet fever, Mr. Downey reported proudly at the time: What would have happened if they had all died was another matter, of course, and so it remained a fuzzy issue that was not to surface for over a half a century.

Dr. Horne returned to the Report at hand, cheerfully citing further staff activities at Orillia. Dr. Wicks had done a survey and reported syphilis as a cause of Amentia, and Miss V. O. Brazier had undertaken the study of the Idiot group from a training aspect. Dr. Horne now moved on to what he saw as his personal achievement: the reorganization and establishment of "Ward Schools" for low-grade and imbecile patients.

Dr. McGhie had previously brought in psychologists from the University of Toronto, for advice on the curriculum. Dr. William McPhee had come and tested the I.Q. of a number of patients and worked with Dr. McGhie on a completely new curriculum (this would necessarily be for High Grades in the Upper Academic School). One of the things that Dr. McPhee had noted was that the teachers had little idea of what happened to the patients once they left the schoolroom and were ignorant of what the children did in Ward Work. Of course, Dr. McPhee was but a psychologist with little actual experience of dealing with low-grade idiots and imbeciles all day long in an overcrowded, underfunded institution, and the necessity to keep them under control, Dr. Horne bristled.

Admirable though Dr. McGhie's recommendations had been — (he had actually had patients learning "Hearts of Oak" from the Public School *Reader Book III* in Upper Academic School!) — one had to be realistic. There was a preponderance of low-grade inmates now in Orillia. Dr. Horne had developed what he called "Ward School" for the idiots and imbeciles, where preliminary training prepared them for the Training Yards. Ward Work could include menial tasks such as cleaning floors, windows, beds, walls, corridors, urinals, sinks and baths, as well as disinfecting clothing, and changing bedpans.

Dr. Horne had also introduced "occupations" in "Ward School" such as the clearing and draining of swamp land open pit (by the railway line) by 100 imbecile boys, and moving sludge from the open pit, so important to the proper running of the sewerage system. The sewage plant, built in 1920 in Mr. Downey's time, was known as the "activated sludge system": compressed air from the Boiler Room oxidized the contents of the tank and the effluent liquid ran into the lake while the sludge passed under the railway track to an open pit. When the wind blew the wrong way, the foulest odours drifted up over the lawns and the flowered terraces, spoiling the view for visitors. What was needed was a new plant — like so much else in Orillia. Low-grade imbeciles were also occupied at the Coal Pile, clearing land, shovelling snow, and doing other physical tasks relative to their level of ability, he wrote proudly. For high-grade boys there was a Special Farm Group, as milking cows and sowing seed required some intelligence.

He would not forget the success of the girls. Colony House had been opened in the town of Orillia on West Street, on July 1, 1931. About fifteen girls were probated at a time, working in homes around town from eight in the morning to six at night. They got half their wages, which were banked for them in accounts, with the rest going to the institution (though already complaints were surfacing in the town that the girls were taking away domestic jobs from the towns-women):

> The establishment of Lorimer Lodge (in Toronto) has greatly assisted us..... This was formerly The Haven, originally the Prison Gate Mission, established to accommodate girls released from prison. It had a nursery for the children of the residents. They took in girls on probation from Ontario Hospitals in Orillia and also Cobourg — a useful outlet for the high-grade girls on probation (who) still remained wards of the government, since they needed supervision until integrated into the community. Lorimer Lodge also took in teenage girls from Junior Vocational Schools in Toronto in danger of becoming delinquent.

Yes, Colony House and Lorimer Lodge were excellent programs for wayward girls.

38.

THE GIRLS WALKED SLOWLY BY after breakfast, wending their way, two by two, led by the nursing attendant. They were going to Sewing in the Industrial Shops, behind Cottage C.

Elvina lived in Cottage O, the new three-storey, brick building, similar to D, as Robbie now knew. Completed a year ago, the bricks were still bright red. It stood near Entrance B, overlooking Memorial Avenue.

The girls, aged between twelve and twenty, wore long, drab housedresses. Sometimes you glimpsed ankles and breasts bobbing under their pinafores. Their hair was cut in the usual pudding-basin style above the ears, and straight across their foreheads. They shuffled along, some stumbling and swaying as if they walked on stumpy legs; others wandered out of line. Girls he now recognized as "Mongols" shambled heavily, making grunting noises. Still, they were girls.

Robbie watched through the windows. You could only look — and whistle — as he hauled wet sheets to hurl into the dryers. One of them turned to look at him; he was sure it was Elvina. He thought he recognized her reddish hair. She pushed out her tongue and made a "V" with her fingers and motioned up and down.

At once the morning came alive. Then the line turned sharply into Sewing, and she was gone. But he had seen her.

Robbie had been transferred to Laundry, now that he was a year older. It was in a low building at the end of a long glass passage. They needed strong boys in there to do the heavy lifting of wet laundry, to push it through the huge mangles and then the dryers. Afterwards, the girls did the folding and pressing at their end of the shop. His back and shoulders ached. He had never worked so hard or done such heavy labour as in Orillia, lugging coal, digging trenches, clearing snow in winter. But he wanted to earn his points to attend the Social in Recreation Hall on Saturday night, instead of going to see the moving pictures.

"Oh, Shine on, shine on, harvest moon... "

He was close at last to Elvina on the gym floor, trying to move his knees in rhythm to the jazzy tunes being cranked out on the old Victrola gramophone with its big trumpet at the front of the room. Some of the cheery aides showed the patients on the floor how to do the Charleston. Why shouldn't they have a little harmless fun? It was part of Social Etiquette, some of the staff said among themselves (especially for the patients they knew were normal). Elvina's hips swayed to the music; she was laughing and gay. Young girls and women approved by the Social Service Committee stood awkwardly along the sides of the gym, known as the Ballroom for the evening, waiting to be asked to dance. The girls had been prettied up by some kind attendants, their short hair curled in the Bobby Shop in Cottage M. Some wore lip colour. Many were in their good dresses (often too large or too tight, handed out by the nurse in their ward). The air was heavy with the thrum of lively songs.

"*Bye bye, blackbird.... Blackbird, blackbird, gotta be on your way, where there is sunshine galore....*"

"Meet outside the lav'tries," whispered Elvina. She was in a flowery dress and wedge-heeled shoes. Out on the landing, you could see the attendants and nurses through the glass doors standing against the wall, their gym keys clipped to their belts. Robbie and Elvina stood outside the lavatories and then quickly, before the monitor spotted them or Nurse Bigley turned (she had the keys to the toilets) they ran down the stairs — *quick, quick* — to the next landing. There, Elvina put her arms around him and put her face close to his. She was laughing and out of breath. She had big, greenish teeth. When she rolled her tongue over his, he was surprised at how giddy he felt. His tongue started to swell. He moaned.

"Got any pin?" She meant pin money. He shook his head.

Elvina could read and write and do figures. She was in Group 25 of Upper Academic School and had been in the Christmas Pageant. She knew how to tell the time, how time passed. She knew years, months, days, and something called "homonyms" and "synonyms."

"Last year, doctors come and stuck needles into all us girls all the time," she said. She pulled out a ciggy from her pocket, matches from down the front of her dress, and struck one against the wall and lit up.

She gave Robbie a drag. His lips felt hot and sore and wonderful. What would she do next?

"It was for Wass'mann tests," she said. Dr. Forrester had been doing a series of Wassermann tests on all the patients. Elvina had heard the nurses talking in the Infirmary, part of research on patients with congenital syphilis. Robbie tried to look as if he understood this. The needle had pricked her arm. She was seventeen.

"I 'ad a baby," said Elvina, "in th' Haven in Toronno." She had been working in the Dominion Box Company when the CAS of Toronto got her. The baby must be nearly two now, she said suddenly, anxious and fretful. She was up for probation soon, to be a domestic. She wanted to go to Toronto, back to the factory, and stab Mr. Ennis.

Orillia

April 20, 1933

Mrs. Henry Hewitt
22 River Street
Toronto, Ontario

Re: Robbie and Edgar Hewitt

Dear Mrs. Hewitt:

I have been in receipt of a letter from Miss Dorkins informing us that you have been given some very unpleasant information concerning our Institution. I trust that Miss Dorkins has relieved you of this worry as I would like to point out that our Institution might be looked upon as a boarding school where every care and attention is given every child. Relatives are permitted to visit and everything that is possible to be done from an educational and health point of view is done for each individual patient with the idea of having them so trained that they can take their place in the community. I wish to assure you that your boys are in excellent health and are quite happy and contented in their surroundings.

Yours very truly,
S. J. W. Horne, M.D.
Medical Superintendent

Henry read the letter slowly out loud when it arrived at 20 River Street. The postman had knocked on the door and called up, "Letter for the 'Ewitts." There had been excitement — the little Hewitt children running around the kitchen. The Newells downstairs had shouted it was not for them, and what the hell was all the commotion about? Old Mr. Crabbe, who lived in a tiny room behind the stairs, had hobbled up the stairs waving the letter. Henry broke open the seal and drew out the letter with the Orillia Hospital letterhead. Only he was able to read.

"Looks like we're in trouble with th' law, Florrie," he frowned. "What the bleedin' 'ell did you say to Miss Dorkins?" he shouted. Florrie was half-deaf.

Florrie began to tremble and cry. "Hear bad things," she wept. "Bad things to th' boys from Mrs. Garr'ty." Florrie was frightened. Mrs. O'Garrity had heard it from Mrs. Demsey up the road on Bleeker Street who had a handicapped boy the doctor wanted to put in Orillia but she had refused. She did not want Alfred put in a cage. How had the great Doctor known what Mrs. O'Garrity had said about the institution? It must be ghosties what let on what Mrs. O'Garrity said.

Henry told Miss Dorkins when she came about. Miss Dorkins assured them carefully that the rumours were unfounded. There were always stories coming out of Orillia. Best to write a conciliatory letter to Dr. Horne on Florrie's behalf. Miss Dorkins glanced at Florrie. She was thin and wan. Strands of greying hair fell in thin wisps from a tight knot held with string at the back of her head. Her pinafore torn and dirty and had spots of grease all over it. She was still nursing the youngest, a feeble-looking mite at her breast. Florrie at once began to blurt out a somewhat incoherent apology that Mr. Hewitt struggled to put to paper. Miss Dorkins sighed. She had over fifty such families like the Hewitts on her roster.

22 River Street

Dear Dr. Horne,

Sorry to give you all this trobe as I got your nice letter to day and was so plese to get it. I did hear some thing that it was only for bad boys that stole money and it wory me a bit but as soon as I seeing Miss Dorkins she made me quite hapy and now Dear Dr. I am so hapy and I am so Sorry for all this trobe and I don't know how am I ever going to Thank you for your good work and kindnes to my Dear boys as they were always good

> boy at home to they mother and I hope they are the same out there. I would love to come out and see them but I am having it kind of hard time no wone working for 2 years So I will try and come as soon as I can. I have a girl Ella 9 years old and They want me to send her out to your hospital please give my love to my boys and tell them I am trying to send them something for Easter.
> Yours very truly,
> Mrs. Hewitt

Of course, the general confusion behind Florrie's earnest promises was only too evident to Mr. Walker, that someone like Florrie Hewitt would never be able to even find her way to Orillia. The letter was once again in Henry Hewitt's handwriting. He must have sat at the kitchen table and laboriously written it on his wife's behalf, scrunched over the sheets of paper, dipping his pen carefully in the inkwell in order not to make blots as he had been taught so long before in England as a boy in Junior III. The Hewitts must have had to buy paper, ink, an inkwell, and a straight-nibbed pen. Or had they used a kind neighbour's writing materials? Or perhaps someone who was literate wrote it for a few pennies?

39.

"I KNOWS HOW TO GIT TO TORONNA," said Elvina. They had kissed, a quick wet one in the basement, before the aide saw; a kiss that made Robbie throb in his work pants again, he said. He would do anything for Elvina, he cried. She was smart. She could read train timetables, something very important for running away, she said mysteriously. When a train came through going south by day (Toronto was south) you lowered the semaphore flag by the station and the engineer stopped the train. But they could not do that. They would have to get a train after dark. Elvina had found this out at the station when she had been in town on a pass with Miss Kidd, the nurse's aide. While Miss Kidd sipped tea and ordered ice cream and wafers in a café, Elvina slipped off. It had been worth the demerit. "There's a midnight freight train that comes through."

Saturday evening was best, after the talkies in the gym. They could stay back in the lavatories when the attendants and aides would be busy with the lines, and then slip down to the tramways and escape through the window by the canteen. Elvina knew the way: she could read the signposts.

Oh, but how exciting it was to be running off with Elvina who knew everything: what time the train came down the track, when the whistle blew, where it slowed right down on the curve before the Orillia Station. She had all her tuck money saved in a cloth bag she had made in Sewing. Both had asked leave to go to the lavatory after the movies, and slipped through a tramway window in the basement while hundreds of patients upstairs were lining up to return to their wards. Quickly they ran down the slope to the hedge far below. The vast Institution glowing in the darkness, a daunting mass behind them. They had then hidden in the bushes. The train came rumbling down the track lighting up the bushes and the cedar hedge, the roof full of strange crouching bodies — rail-riders. Robbie and Elvina jumped separately onto the moving car. Elvina's skirt got caught and ripped on a girder. Some men on top helped haul her up. "On the lam," they cried cheerily. "Here's a lassie."

"Keep yer 'ead down for th' tunnels," warned a desperate-looking older man clinging to the rails of the boxcar. He had an unshaven, pock-marked face, and his teeth had glinted green in the darkening twilight. "Escape from hell," he grimaced.

Dr. Horne went into swift action. He checked the Minute Book, a heavy leather-bound volume in which was recorded each day's activities at the hospital: Morning Reports sent in by supervisors at the various Cottages at nine a.m. after Roll Call giving the number of patients on the Ward, and again at nine p.m., including any reports of fits or burials. Mr. Bayliss, Night Attendant on D, had first noticed Hewitt's absence at Roll Call after the boys on the ward had brushed their teeth. His brother Edgar had been taken into the Punishment Room and roughed up a bit: "You knows where 'e is! Tell us!" But to no avail. Edgar had sobbed he did not know anything, but was kept tied up for safety in the Punishment Room. Mr. Bayliss had called Emergency at once by pressing the red button at the Nursing Station. Nurse Moffatt had done likewise over in Cottage O concerning the Thomas girl. It was obvious the two had absconded together.

The grounds were searched including the bushes and the beach hut by the lake, as well as the Smoking Rooms in the basement. Monitors checked the canteen and tramways where the broken window lock was discovered. Mr. Walker, Administrative Assistant, rang the police in town to check out the bus shelter and train station. That was when it occurred to Mr. Walker that the culprits may have actually jumped a freight train.

Orillia, Ontario

June 4, 1934

Mr. Henry Hewitt
20 Oak Street
Toronto, Ontario

Dear Sir,

I regret to inform you at this time that Robbie eloped from the hospital some time before evening Roll Call. A thorough search of the grounds and vicinity was made, but no trace of him could be found. If you should hear of his whereabouts, will you kindly get in touch with us immediately.

Yours truly,

N. L. Walker, M.D.

(for Medical Superintendent, Dr. Horne)

The train sped through the dark countryside, waves of smoke and cinders blowing back over the silent, desperate rail-riders. It was cold. Robbie was excited and clung to Elvina whose face was tense.

Of course, the Station Police were waiting, on the alert at Union Station in Toronto. Robbie and Elvina were quickly spotted clambering down, trying to slip through the train yards, unaware how easily identifiable they were in their institutional clothing, their faces and clothes covered with dust and cinders from the tunnels. The Station Master had been contacted by Dr. Horne himself: "Two elopers possibly jumped the train around 11:00 p.m." These types had a certain street sense and cunning, and Hewitt would have followed the Thomas girl, who was of high-grade intelligence but of dubious morals.

Clinical Record: Hewitt, Robbie. Case #5734.

June 5, 1934

Robbie Hewitt eloped yesterday evening before Roll Call, with Elvina Thomas (Case #5656, Cottage O.) A search was made of the vicinity, but they were not located. They were picked up in Toronto and placed in #12 Police Station. The hospital car brought them back to the hospital this evening.

D. B. H.

Robbie lay, his feet shackled, on the narrow bed in Punishment Room One, off Ward D. He could hear the familiar voices of the boys in the dorm beyond the door, preparing for bed, Night Attendant Bayliss calling, "Get along, you pricks, get along."

Robbie tensed, pulling at the iron shackles joined by a heavy chain between his feet. His head and arms ached from the scuffle with police officers, and his buttocks and back burned from the whipping he'd had from Bayliss on his return. He recalled a police cell, iron bars in rows, and that he was locked in, he had realized, just like in the dorm, in the "waiting area" they had said. Elvina was someplace else because she was a girl, just like in the hospital too. They were to stay put until the attendants arrived from Orillia. There was a piss-pot by the small window in the Punishment Room, a plate of dried bread and a cup of water on the floor. "That'll learn'yer, boy," Mr. Bayliss had smirked. He and a monitor from Cottage C had put on the shackles, one holding him down. This boy had to be watched.

Elvina had been taken away as soon as the staff car from Toronto had drawn up to the Administration Building, met by a worried Dr. Horne, Mr. Walker, Mr. Zarfas, the bursar, and Nurse Moffatt. Elvina had fretted. Her probation to Lorimer Lodge would now, of course, be rescinded, Mr. Walker informed her grimly. "Foolish girl!" he admonished.

"I'm eighteen, I c'n go where I please," she had said sulkily.

"Well, you'll find out different, Miss!" said Nurse Moffatt. Elvina would remain for the time being in the Infirmary to be checked over. Who knew whom Thomas had been with even in the short time she had been on the loose? This girl already had one child out of wedlock at fifteen. Tense and tight-lipped, refusing to cry, Elvina had been led away.

Robbie tossed restlessly on the narrow bed, the shackles rubbing his ankles. He tensed as night began to deepen in the small room. The restless breathing of boys half-asleep in the dorm on the other side of the door did not help. Presently, he heard the tread of Mr. Bayliss's feet. Then came the twist of a key in the lock, the turn of the handle on the door. Bayliss's body looming softly for such a big man. Robbie turned towards him. Pointless to cry out, "No, oh no, sir, please..."

Dr. Horne scanned the Register of Elopement before signing, "Robbie Hewitt ... an eloper." There had been 28 escapes the year before, in 1933 — six of them girls. One girl, a Mary Dewson, High-Grade Moron, was marked: "never returned." Thirteen in total had not been recaptured. Of course, elopements were not uncommon at Orillia, especially during the spring and summer season. Closer watch must be kept during the summer months, and strict segregation must be imposed at all times, with exception to supervised functions such as Prayer Service on Sundays, Socials, and visits to the Orillia Opera House.

The heavy, thick, wood-bound Register of Elopements was laid out in columns dating back to 1917, when a Frank Rice had absconded on June 23. The columns were under concise headings: "Register No.," "Name of Patient," "Warrant or Certificate," "Date of Elopement," "Date of

Return," "Religion," "Time Out," "Married or Single," etc. He checked for that year, 1934. Fifty patients eloped to date, 27 so far not caught, 14 being girls, he frowned (they apparently escaped in pairs, according to the Register). The Hewitt boy and the Thomas girl had been among the unlucky ones, or less astute, easily recaptured, thanks to Mr. Walker. Quick thinking on Mr. Walker's part, noted Dr. Horne, to have checked train schedules.

A note should be made in her record of the cunning of the Thomas girl, who could read.

Hospital for Insane, Orillia

Report of Recapture of: Robbie Hewitt

1. Date of elopement:	June 4, 1934
2. Date of Recapture:	June 5, 1934
3. Where Recaptured:	Toronto, Ont.
4. Amount of expenses connected with the recapture:	80 cents

5. By whom recaptured and in what manner:
Word was received from Toronto and an Attendant was sent down to bring them back.
6. Has any ill result followed elopement? No.

Dr. Horne viewed for himself the latest missive in the Orillia mailroom from Mr. Hewitt, a most high-handed letter that actually contained a veiled threat. Dr. Horne's face tightened.

Dear Sir:

Received your letter dated the 4 June and one [on] the 7 [June] regarding my son Robbie and was very much surprised at his behaviour. I am at loss to account for his actions. Maybe he is longing to see his parents. A year and ten months is a long time without seeing any one of us. If I was in better circumstances I would visit Robbie and Edgar. If they had a holiday at home it might help to make them more contented. But sooner than let them stay with you and turn out to be criminals I would rather let them come home and take full responsibility They are not Bad boys nobody can convince they are only Mentally backward.

I am an Ex Service man and I know what discipline is. I had often felt like revolting against it myself. I am afraid I will have to hear more favourable reports. Otherwise I will demand their release from your care. Hoping they will not cause you any more trouble in the future.
I remain Yours
Truly,
Henry Hewitt
20 Oak Street, Toronto, Ont
formerly 22 River Street

P.S. I no a friend that has a car that would take Them home on a Holiday.

A firm, clear response was, of course, in order here that would put an end to Mr. Hewitt's grandiose idea that he (an unemployed labourer of low intelligence with no stable home) could simply remove his children at will from the institution.

Orillia, Ontario

June 18, 1934

Mr. Henry Hewitt,
20 Oak Street,
Toronto, Ontario

Re: Robbie and Edgar Hewitt

Dear Sir:

In reply to your recent letter regarding your sons Robbie and Edgar, I am glad to inform you that they are getting on quite nicely here in hospital and have made fairly good progress at school. I might state that we are giving the boys every possible attention here in hospital and are doing all in our power to better their condition. They are now occupied in Landscape Gardening.

I may state that, at any time you have the opportunity, we would be only too glad to have you call and go through the building where your sons are at present domiciled. I believe

that both Robbie and Edgar are fairly contented, and I think it was more through the influence of another patient that Robbie eloped recently from hospital.
Hoping this clears up this matter, I remain,
Yours truly,
N. L. Walker, M.D.
(for Medical Superintendent Dr. S. Horne)

Yet another letter from those Hewitts in Toronto! This time, from the mother. Mr. Walker frowned, taking in Florrie Hewitt's latest missive, with all its unfortunate punctuation and spelling errors. It had been stamped in the Orillia mailroom: "RECEIVED JUNE 26 1934, ONTARIO HOSPITAL ORILLIA," with the familiar black circle. He showed it to Dr. Horne. Why couldn't this woman understand that the boys were in residence to stay, and were not to have their training continually interrupted?

10 Sumach Street

June 26, 1934

Dear Sir,

Regarding Robbie and Edgar Hewitt I am asking you would you kindley let them come home for a Holliday I am willing to pay There fair as it would make me hapy as I hope they wont have to stay in Hospital very long as Robbie could be some suport to me now. I am just longing to see The Boys, and I Think it would do them good to get a Holliday at home I get a penshion.

I would be greafull if you will kindley let them come, I am shure They will be taken great care of as They have a good home and a good father and we are Just longing to see them.
From Mrs. Hewitt

Dr. Horne was taken aback by Mrs. Hewitt writing at all, being illiterate. It was obvious that Mr. Hewitt had put her up to it as a mother's plea might appeal to the heart-strings, a sort of last resort. Of course, it would not work. This family lived in circumstances clearly indicated in the boys' records from the CAS of Toronto as a virtual hovel. Yet she had persisted. He instructed Mr. Walker to reply unequivocally: "I think you would be well advised..."

Back in Toronto, Henry read Dr. Horne's letter aloud in the Hewitt kitchen: "...advised to leave the boys here for the summer ... require strict supervision..."

"Bleedin' 'ell, they ain't coming, Flo!" Henry tossed aside the letter. Florrie let out a wail as she threw some oats into the pot with the rabbit Henry had caught down by the Don River that had been on the stove simmering all week. Young Oswald, now age nine, had caught a little robin that morning and wrung its neck. He had brought it in still pulsing and Ella had chopped off its head with the cutter on the stovetop: "Me! Me!" she had clamoured, all excited. After Dada dipped it in the boiling water, she had helped pluck out the feathers and Mama had thrown it in the pot with the rabbit. Now Ella stood uncomprehending with her brothers and little sister, as her mother wept.

"Wished we not sent 'em, 'Enry. Mebbe Miz Dork'ns 'elp."

"I'll git them back, Flo."

It was not uncommon for parents and even ex-patients to write letters to the Superintendent, of course, as Dr. Horne well knew. Parents sometimes pleaded for the release of their child, others complained of treatment. Dr. Horne prided himself on the many letters of thanks he received from parents of high-grade ex-patients, the successful ones (who were, conceivably, "normal" from the outset. Of course, it was poverty, legal troubles, or homelessness that had more to do with their committal than retardation). These ones were full of praise for the institution, and grateful for the vocational training they had received at the institution. Indeed, the same training that Henry Hewitt had secretly hoped for and expected for his own boys.

But how to explain Mrs. Hewitt's persistent letters? What was she doing getting pen and inkwell and paper for a second time and approaching her husband, one wondered, or perhaps a neighbour — Mrs. O'Garrity? — to write again for her boys, the nearest she ever seemed to have come, according to the records, to giving voice to anything. Florrie Hewitt, long forgotten in the slums of Toronto of a past that once was, one of thousands of illiterate women, worn down by child-bearing and ill-health, was a forgotten statistic lost to the records. But something about Florrie here surely shone briefly through the grime and wretchedness of Lower Sumach Street.

40.

THE INSPECTION OF ORILLIA on July 31, 1933, by Dr. McGhie himself, former superintendent of Orillia from 1927-1930, and now Deputy Minister of Health, had given Dr. Horne much cause for concern, like most inspection reports over the years. Dr. McGhie had drawn attention to the ongoing problem of eneuresis (chronic bed-wetting) among the boys in the Male Wards in Cottage A:

> Notwithstanding that patients were taken up regularly during the night, the problem of eneuresis is not being checked to an appreciable extent. The attendant-in-charge was of the opinion that when patients were taken to the bathroom the shock of stepping on the cold tiled floor in their bare feet resulted in the visit being futile but that a return to the warm bed had the opposite effect.

But what had been the solution, Dr. Horne had wondered. Heated floors to match the warmth of the beds, on Orillia's pitiful budget?

On a different note, Dr. McGhie had praised the supervision of Cottage D for Boys. He had noted that a "special type of boy was housed there. Staff appear to be interested in the job of training rather than simply housing the boys under care." Praise indeed! That would be Mr. Atherton, a good sort of fellow on the wards, Dr. Horne had thought warmly.

Dr. McGhie had, however, unfortunately made further unfavourable comments about the running of the institution, this time concerning the mattress-making department in Trades, drawing attention to "soiled mattresses." He had noted that employees in charge said they could make double the mattresses if they had the cooperation of the laundry in sterilizing the hair. Dr. Horne had made a mental note to look into such practices as the washing of hair and ticking for mattresses, though the laundry was overloaded as it was, and was hair in the same category as sheets and towels?

Dr. Horne dipped his pen in his inkwell. It was time for the Superintendent's Annual Report on the Institutional Activities of Ontario Hospital, for the previous year 1933, in response to Acting Deputy Minister of Hospitals, Parliament Buildings, Toronto, Dr. B. T. McGhie's earlier report for that same year.

First in importance was the catastrophe at Orillia: the fire. It had in fact been a year of conflagration at the hospital, he mused. Only a month after Dr. McGhie's inspection, a fire of unknown origin had started on August 20, 1933, in the attic of the Recreation Hall, highly suspicious. That had been followed, on September 30, 1933, by a second fire "of incendiary origin" that had partly destroyed the roof in the piggery: "Fear some pigs lost. Our pigs are a special breed imported from Scotland." Here Dr. Horne paused, reluctant to admit the end of his endeavours with Colony House in Orillia, which had burned down at the end of 1932. That had been the year of old Dr. Beaton's death in Orillia at age ninety-four. He had loved the town, staying on there after his retirement, and contributing to the building of the sanctuary in Orillia Presbyterian Church. Colony House had subsequently been taken over by Lorimer Lodge in Toronto.

He hastened to assure Dr. McGhie, that the religious aspect of life at the hospital had not been compromised by the fire. Sunday Schools had been established in the Cottages, though limited to thirty for the year. As well, the more pleasant aspect of life for patients in the Orillia Hospital had continued: "Children from "K" "L" and "M" and Infirmary attended two Shirley Temple pictures at the Orillia Opera House."

He was proud, also, as always, of the magnitude of the Physical Instruction and Recreation Programme — 37 baseball teams, swimming, basketball; in winter, skating, and tobogganing; moving pictures and Orillia Band concerts in the Recreation Hall. It was little wonder that Dr. McGhie had commented in his Report that amusements for the patients were "greater in variety than most had at home." Most of all, he took pride in his success with the Probation Program begun under Dr. McGhie himself during his superintendency:

> We maintained our efforts in having patients placed on probation to the point where we have a waiting list of employers who are anxious to have our girls

> for domestic work. In this connection Lorimer Lodge has been of untold assistance in placing our girls in Toronto.

He was able to note further under Institutional Activities the gainful work of the residents:

> Our Ward School expands. Patients in Cottage D who have gone as far as they could in Academic School are doing Ward Work — weeding, stoning, raking, berry picking, trenching, coal shovelling, clearing land and swamps is done by this grade.

He continued in the same vein, stressing the labour of both the High Grades and the Imbeciles:

> The acreage of the garden was increased by eight acres which demanded a large number of high-grade boys. A large number of imbecile patients were placed with the Landscape Gardener, Farm, and at the Coal Pile.
>
> During the holiday season our school boys were kept well occupied at various tasks such as picking berries, weeding, etc., working with the utility men.

Yes, life in Orillia was certainly a mixture of work and play. He reported once again on the ongoing construction of new buildings and such with the help of patients.

> Construction of new buildings.... The rough work was done by the Unemployment Relief but the final grading, levelling, and seeding done under the supervision of our Landscape Gardener with patient labour.
>
> One mile of flagstone has been laid. A new bowling green is well under way, and five baseball diamonds were surfaced by our Junior boys.

Dr. Horne turned now to the vital issue of segregation of boys from girls, absolutely essential in a place like Orillia:

> The occupation of Cottage "O" for high grade girls of teen age has materially assisted us with segregation problems. This Cottage fully occupied by May 4th, 1933. One hundred and fifty beds added to accommodation at Orillia.

> Separate beaches now for boys and girls. This new beach has 300 boys and girls swimming with proper supervision.

And, appropriately he thought, the Social Services Department gave talks and lectures with Senior Boys and Girls on proper behaviour and table manners.

On the other hand, congestion of sleeping quarters was regrettably unchanged since Dr. Beaton's day. At present, patients were sleeping on the floor and there were over 1,000 on the waiting list. (He received one new application per day on average.) He noted that proper ventilation was also needed on the boys and girls' side in the Infirmary.

Nevertheless, that said, Dr. Horne had been delighted to report on the number of visitors to Orillia over the past year:

> A total of 304 persons visited the Institution. The most noted was the visit of their Excellencies the Earl of Bessborough and the Countess of Bessborough, on October 30th, 1933. The Vice-Regal Party visited the school and entrained from the Hospital Station.

Dr. Horne had been particularly gratified by the presence of their Excellencies — an Earl and Countess but also of the Mayor of Orillia and the numerous townspeople who had flocked excitedly to the Hospital in December for the Annual Christmas concert and pageant — this year *Little Red Riding Hood.*

One could not but help entertain a certain sense of self-congratulation. There was a time, he reflected, back in Dr. Beaton's day when the townsfolk of Orillia had regarded the Asylum as a "pest house" and the inmates, as "absolutely dangerous creatures."

41.

DR. HORNE STARED IN DISBELIEF at the letter from the Department of Public Welfare at Queen's Park, Toronto. It concerned the Hewitt boys. Apparently, Mr. Hewitt had somehow found his way to the correct government agency and — astounding — made a complaint to the Commissioner. The devil! Furthermore, here Dr. Horne grimaced in anger; he was requested to provide an explanation in answer to Mr. Hewitt's claims.

Department of Public Welfare
Stewart Building
149 College Street
Toronto, Canada

Dr. Horne,
Medical Superintendent,
Ontario Hospital
Orillia, Ontario

Re: Robbie and Edgar Hewitt
Dear Sir:

We are extremely interested in the above-mentioned family whom we have known for some time. We understand that, recently, Mr. Hewitt received a communication from you in regard to the elopement of Robbie from Orillia, and with that letter, he received a second letter stating that the boy had been returned to the Hospital. This information has worried the father considerably, as he feels that Robbie could not be happy in his present environment.

In order to assure him that Robbie and Edgar, who is also in the Hospital, are making satisfactory progress, we promised him that we would write you for a report on this matter. From the home situation, we feel that the two boys would be better cared for in the Ontario Hospital and we would like your approval of the present arrangement. We would be interested in a report of the diagnosis and prognosis of both boys.

Yours very truly,
A. W. Laver
Commissioner

The response to Mr. Laver would, of course, be terse and to the point. Dr. Horne was not going to be bullied by an illiterate.

Orillia, Ontario

July 19, 1935

Attention: Moss Park District
Mr. A.W. Laver,
Commissioner of Public Welfare,
Department of Public Welfare,
149 College Street,
Toronto, Ontario

Re: Robbie and Edgar Hewitt
Dear Sir:

In reply to your letter of July 13, regarding the above named boys, I may state that both Robbie and Edgar are at present residing in the hospital. Both boys were admitted on August 18 1932, and have been in residence since then. Edgar was diagnosed as a High-Grade Imbecile — CA: 12.7; MA: 5.6; I.Q.: 43, September, 1932. He is a weakly sort of boy, though active and inclined to be somewhat rough in his play. He has a slight speech defect, and since his admission to hospital, has been attending our academic school but his progress has been rather slow and he was demitted. Since admission, he has improved some both mentally and physically but not to the extent that we would advise his leaving the hospital.

> Robbie Hewitt, a brother of Edgar, is diagnosed as a High-Grade Imbecile – CA: 14.0; MA: 6.6; I.Q.: 46, August 1932. Since admission to the hospital he has been receiving some academic training and he has made some progress, but this has been very slow, and he soon reached his limits. The aetiology in both these cases is heredity.
>
> As to the prognosis, I am sorry to state that I am unable to give a definite prognosis at this time as I feel that this entirely depends on their ability to grasp the training which is afforded them here in the hospital. At the best, I do not believe they would be any better than farm labourers.
>
> Yours very truly,
> N. L. Walker, M.D.
> (For Medical Superintendent, Dr. S. J. Horne)

It was hot out on the terrace. Robbie lifted the hoe and it thud dully into the dry earth. Thud, thud, thud. They were to weed the beds in the hot sun. He sweated, his neck red and burning. Jack Daly, his buddy now in the dorm since Fletcher had transferred to Cottage C, was raking leaves; they were then to sift in cow manure from the farm that had been brought in buckets by Group 9. Some boys in Group 5 from Cottage C had been swimming in the lake after their farm labours, down on the boys' beach accompanied by attendants. There was a boys' beach and a girls' beach, carefully separated. The boys tried to see what was going on with the girls across the sandy shore, but they were carefully hidden behind screens. Then, they came out half-naked, standing sissy-like at the edge of the water, and covering their chests in a criss-cross with their hands the way girls did. Robbie could not stop looking when he got the chance when kind Mr. Atherton took his group. He tried to see if Elvina was among them, but she was not. She is gone, he thought. To a place called Cobourg, she had whispered once quickly in line, a long time back.

He could hear screams and squeals and splashing far below; the voices were carried up the slope. It reminded Robbie of long ago — so long ago now — when Dada had taken him and Edgar and the little ones out on the free tram the city ran to Sunnyside Beach in Toronto, everyone packed in the wooden car, until the conductor in the centre called out "*Sunnyside!*" The regular streetcar ride was seven cents for adults and four cents for children. You got off at Roncesvalles. The excitement and thrill of the great lake at the edge of the sand you had not known was there before was strong. Before, all you knew were the row houses and broken walls and dusty bins and frowzy trees and factories and their smoke. The lake water was dark blue, crested with waves, and birds that Dada said were gulls. There was the beautiful white Palais Royale, the swimming tank, the carousel, the helter-skelter, and the loud gay music blaring into the ears of bathers and day trippers up and down the boardwalk. How grand! How wonderful! Dada had extra pennies for ice cream cones and even — joy! — cotton candy for them to share, a sticky mouthful each. Then Dada forgot the slump; you just jumped in the tank and swam in the bathing costumes Miss Dorkins had brought them, all of them in the tadpole end as no one could swim. That is, except for Dada, who wore a funny wool bathing costume down to his knees with wool straps extending over his shoulders. You could be arrested by the cops if you were half-naked to the waist, said Dada. "Bleedin' rubbish if you arsk me."

They went home on the return streetcar run by the city, at the end of the day, tired and red-skinned and joyful. Mama had stayed behind to nurse the baby, Sophie, who was poorly. "Summer diarrhea," he had heard Miss Dorkins say, with a strange sigh. That was something you died from, something to do with the crap-house in the yard and the flies (he and Edgar would catch them and pull off their wings on hot afternoons) and the hot small room they lived in, dark and dank. But he longed for it. He longed for Mama's roast sprats and for the old mattress at night, his arms around his brothers and sisters.

Clinical Record: Hewitt, Robbie.
July 22, 1935. Cottage D
Was transferred from Coal Pile to the Landscape Garden this month.
Easy-going lad. Suffers from occasional enuresis.
T. Mac.D.

July 25, 1935.
Robbie says he likes his work in the Landscape Garden. He is doing satisfactory work. Mixes well. Has eloped twice this season and shows a continual tendency to continue his elopement. A good worker. He is out on the lawns now; very untidy.
D. P. L.

July 26, 1935.
This boy eloped again yesterday from the Terrace accompanied by Jack Daly at around 4:00 p.m. He was returned to Cottage D at 6:00 p.m. by Mr. Atherton.
D. P. L.

Dr. Horne looked out over the grassy slope and terrace of the hospital from his office window, irritated but also resigned. The Probation Bond had been duly issued for Robbie and Edgar Hewitt (Authority: R.S.O. 1927), Form 117. Mr. Hewitt, of moron intelligence, had failed to grasp the fine opportunities here at Orillia Hospital for the boys, and that they could be of permanent benefit to the hospital, looked after for life.

He had persisted that Robbie "must of not liked something 'bout the place. Boys don't run away from a place fer nothin'. You can't keep 'em here, I gort my rights as a father."

So they were gone, demitted on Bond, one of the lucky few. The boys were never to return to Cottage D, to the Coal Pile, or Group 15 Lower Academic School in which they had spent so little time. You could be released if the parents so willed it on a Bond, but so few did. The Demission lists in the yearly reports attested to that. Out of 1,805 patients in residence in 1934, only 88 were discharged. It was not necessarily a life sentence, permanent custody. Parents could exert pressure, could fight, and Mr. Hewitt had.

Henry Hewitt, as father of Robbie and Edgar, "inmates of the Ontario Hospital, Orillia," went the Bond, had promised Dr. Horne "to keep oversight" of his sons while they lived in the Hewitt home (now moved yet again, back to rooms on Sumach Street, noted Mr. Walker), for the period of one month. Mr. Hewitt was further required, according to the Bond, to send Mr. Walker a monthly report of the mental and physical condition of the boys. His neglect to do so would mean the forfeiture of the boys' readmission to Orillia.

Was it surprising that no monthly reports had followed? Who knew what was happening to those boys — not bad lads — down in the slums of Toronto? By the end of winter, despite a reminder sent to Mr. Hewitt that unless the rules were obeyed and some indication of the boys' progress received, the Hewitt boys would lose their place and be permanently discharged.

Dr. Horne sighed. One was not always successful in this line of work. The entire probationary program (minimal at best) was due to the effort and insight of previous Superintendent Dr. McGhie who, not unlike Dr. Beaton in the founding days of the Idiot Asylum, actually saw Orillia as a place of opportunity where patients would eventually be released, well-trained, back into the community. Mentally retarded children, in Dr. McGhie's opinion, differed "only in degree and not in kind from the normal and superior." That was the ideal. And the ideal was often far from the reality.

Elvina Thomas, for instance, had had a different fate. She had been strictly contained on Ward M-3 and then later transferred to Cobourg. A survey of girls on probation at Orillia, conducted by Marion Haugh, a Social Service Internee at the hospital in 1933, had shown that out of 39 girls in one group, admitted by warrant or from the Juvenile Court, sixteen were unmarried mothers, with one having seven illegitimate children; eight had been admitted for abnormal sexual tendencies; three were charged with promiscuity; four with moral weakness; and one with nymphomaniacy. That was what one was dealing with.

Dr. Horne thankfully closed the Hewitt file, hopefully forever.

Ontario Hospital at Orillia
NOTICE OF DISCHARGE

To be sent in duplicate to the Deputy Minister of Hospitals, Toronto, immediately upon discharge of patient

Patient's full name:	Robbie James Hewitt
Date of Discharge:	September 5, 1935
Legal domicile: City, Town, Village or Township, and County:	Toronto, York County
Paying or Indigent:	Indigent
Date of admission:	August18, 1932

If ordinary paying patient how much is owing for maintenance and when will payment likely be received in full settlement?
From last information available how was patient progressing? Very well.

Feb. 2, 1935
S. J. Horne
Superintendent
O. Zarfas Steward

42.

THEY WERE BACK. Tall, handsome, healthy boys with lots of fat on them, Mama and Dada cried. Robbie and Edgar swaggered about, young men now: Robbie was seventeen, a man, and Edgar sixteen. They cuffed their little brothers and sisters amiably, and tickled the baby Charlotte, who had been born while they were in Orillia. Everything was the same: the same sort of house with its small room reeking of onions. The Hewitts had moved back to Lower Sumach Street into a row house. Everything seemed cramped to the boys after the high-ceilinged wards of Orillia.

They were up at dawn expecting to do jobs, to pick up coal from down by the docks, to chop wood, to even clean out the privy. There was still the old battered handcart on three wheels Oswald now used to scour the back streets picking up refuse and odds and ends to pawn, and pieces of coke. The boys wanted real work. "Orillia done them some good," said Dada. But there were still no jobs in Toronto, "due to the Depreshun," he mourned. "Have ter go down to the Employmunt Bureau an' see what you c'n git for th' day," said Henry. Hundreds of men stood in long, grim lines each morning at the Public Works hoping for a day's work in construction or road works. "Bleedin' shame when 'ealthy young lads are willin' ter work. Boys'll have t' join the soup line at the Mission, worse comes t' worst."

Mama had a pot of stew on the stove that she threw stuff into, any old thing that came along, even a chipmunk. The boys were hungry. They were used to three meals a day, and lots of bread, but George's Bread van, with his big dray horse no longer stopped at Lower Sumach Street. At night, Mama pulled out an old cardboard box with sacking for the babies. Robbie lay restless, excited, on the mattress in the corner of the kitchen he and Edgar shared once again with their brothers and sisters: Oswald, Cedric, Violet, Agnes, now a toddler falling about the floor, and the new baby and Wilfred who peed the mattress, and Ella. Their parents were on the other side of the curtain. This was a new Ella, no longer the thin eight-year-old sister they had left behind, but a big girl of eleven. Robbie saw her little pointed breasts and the shape of her buttocks through her nightie. Ella lifted it up when he said to. She saw his big cock coming up with thick, black, curly hair like Dada's around it, and Edgar's which was longer and pinker in his hand, as they rolled beside their sleeping brothers and sisters. Edgar remembered something from Ward D, and turned his bum towards Robbie, getting up on his hands and knees and bending his head. Robbie mounted him, and they shuffled just like dogs out in the yard, thought Ella excited. They were panting until Robbie gave a yelp "Ugh-huh." Then it was her turn.

"Don't let me catch you at that agin, girl!" Dada had slapped her, hard — Robbie had hastily dropped his nightshirt.

"Yes, I give 'er a good slap across 'er face for it," Mr. Hewitt confided to a horrified Miss Dorkins. He said he was worried Ella was becoming a "sex delinquent," a potent term he had learned at the Clinic.

"Absolutely essential this girl be put in Orillia," Miss Dorkins contacted Dr. Malcolm at the Toronto Psychiatric Hospital Clinic at once. Offspring sleeping eight to a bed; a seventeen-year-old in the same bed with a prepubescent eleven-year-old sister, all mentally defective.

It was obvious little had improved in Ella Hewitt's I.Q. or demeanour since her previous testing in 1929 and 1932. "She was almost helpless," a Miss Vincey had recorded in the last test. "Left-handed, with a noticeable speech defect," and an I.Q. of 45.

Now, in July of 1936, Dr. Malcolm rated the girl's mental age as still only five years: "Tall for her age. Brown hair, blue eyes with strabismus. Slight dorsal kyphosis, slight scoliosis. Body not clean. Nose, negative. Tongue protruded from midline. Gait normal, hands cold and clammy. No real stigmata. I.Q. of 51."

"So it *'as* gorn up then, Sir," Mr. Hewitt seized eagerly on the numbers.

"Well..."

Dr. Malcolm and Miss Dorkins looked cautiously at Ella, a big, dull-looking girl sitting unconcerned in the examining room.

"Tain't fair she ain't learned 'er letters, she never 'ad no schooling at Sint Mary's," protested Mr. Hewitt. "She was sent 'ome without no explanashun in kindergartin."

"Yes, well." Dr. Malcolm glanced at Miss Dorkins. How to explain to this Mr. Hewitt that his daughter had not ever been eligible for an Auxiliary Class, not with her level of developmental delay (mental age of two at age five and now a mental age of five at age twelve!). Dr. MacMurchy, who had been Inspector of the Feeble-Minded for Ontario, a position now defunct, had been emphatic about that: the cut-off point was an I.Q. of 50. Ella had not gone to school until age seven, and then had lasted only two months in kindergarten, being "excluded." She still played with mud pies outside, according to reports, and older girls her age would not play with her. It seemed she banged her head against the walls and tore her clothes when told what to do at home, though she was obedient to outsiders. The older sister, Henrietta, had already borne one illegitimate child, now about five years old and deemed mentally deficient (and therefore not adoptable), though the Hewitts did not know this, nor where she resided. Henrietta, according to the confidential "Family History" form, had ended up marrying a delivery boy, Percy Wilkins, while on weekend leave from the Cobourg asylum. The two lived in rooms on Shuter Street, where her parents had once lived, surviving on pogey.

Now the younger girl, Ella, twelve, was going the same way. Incorrigible. She had admitted to one sexual experience with her older brother Robbie — and possibly Edgar — in 1935 (and who knew how many more) at age eleven. This girl needed segregating in Orillia *at once.*

Mr. Hewitt nodded humbly. "Y-yes, yes, Sir. I know she's a bad girl."

As a member of the Eugenics Society of Canada (ESC), Dr. Malcolm, along with other colleagues at the Toronto Psychiatric Hospital, was in favour of putting a curb on girls like this. The ESC in its pamphlet, "The Aims and Objects of the Eugenics Society in Canada," advocated for eugenic sterilization legislation, for eugenics was "the science of improving the human stock." Dr. Farrar, Director of TPH, and Dr. Hincks, accompanied by American colleague Dr. Paul Popenoe, Director of the Human Betterment Foundation of Pasadena in California (which had the highest number of sterilizations to date in the United States: 5,820 surgeries performed up to January of 1928), had been outside witnesses to the Royal Commission on Mental Hygiene in British Columbia in 1925, in support of "preventative treatment" such as sterilization for mental defectives. The CNCMH had stressed that heredity was the biggest factor in aetiology. Dr. Hincks, in his surveys a decade earlier in Alberta, had pointed out that sterilization was the cheaper, more humane method of restricting the breeding of the feeble-minded. Dr. Malcolm recalled Dr. Hincks' own successful CNCMH travelling exhibit across Canada in 1924, with photographs on display of "Imbeciles," "Mongolian Idiots," and "Morons."

Now Dr. Farrar, who favoured eugenics, was continuing to watch developments in the western provinces with interest. Alberta, which had passed its *Sexual Sterilization Act* in 1928, had successfully sterilized 300 feeble-minded and insane persons, mostly females. This was on a voluntary basis, of course, Dr. Malcolm assured Miss Dorkins.

Miss Dorkins wondered how "voluntarily" a girl like Henrietta Hewitt would go to a salpingectomy. She tried not to think of Henrietta, who perhaps had been "done" in Cobourg to get her final release (one could not know for sure, certainly not from Henrietta herself). Would Henrietta have understood if she had been led to the operating table by the nurse who might have said, "This won't hurt," that she wouldn't ever have little babies. And would Percy Wilkins know that?

Dr. Malcolm frowned, irritated.

The Act allowed for the sterilization of feeble-minded girls and women with their breeding life ahead of them, as well as the mentally ill. As Dr. Farrar, the Director of TPH himself had pointed out, the expense to the taxpayers of maintaining big institutions like Orillia had to be reconsidered. The sterilization of people of inferior stock made economic sense for those who were unable to use birth control techniques, he had explained in his article, "Sterilization and Mental Hygiene," published in the *Canadian Public Health Journal* in 1931. Dr. Farrar, himself an American, was editor of the prestigious *American Journal of Psychiatry* and taught a whole new generation of young psychiatrists coming up through the ranks at TPH, enthused Dr. Malcolm.

Miss Dorkins hesitated. As a social worker she knew that CAS Toronto executives, such as the honourable Miss Vera Moberley, secretary of the Toronto Infants Home, supported sterilization. And there was that evil Mr. A. R. Kaufman, financial secretary of the Eugenics Society of Canada and anti-Catholic, of Kaufman Rubber Goods Company in Kitchener, specializing in condoms, cervical caps, sheaths, and pessaries (all banned by the Holy Father). Mr. Kaufman had recently won the much publicized court case to distribute contraceptives on the grounds of *pro bono publico* ("for the sake of the public good"), even though Section 207(c) of the Criminal Code forbade the sale or advertising of contraceptives. He believed in sterilization for those suffering from epilepsy, syphilis, tuberculosis, heart and kidney conditions, congenital deafness, blindness, or nerves. This terrible man had actually arranged for the sterilization of his own female employees or supplied them with diaphragms. Mr. Kaufman's nurses were now free to travel around the province handing out diaphragms and spermicidal jelly to working-class women.

Sterilization was, by far, the most reliable solution, persisted Dr. Malcolm and it was more than time for Ontario to follow suit. The Toronto Board of Control had sent delegates to Queen's Park requesting the sterilization of imbeciles. According to Mr. Arthur Laver, Toronto City Relief Commissioner, out of 30,500 social cases families in Toronto 2,277 were "clear cases for sterilization." In November of 1935, the reeve of Newmarket, Dr. Dale, had called for sterilizing the children in the York County shelters: "If we are forced to keep such children in our shelters instead of having them admitted to Orillia, we should at least have the right to sterilize them and protect our social order." The Mayor of Fort Erie wanted *all* unemployed fathers on relief sterilized.

Miss Dorkins again looked sombre, unsure. What about Pope Pius XI's encyclical on Christian marriage, *Casti Connubii*, to be read at mass in all the Catholic churches: "How great is the dignity of chaste wedlock"?

43.

To The Editor of the *Star* (1933)

Sir—Thank God for such men as Lieut.-Gov. Dr. Bruce who have the courage to come out publicly and advocate drastic changes with regard to mentally unfit. We give endless thought to breeding cattle, horses and dogs and none at all [to] ... that infinitely more important animal, man. Tubercular men and women are blessed by churches which ought to be ashamed of their attitude toward marriage while half-witted girls career over towns and villages making an annual event of reproducing their kind. The soundest stock of the nation, professional and high-class artisan, have to limit their families to one or two because they are taxed out of existence to pay for the unregulated excesses of the unfit.
Signed, COMMON SENSE

MISS DORKINS TRIED NOT TO THINK of Mr. Hewitt rolling on top of Florrie Hewitt in an animal embrace. She had been following the issue in the newspapers with concern for the past few years. In one letter to the editor of the *Mail and Empire,* back on June 23, 1933, entitled "Road Hog Sterilization," the writer claimed to have been driving from Toronto along Dundas Street when the road had become "crowded with cars jammed full of morons":

> I took to the ditch as the load of flat-headed women, cigarettes in red mouths, tore onward....
>
> When Colonel Bruce spoke on sterilization of the unfit did it occur to him, I wonder, whether it would not be a good thing

to start the campaign along some of our roads in the evening?
Hamilton, F. B. B.

This had been followed by Father W. Morrison's address on May 14 to the Holy Name Society at the Catholic Cathedral, in London, Ontario, entitled: "Rights of the Church: London Press Takes Strong Issue with Lieut.-Governor — Attacks Theory of Sterilization," and also reported in the *Mail and Empire*. The sterilization of mental defectives was "absolutely contrary to the teaching of Almighty God," he had declared. "We're sick and tired of theories propounded by fanatics, faddists, and extremists. Sterilization smells like a barnyard." Birth control he had pronounced as "child murder."

Miss Dorkins had read on, gripped, trying to put out of mind poor Florrie crying that "her insides was come out" after the birth of her eleventh feeble-minded child. Catholics had been reminded during mass in churches across the province of the injunctions in the Papal Bull, *Casti Connubii*, when the Holy Father had reminded everyone of the true way of Christ, warning of the "grave eugenics crime."

Re: Sterilization of the Unfit:
To the Editor of *The Mail and Empire:*

Sir — Every woman must resent with righteous indignation the attack made by Father Morrison of London, on the position taken by the Hon. Dr. Bruce in his advocacy of sterilization of the unfit.... Father Morrison declares that only the Roman Catholic has a right to pronounce on matters of faith and morals. With a magnificent courage Dr. Bruce has spoken. It is well known what he must be subjected to at the hands of the rulers of creeds....

Miss Dorkins personally attended the Catholic Cathedral on Bond Street in Toronto. She had read in the *Star,* on May 15, 1933:

ANGLICANS DIFFER ON STERILIZATION:
Church Has Taken No Official Stand on Treatment of Mental Defectives

The Anglican Church has never taken any official stand on the question. It has never come up at any of our conferences and synods," explained Rev. Canon Plumptre.

Rev. Plumptre's wife, Adelaide, had agreed. She was a member of the CNCMH with Dr. Hincks, Director, whose father had been a Methodist minister but whose wife was Anglican, Miss Dorkins tensed. Enough said.

Meanwhile out west, Alberta planned to end the "consent" clause in the *Sexual Sterilization Act* of 1928. The Bill as it stood was far too lenient. A Eugenics Board consisting of two medical practitioners and two members appointed by the Lieutenant-Governor, authorized the operations. If the inmate was unable to give consent, consent had to be obtained from the spouse or, in the case of the unmarried, by parents or guardian. But family consent, tedious and time-consuming, surely was not needed. The aim was to get the 25,000 lunatics in the country under control and produce a nation of "human thoroughbreds." As Agnes Macphail, first woman Member of Parliament in Canada had declared, at a meeting of the United Farm Women in 1935: "You farmers — would you want the worst type of your cattle to be seed-bearers?"

Meanwhile, the sterilization debate had heated up again, as Miss Dorkins noted, with the publication of Dr. Helen MacMurchy's terrible book in 1934: *Sterilization? Birth Control? A Book For Family Welfare and Safety* that Miss Dorkins made it her business to read.

"It is unnatural, it is repugnant to a member of the medical profession," Dr. MacMurchy, now retired, had written of birth control, while advocating at the same time the sterilization of the feeble-minded, noted Miss Dorkins, confused. The Holy Father had condemned birth control as well as sterilization, did not Helen MacMurchy understand that?

"Dr. MacMurchy Would Halt 'Propagation Of The Unfit'" blazed the headline in the *Star* on June 24, 1934.

Never one to mince words, Dr. MacMurchy described in detail the two simple operations used for unsexing both the feeble-minded and mentally unfit. She had, of course, read the booklet, "Sterilization Without Unsexing," put out by Dr. Robert Dickson in New York and published in the *Journal of the American Medical Association* in 1929. Dr. Dickson had cited a choice of methods: heat to the testicles, which arrested the production of spermatozoa; salpingectomy for females, though "oozing is sometimes hard to control," he had noted; and, as an alternative, ligation for females, although the crushing method did have a high per cent of failure. He pointed out that a considerable amount of operating was in the hands of psychiatrists in state hospitals.

Dr. MacMurchy first felt the need to explain for the uninitiated, such as Miss Dorkins, how exactly procreation took place: sperm cells had to do their floating along a duct called the vas deferens until they reached the tip of the penis, the organ "which places the sperm cells where they will meet the ovum-cells," as she delicately put it. This modern operation for males went by the name "vasectomy" and involved merely cutting out a part of the duct — *snip, snip* — "and nothing else," Dr. MacMurchy explained.

There was no pain to speak of, promised Dr. MacMurchy, merely a wound about one inch long. The sterilized mentally deficient man stayed in bed one or two days and could be back to work in the hospital within three. "But he cannot have children."

Admittedly, a salpingectomy was more serious for females since a general anaesthetic was needed. But even a salpingectomy involved simply cutting out part of the Fallopian tube on each side, a simple task again — *snip, snip* — and the girl would no longer be able to bear children.

"Absolutely abhorrent to nature and God," averred the Holy Father, Pope Pius XI. Dr. MacMurchy's book was condemned by a Jesuit priest out in Montreal — no actual name given by the *Star*, noted Miss Dorkins — who claimed to be writing on behalf of the church, and described the book, cited in the *Toronto Star* on June 27, 1934, as "the vilest of propaganda" and sterilization as an example of "the rapid growth of materialism in social work."

But part of her would always admire the great Dr. Helen MacMurchy (Presbyterian notwithstanding). The photograph in the *Star* showed the doctor wearing a gracious string of pearls, a monocle held at one eye, and a brimmed flowered hat cocked sideways jauntily.

She had retired in 1934 from the Child Welfare Division of the Dominion Department of Health, after receiving the OBE — Order of the British Empire — the highest honour (that would be for her work for children's welfare, thought Miss Dorkins).

The University Women's Club of Toronto had held a tea in Dr. MacMurchy's honour attended by notable professional women of Toronto such as Dr. Margaret Patterson and Charlotte Whitton. Pouring tea were Dr. M. E. Addison, Dr. Rowena Hume and Dr. Elizabeth Stewart. Miss Dorkins had read the write-up in the *Star,* absorbing every detail of the beautiful old mansion at 162 St. George Street, with its gracious vestibule replete with grandfather clock and aspidistra in the corner. Dr. MacMurchy's two sisters, both illustrious, had been present: Lady Marjory Willison *née* MacMurchy (who had married Sir John Willison in 1924, no doubt setting the standard forever for the MacMurchy women), and Bessie MacMurchy, prominent in the First Presbyterian Church. The two sisters, Bessie and Helen, lived together in their lovely home at 122 South Drive, Rosedale. Dr. Helen MacMurchy herself had remained unmarried, a spinster to the end. Miss Dorkins, now in her late forties, felt vaguely comforted by that.

Yet, at the same time, in November, Dr. MacMurchy sent a spirited letter to the editor of the *Toronto Daily Star* concerning the Toronto Housing Report of 1934. Dr. MacMurchy condemned "the vermin, the unmentionable, indecent and insanitary conditions" of the housing of the poor in the slums as "a disgrace to Toronto and a blot on her fair name."

Dr. MacMurchy wanted 200 new, cheap, and decent houses built in the area bounded by Sackville, Oak, Sumach and Dundas Streets: "Other slum areas to be dealt with in turn."

Premier Mitchell Hepburn of Ontario promised to look into the sterilization of the unfit and a possible *Sexual Sterilization Act* after a delegation on February 4, 1935, from the Eugenics Society of Canada, led by Dr. Hutton and Rabbi Eisendrath, demanded action. Rabbi Eisendrath had urged his congregation at Holy Blossom Temple, Toronto, to use birth control to limit their offspring and so produce superior children. The ESC wanted to encourage the fittest germplasm. This, despite the failure of their colleagues in England in 1934 to get the Brock Report accepted. The Brock Report had advocated eugenic sterilization of mental defectives and was rejected by the British government in favour of only medical sterilization. However, Dr. Hutton who was a correspondent and colleague of Marie Stopes in England, and who exchanged views on such matters, knew that castrations were carried out in the Poor Law Hospital in Gateshead, London, to curb excessive masturbation in some inmates. Something had to be done in Ontario, in Canada.

But opposition had annoyingly come from the Deputy Minister of Health, Dr. McGhie. Though a member of Eugenics Society of Canada, he had once again taken a contrary position, opposing the idea that mental deficiency was necessarily caused by retarded parents. He actually claimed that only a third of the feeble-minded at Orillia had mentally defective parents; most were the offspring of normal parents, and, therefore, sterilization would not put an end to retardation. He cited statistics showing that out of 60,000 to 70,000 mentally retarded people in Ontario, only 2,000 were actually institutionalized. Which meant, startlingly, that the vast majority of retarded people lived amongst them unnoticed by social agencies, without ever entering an institution.

He was backed by Dr. R. O. Earl, Professor of Biology at Queen's University, who also claimed that recent research showed that the majority of the feeble-minded had normal parents. Even the sacred I.Q. test was under attack. Dr. W. E. Blatz, foremost child psychologist at the University of Toronto, maintained that most eugenicists had little true scientific background and were ignorant of genetics and came from welfare work rather than medicine. Moreover, Walter Lippmann, an influential syndicated journalist and founding editor of the *New Republic* in America, publicly denounced claims that I.Q. tests could measure "inherited" intelligence, and actually called the tests "quackery" and a form of "New Snobbery."

In the end, Premier Hepburn hedged, no doubt due primarily to the agitation in the Catholic Church led by Father McNally in Hamilton. Miss Dorkins found herself torn between loyalty to the Holy Father and awareness that what the Premier feared was the loss of Catholic votes in Ontario.

At the Toronto Conference on Social Welfare, which Miss Dorkins had attended in April that year in 1934, Lieutenant-Governor Dr. Herbert Bruce had pointed admiringly to the success of the Nazi sterilizations in Germany in his speech. And in another speech to the Eugenics Society of Canada in 1936, Dr. Bruce praised Germany's sterilization of 30,000 "misfits" to date.

Meanwhile, up in Orillia, Dr. Horne had been following the fracas, bemused. He knew, of course, that sterilizations on the feeble-minded and those of unsound mind had been carried out quietly for years in Ontario. On February 20, 1935, he had received a letter from Dr. H. S. Atkinson, the Medical Superintendent of the Manitoba School for Mentally Defective Persons, in Portage La Prairie, lamenting that the overenthusiasm of supporters for sterilization was creating difficulties for the medical profession. The radical statements emanating from that group, agreed

Dr. Horne, had done more to retard a sterilization law than anything he knew of. Dr. Atkinson had written: "I believe if we keep the question on a reasonable basis that sooner or later it will become acceptable to the general public."

However, both Dr. Atkinson and Dr. Horne agreed that sterilization had its limitations, and that the feeble-minded were being blamed for problems that were not their fault.

City of Brantford
Ontario
Industria et Perseverantia

August 1, 1936
Dr. Sidney Horne, Supt.
Ontario Hospital
Orillia, Ont.

Dear Doctor Horne:

I beg to enclose a copy of "A Brief for Sterilization of the Feeble-minded." I have a notion that you fellows in the mental service are really behind this sterilization. If you would like more copies of this brief, please let me know and I will send them to you. 10,000 copies have been printed.

Yours very sincerely,
William L. Hutton, MD
Medical Officer of Health

This was followed by a spate of requests from Children's Aid Society officials, mayors of small towns, even ministers of various churches, for information on eugenic sterilization. Yet Dr. Horne had no definitive answer. Members of the Royal Commission on the Operation of the *Mental Health Act* in 1938 had been horrified to discover a number of young women in the institution in Cobourg who were of normal intelligence and had been incarcerated for no other reason than that they were poor and pregnant.

The Commissioners had suggested that if sterilization was permitted, a large number of these women could be released. Of course, they would still have a sex problem in the community, they agreed, however, it would not be "the same problem." Quite.

When Dr. Horne, therefore, was asked by Dr. McGhie, in 1944, to evaluate a *Sexual Sterilization Act* for Ontario and how it might affect the institution, he undertook a survey of the high-grade girls in the wards of the "improvable" type. These "improvables" were of limited degree of intelligence, but could earn a livelihood. However, he noted realistically, "the salient fact" in preventing their return to community life was the possibility of further pregnancies. So, they were kept locked up. If these girls were sterilized they could be released early in life, he urged, making their lot "much pleasanter."

At present there were 52 such sexual potentials in Orillia. "This group is of the moron level, and none greatly in excess of twenty years of age."

In January of 1944, 64 girls were transferred from Orillia to the hospital in Cobourg. Eugenic sterilization, Dr. Horne concluded in his survey, could be an effective policy for such girls, possibly carried out through the mental health clinics. "One cannot help but feel that a *Sexual Sterilization Act* for the province of Ontario would in some ways lessen the burden of the taxpayers."

44.

ELLA WORE A BROWN CLOTH COAT purchased by Miss Dorkins from the St. Vincent de Paul store in Toronto. She had an old pair of ill-fitting shoes handed down from Henrietta, and scratchy black stockings that were itchy in the August heat that summer of 1936 when she was put away. The stockings were from Mama, who had cried.

The new girls were going down a long tunnel to Ward G in the Infirmary for the mandatory tub bath. The new patient's few possessions—a pink hairband and a comb—were taken by the nurse and put in a box marked with her name, "Hewitt, Ella."

Nurse Marsden duly entered the new girl's clothing on the Ontario Hospital form. These paltry items were also put in another box marked "Hewitt" and placed on a shelf. The bulk of the newcomer's clothing henceforth would be institutional, drawn from a jumbled array of standard government service. Clothing had been supposedly furnished by the father, Henry Hewitt, and not much of it. Nurse Marsden noted that the new inmate had no kimonos, no night-dresses, no flannel drawers, no sweater-coat, no blouses, no corsets, and no corset covers.

Ward Admission Record: Hewitt, Ella. Case #5734
Bathed at 1:45 pm.
Body very dirty. Vermin present (pediculi capitis) — lice and nits.
M. Marsden.

"Undress and stand in line until you are called," said a woman's voice. The woman was dressed in a white uniform and had a banded hat on her head. Was it the next day or the next week?

During the tub bath Ella Hewitt had seen other naked girls in line waiting, with newly shorn heads. The nurse held the shears in her hand, and your hair fell to the floor. The girls held their hands instinctively over their chests, over their nipples; the girls with larger breasts tried to prevent them from bobbing up and down.

"Don't be silly," said Nurse Marsden sharply. "You're all girls here," pulling their hands down.

A man in overalls came in with an armful of towels; he smirked when he saw the girls. "On that pile, Saunders." He dropped the towels and strolled out, with a slow swagger. The doctor came in at last. He had on a long white coat, and a stethoscope round his neck. The metal piece was cold on your chest and back. Dr. Stroud breathed close to you, and his whiskers tickled. He had a red face, and long yellow teeth like tusks. Ella breathed in sharply. "Up on the table, on your back, feet in the stirrups, spread your legs. It won't hurt."

The nurse motioned to a high, narrow table with metal horseshoe shapes you put your feet in, your head thrown back, your thighs spread apart. The other big girls stood behind the screen in a line, shuffling. "Nothing to cry about."

Height: 60 3/4"; weight: 74 lbs.

"Small identifying scar on left leg," wrote Dr. Stroud, noting that such a marker would be useful for identification in the case of elopement.

Eyes: blue, hair brown.
Tonsils enlarged. Fauces clear.
Tongue protrudes midline, he noted.
Genital and urinary system: normal
Head measurements (always indicative):
circumference 53 cms; A.P. (Anterior/Posterior) 17.8 cms, lat (lateral). 13.5 cms.
Family history of syphilis: unknown.

Dr. Stroud glanced through the usual documents forwarded from the Toronto Psychiatric Hospital: history forms, financial statements and two Physicians' Certificates of Incompetence. The patient was referred by the public health nurse and a social worker, Miss Dorkins, of St. Vincent de Paul Catholic Children's Aid Society. He took up the Mental Defective Patient's History Form (Department of Health) signed by the father, Henry

Hewitt, before making his final decision as to the new girl's placement within Orillia. It was three pages in length, revealing much of what he needed to know. He skimmed shrewdly, as others had done before him. He could hardly decipher the physicians' tiny flourishing black script on the two Certificates of Incompetence completed that July, 1936. Under "Facts Indicating Insanity observed by myself," Dr. MacLeod had scrawled of the patient: "...never went to school, has no knowledge of Current Events, cannot name the days of the week nor the months of the year. Can add 2+2=4 but cannot make 3+3. Intelligence rating today is 51."

The "today" certainly said everything.

Dr. Stroud turned to the second Certificate:

"Stays at home and does scrubbing," stated Dr. Pryce. Older children will not play with her."

"Uncleanly. Rash on face."

The whole family was of low mentality. Two older brothers had already been patients in the hospital (1932-1935), and were both now unemployed at home. A baby sister, Charlotte (born 1934) had died at age two of chorea; another infant, Sophie (born 1928) had succumbed to summer diarrhea; one had been stillborn; and there had been two miscarriages (so-called). Oswald, age fifteen (born 1921) was backward; Violet, age five (born 1931) could not speak intelligibly, and had rickets. The toddler Agnes (born 1933) was doubtless the same.

Dr. Stroud noted that Ella had had rheumatic fever in 1934, and survived. It was the social worker, Miss Dorkins, who apparently had spotted the girl at home and recognized the symptoms of raging fever, swollen joints, and sore throat. Ella had been in the Hospital for Sick Children in Toronto, for six weeks, where she doubtless had been given the best medical care, including antibiotics for the streptococcus. Another example of mental defectives being needlessly saved by modern medical science instead of being allowed to die naturally according to the survival of the fittest, he thought, annoyed. Quiet euthanasia of defective newborns and withholding treatment to the feeble-minded was a regular occurrence in American hospitals. And rightly so.

He skimmed the rest of the report, particularly the Hewitt girl's "Moral History." The new girl apparently had no court record. She was "disobedient" to her mother, banging her head against the wall in temper tantrums (that would soon be dealt with in Orillia) but "obedient to outsiders." No history of stealing or petty thievery, but "admitted" that she had had one "sex experience" with her older brother at age eleven, not surprising considering the slum environment. However, under "Habits" she reportedly could dress and undress herself, did not cry out at night or wet the bed, and did not masturbate. Mr. Derwent, the psychologist at Orillia, who had examined Ella that morning in the infirmary had actually described her as a "bright appearing child" but undernourished, though testing as a High-Grade Imbecile, I.Q. 47. Dr. Stroud had no doubt of that — appearances were often deceptive with this kind. Previous testing at TPH in 1928 and 1932 showed her I.Q. to be 51 and 52 at best, and another test done by the Mental Hygiene Division in 1933 at age nine gave her an I.Q. of 45 with a mental age of four. There you had it. He noted with alarm that the patient regularly tore her clothes at home and was "attracted by fire." Essential this be flagged. (One but thought of the fire in the Dunn Farm piggery a few years back, cause still unknown.) She was healthy and therefore useful (reportedly did the scrubbing). He had no hesitation designating Ella: Cottage O. Ward Work.

Dr. Horne checked over the Minute Book that day for new Admissions. Another Hewitt. "This family is not unknown to you," Dr. Malcolm, trusted colleague down in the Toronto Psychiatric Hospital, had written dryly. Ella was the younger sister of the two Hewitt boys in residence in Cottage D two years earlier.

He noted without surprise the details of the family circumstances: Henry Hewitt, now cited as "Unemployed," received a pension allowance from the Department of Pensions and National Health (DPNH), "a mere $51.95 per month on which to support eight children, as well as a meagre $14 per month from his DSCR (Department Soldiers' Re-establishment) pension (3rd Batt. C.E.F). This meant the Payment of Maintenance — the statutory rate being $7.00 per week — attended to by the steward, Mr. Zarfas, would be underwritten once again by the Public Trustee at Osgoode Hall in Toronto, in lieu of Hewitt, who had not a dime to spare.

Dr. Horne turned to the form marked "Confidential": Ella Hewitt, prepubescent female, High-Grade Imbecile, disobedient, parents no longer able to manage her at home, sexual delinquent. Had had — Good Lord — "incestral relations" with her older brother, Robbie.

45.

THERE WAS A FLIGHT OF STEPS going down and an iron railing you held on to. Then came the clatter of hard shoes and a swish of house-wrappers, a sort of wrap-around pinafore that kept your clothes clean underneath, during Ward Work. There was pushing, and great excitement from some of the girls as they were on the move, gasping and grunting as they stumbled down.

"Quiet lines!" called the Supervisor Nurse Marsden, ahead. Ignored, of course. Ella gripped the rail, frightened of the steep stairs, high walls and far-off ceilings above. She could smell the dampness, feel the coldness. You moved in lines everywhere, from exits to doors to rooms to the outside, where, in line, you followed a narrow, gravelled roadway leading from Cottage to Cottage. A row of wrought iron railings ran along the property to keep them in.

Someone stumbled and was pushed forward. Was it herself? She felt her leg scrape the wall, the edge of the step hit her shin. "Watch it there! Idiot!" The big heavy girl in front of Ella was not holding onto the rail properly, not obeying the rule. She yelled excitedly and shook her head; had she understood what was being said to her? Ella struggled to her feet, frightened. Where were they going? To the dining room? It was time for breakfast: porridge, bread and butter, and a cup of tea.

They sat at long tables covered with shiny oilcloth, and your food was dished out by monitors after "Grace," said by the head monitor, a big girl at the head table, an important girl from Cottage M who could go into town by herself. She said words Ella understood as, "Thanks be to God."

Some of the monitors could not count, and gave the wrong number of ladles of porridge — too much to some girls and not enough to others.

"You should have said something."

"It's minor. Just a scrape," said the attendant; she wore blue and a different cap. Nevertheless, blood. And she was a new patient, too, only in her first week. "Best take her to the Nursing Station, Hilda."

"How old are you?"

Ella shook her head. The nurse smelled of carbolic soap and cleanser and iodine. The Nursing Station had screens around it and a desk and some shelves and a buzzer that the nurse could press to contact anyone anywhere in the hospital in case of an emergency. There was a list of numbers and words Ella could not read pinned on the wall.

"Don't you know, a big girl like you? This will sting." The nurse had stiff hairs on her upper lip and reddish eyelashes and a wart. "Next time watch your step. You're from Toronto?"

Was that where she was from? Toronto, and now Orillia.She now realized she had fallen down the stairs. "Bin push," she said stubbornly.

"Oh, aye, I've no doubt."

"Wan' go 'ome," she said suddenly to this kindly nurse.

"Oh, they all do, at first. But you'll get used to it. Damn lucky if you arsk me, three free meals a day, all the bread you want, more than the poor little blighters on relief in town get. You're here to stay."

She did not say "forever." The girl would find out soon enough.

ACCIDENT AND INJURY REPORT
Ontario Department of Health, Hospitals Division
Form No. 88 10M (L. 961)
Name of Patient: Ella Hewitt Age: 13.4 yrs
Date of Accident: September 10/37 Hour: 8:30 a.m.
Date of Report: Sept. 10/37

Report of Ward Supervisor
Patient fell down several steps scratching her right shin considerably.
Witness of Accident: None.
M. Marsden.

Report of Chief Supervisor or Superintendent of Nurses
Oct. 2/37. Area cleansed and iodine applied.
Signature: B. Stoddart.
Report of Physician's Investigation —Fell downstairs scratching right shin.
L. Stroud, M.D.

Superintendent's Findings, and Action Taken
Names of Relatives Friends or Notified Committee — None.
Superintendent S. J. W. H.

Ella heard the keys jingling, then a turn in the locks at the end of the Ward at night. Nurse Marsden clipped them back on her belt at the waist, the powerful keys only the staff had. She soon learned that. The keys locked the big fire doors marked "exit" and a sign she could not read. She showed Ella how to clean her teeth with the powder and to hand the toothbrush back to the attendant and keep her bum on the edge of the lavatory can to pee.

There were rows of iron beds with a sheet and blanket; you put your clothes underneath. There were shelves at one end of the long dorm filled with more clothes; in the morning you just put on whatever was handed out to you from the assortment of blouses and skirts and cotton drawers.

"You from Sumach Strit?"

Ella nodded. She knew Effie, Effie Lumsden. The Lumsdens had once lived in rooms somewhere behind the outhouse in one of those layers of collapsing houses in back of Sumach. Her brother Ernest was supposed to be admitted, said Effie, but they changed their mind. Ella had little memory of Ernest (her future husband, if she but knew); there had been so many Lumsdens like the Hewitts, thin-faced and hungry, running about the yards. Effie was thin and freckled, her face screwed up tight and anxious like her mother's, Violet Lumsden. Effie's shorn hair stuck out like thistledown. She wore a grubby dress made of sacking that went down to her ankles and was tight at her neck. Over the dress, she wore a coarse apron. "You in school?"

Ella said "Ward," the only word she could remember from Dr. Stroud who had examined her on the high table and put his fingers up her like Robbie. "Satisfactory," he had said mysteriously.

"Aw, you be doing scrubbin' an' sweepin. An' laun'ry."

"Stop that whispering down there!"

The attendant came bearing down. The girls in their night shifts had pushed forward at the sinks, making a commotion. You held out your hand and a monitor put white powder on it and you dipped your toothbrush (*Hewitt, Ella*) in it, then wet it under the tap and brushed your teeth and spit. Some girls trembled, and spilled the powder or could not put the brush to their mouths straight. The attendant slapped one girl hard over the head. "Pay attention! Ethel, clean that." Every girl spat into the bowls that were rimmed with old spittle and grease and blood. A girl had suddenly screamed and jumped off the toilet can, tearing her shift. "Get 'er, Ethel!" There was a struggle. The girl rolled over the floor. Someone, an aide, brought strips of wetted cloth and the shrieking girl was swiftly bound, her arms and legs tight to her sides, and tossed into the Punishment Room at the side of the dorm. Nurse Marsden slammed the door and locked it. Her keys bunched at her waist. Most of the patients had carried on spitting and peeing into the cans.

"Lights out!"

But not silence. There was the heavy thrum of breathing from eighty-odd girls, and moaning from Hortense who was locked in her cage-cot for the night. She was a big, heavy girl who was brought out only for meals and toileting and some play. She could not speak but made grunts like an animal, said Effie. Effie thought she was maybe thirteen now, "an ep'leptic what 'as fits," she whispered. "An' she mad, a lunatic." Effie had been in Orillia school for three years because she was now fourteen. Then Nurse Marsden said she was to do Ward Work, like cleaning and folding in the Laundry, she whispered. Their beds were so close they could touch. She had been in the Children's Dorm first, in another Cottage on the grounds.

Some young women leashed to their beds tossed and moaned in the dark. Why was that? So they wouldn't run away, Effie whispered. There was a long dormitory and a Nursing Station in the centre; an attendant sat there with a clipboard watching over you. It was strange to sleep in a narrow bed by herself; Ella feared she would fall over the edge. Strange was the darkness. No light came in from the street lamp outside on Sumach Street, no rumble of trams. But she was not home on Sumach Street; she was in Orillia, high up in a dorm on the third floor of Cottage O. Ella knew it had something to do with lifting up her nightie to Robbie. "She'll be a different girl in Orillia, Mr. Hewitt!" Miss Dorkins had assured Dada who had suddenly wept.

There was the strange call of something outside, low and muffled. She had not known birds to cry at night, but here they did.

Hortense rattled her cage bars and pressed her face against the rails. "Settle down, there!" called a voice from the Nursing Station in the dark.

A greenish light fell through the high window in the dorm early morning at a slant. The end of the Ward in a partitioned section smelled, worse than the privy on Bleeker Street. The nurse let Hortense out of her cage-cot by unhooking the side. Hortense scuttled joyfully on all fours down the aisle between the beds like a crab. "Mind she don't get out!" There had been that one time during a fuss on the Ward when Hortense had scuttled out unnoticed, scrambling breathlessly down the stairs to the very bottom. She had cleverly lifted herself up and pulled at the knob and the door had opened — Oh, wondrous moment! — and she had crawled into the dazzling light of outside, gasping and reaching for the sunbeams over the trees. "God's alive, there she is!" She was dragged back inside, of course, the door slammed shut on her forever. Well, what else were they to do with overexcited, frenzied ones like her? said an attendant to beautiful new Nurse Beatrice Mossom in for her morning shift. The staff had no time to do *everything* with eighty-odd youngsters to oversee.

By day some of the older girls were tied to commodes — strange, square wooden chairs — grunting and pulling against their straps. Their heads bobbed as they strained. There was a smell of feces and old blood. It was essential to keep these ones on the commodes during their courses, said Nurse Marsden to young Nurse Mossom who was "in training" in the Nursing School on the grounds, and quickly became known as Nurse Beatrice to her charges. Ella longed to touch Nurse Beatrice, to follow her but it seemed she lived in the Nurses Residence next to Cottage D. She had a beautiful, shining face. On top of coiled, fair hair sat a lovely cap. An angel, Ella thought, like the one she had seen on the Christmas tree at the Clinic at TPH.

The incontinent and non-verbal girls let up a roar and fussed, jerking against their leashes. They made plenty of noise for non-verbals, said Nurse Marsden. They were herded together on the tile floor at the far end of the Ward. They sat miserably, these ones, girls and teenagers, their legs splayed, while their blood ran for three or more days. These ones could not handle pads and pins, so it was quicker to just hose them down at the end of their courses and the blood could drain down the drain, explained Nurse Marsden to Nurse Beatrice, who tried to look stoic. Loyalty to one's Department Head was paramount, as stressed in Nursing School. She had struggled to learn lavage, catheterization, oxygen therapy, preparations for vaginal and rectal examinations, cystoscopy, poultices, fractures, and bladder irrigation, conscious all the while that a good nurse was, at all times, expected to be fresh not fagged. She was also expected to be patient and intelligent — of above average ability —

and of sound character, all for a starting salary of $50 a month, including maintenance. But young Nurse Beatrice loved Orillia, was proud of being a nurse, and of following after other members of her family who had worked the wards. She wanted to do her best by the patients.

"When did you last have your courses?"

Ella shook her head and did not answer. If only it were Nurse Beatrice, but she had gone to another section to do a catheterization.

"A dull expressionless child with chubby cheeks," the records had said. Nurse Marsden frowned, irritated. She pulled a white rag from the cupboard in the Nursing Station and rolled it in a pad and motioned between her legs (the Hewitt girl, she already knew from consultation with Dr. Stroud, was a High-Grade Imbecile).

"Menstruation."

Blood. The bloods Mama had that made her glad.

When did the bloods come? When the winds rustled through the bare trees and the lake turned grey at the bottom of the slope, a dangerous slippery place after rain, and there was no more swimming, and the change rooms and bathing station were boarded up for winter. Ella understood she was to answer.

The nurse's aide had a clipboard. On it, she carefully made neat ticks — this was important — against long columns filled with girls' names, about when their courses started, when their courses ended, and how many pads were given out and used per day.

"You must tell the staff as soon as it comes on," said Nurse Marsden. "If it comes at night, inform the nurse or monitor first thing on rising." This one, Nurse Marsden knew from the records, was "sexually promiscuous," and needed watching.

After breakfast the staff handed out cotton pads back in the dorm upstairs, and two safety pins and a waist band. "Don't lose the pins, or swallow them," someone said. Ella nodded. She understood vaguely she was to line up and hold out her hand after breakfast; her *name* and *day started* would be recorded, said the voice. Each pad was to be counted. It was essential to keep accurate records. It was the only way one knew if a girl missed her courses (or was pregnant). Little opportunity of that here, of course, said Nursing Attendant Berkeley, with a smirk. Nurse Marsden's lips pursed. Some of these girls would always find their chance.

There were buildings all around. No one thought to tell her what they were. She saw boys always coming out of the long building next to hers. It had a big letter in it that eventually Nurse Beatrice said was D. She did not know that Robbie had been in there. Cottage C (where more boys lived) had big white verandahs with lovely glass windows. Boys emerged in rows dressed in coarse pants and loose vests, following their attendant. Some looked like men but were the size of children; "dwarfs," she had heard. She knew Cottage L was full of old women, and that another big building was filled with old, ugly, frightening men. They wandered around the grounds at will, toothless, spitting phlegm to the ground or chewing on their toothless mouths or scratching their crotches. "Aw, they can't do nuthin' to ya," said Effie. A narrow road around the grounds joined these buildings to the big Administration Building. She saw a pretty white house set back in the grass. She pointed to it, and grunted something that sounded to Nurse Beatrice like, "Wazzut?" "That's the Superintendent's House, Ella." It had a deep verandah, and all around it were curly vines and dark bushes.

They had reached Cottage L where they were to hand over new laundry for the patients changing beds, part of their Ward Work, for Deputy-Supervisor Nurse Bigelow. Ella was fearful but curious as they entered, as it was a foul-smelling place. Shrieks and moans came from what she now knew were the Punishment Rooms off to the side. Nurses came bearing down the aisle with wet cloths, their faces determined. Nurse Pritchard was flushed; it was heavy work trussing up a naked, wild, old woman. "Mrs. Dinsmore again," she panted to Nurse Beatrice. "Put them there," she motioned to Ella and Effie and another girl carrying towels. There was a stench of urine and feces and grime and sweat.

On the way back to Cottage O, Ella could see through the railings onto a long, winding road disappearing into trees. On one end of was supposed to be Toronto; the other end led to the town of Orillia where well-behaved patients who had not disobeyed had been taken on Saturday night as a treat. They had gone to see a talkie at the Orillia Opera House. She had sat with the girls from her dorm in the vast darkened theatre after the lights went down and watched a little girl called Shirley Temple with a mop of curls on her head, nothing like the haircuts in Ward O, sing and dance and be wonderful in a way Ella had never known. The two nurse's aides and Nurse Marsden, who were sitting with their patients, had cooed "Aah!" and "Oh" and "Isn't she a darling?" You had to be trusted to be let into town by yourself. Boys could earn a "pass" but girls always had to have a nurse or a chaperone accompanying them unless they were "on probation," said Effie. That was when you were older and lived in Cottage M.

"What'z at?" asked Ella.

"When you is sixteen," said Effie.

There were three floors to Cottage O she now understood. There were very little ones on O-1 on the ground floor, where sometimes she had to help out the attendants by changing soiled diapers or feeding the children who would not cooperate. There was a Day Room filled with cots and low iron beds, as well as some toys provided by local Women's Auxiliary Club. In another cleared area, a teacher's aide and a nurse's aide were working with a few children who sat nodding and struggling to follow. A nurse played a tune on a gramophone like "Across the Meadow" or "Little Boy Blue" and the small children clapped hands and banged sticks. One had a little drum. Something was very wrong with some of them, Ella thought, worse than Oswald had been as a little boy at home. Their little bodies sagged and seemed to crumple as they tried to grip their rhythm sticks. "Hold her hand, Ella, hand over hand," said the aide, Vera. "Watch she don't bite." The little girl of about four did, of course, but was it deliberate? Her head tossed and rocked, and her mouth opened and gasped. She lunged again. "Stop that, Susie, or you'll git tied up agin!" called Vera sharply.

Ella listened wonderingly to the songs, enjoying tunes she had never heard. "*Little boy blue, come blow your horn / The sheep's in the meadow, the cows in the corn*," sang Miss Dunstan hoarsely. A small girl rolled towards Ella and sat her in her lap. The little girl as small as baby Charlotte had been clung to her neck with hard little spasmic fingers, and she put her head on her chest. Ella pressed her nipple to the little girl's mouth through her thin blouse, just like Mama. Oh, it was nice. "Look at '*er*," a nursing attendant nudged another and they sniggered.

"Enough of that, Hewitt." Wards O-2 and O-3 were reserved for older teenage girls like herself. She was now a teenager since her courses had come; she wore the pads inside her drawers for her courses that came and went, she never knew when. "They can't *count*!" said Nurse Beatrice despairingly.

"That's why they're here," said Nurse Marsden.

She had gone to pee in the lavatory — there was a row of them open to the nurse on duty. Her drawers had blood in them like Henrietta's at home. "Bloods!" she had pulled up her panties and pointed to the nurse.

"What, there?" The nurse attendant on duty did not know her name; she could not be expected to know *every* patient in this hospital. Girls were spitting tooth powder everywhere, getting out of control, the idiots. She knew the girl was new by her hair that stuck out like straw.

"Bloods."

The nurse looked at where the girl's finger was pointing. "Your courses have started? What's your name?" She got down a clipboard from the Nursing Station. "Speak up, girl, name and group."

"She's Ella 'Ewitt, Miss. West Wing."

"Can she talk?"

"Yes an' no, Miss."

The nurse rolled her eyes. She wrote something on the clipboard. "It's Day One of your menstrual cycle, Ella." Ella nodded as if she understood "cycle." Henrietta and Mama had wore the rags 'til they was done. "Stand up in dining hall in the morning at breakfast and put up your hand — high — like this," and here the nurse demonstrated for Ella before continuing, "so the monitor can see. Say your name and you will be given a pad, and then another at lunch and one at night. Here is a belt and pins." Could this girl, an obvious imbecile, snap a safety pin?

Ella wanted a boyfriend like Effie. There were boys everywhere in this place. You saw and heard them but only at a distance in groups and lines crossing the grass or marching with shovels up the hill somewhere. She heard them and smelled them, that *boy* smell, especially on Sunday morning at service in the gymnasium, suddenly called "Recreation Hall" by the attendants. Girls and women sat to the left, boys and men to the right, separated by a central aisle, the attendants and nurses standing along the walls or sitting at the end of the rows. But you could look across the chairs and give "looks" and wave fingers. She heard the older boys' deep, croaky voices joining in to sing "Saviour like a shepherd lead us," following the Orillia Choir on the stage. There were wonderful older girls in the choir with lovely brushed hair curled round their necks. They wore their best dresses, and the boys wore uniforms, looking like little soldiers. One young man played a drum, and others in the band played instruments, led by an attendant who waved a stick. They had learned by tonic sol-fa, since few could read. On Sunday afternoons, she could see the faces of boys' faintly pressed against the windows of the cottage opposite Cottage O, their eyes peering through the grilles, these anxious boys in the drizzly afternoon.

On work days Ella watched for them, for one particular boy. What was his name? She could hear their deep loud voices across the grass, or the silvery voices of the young ones being taken by their nurses over to the gymnasium in the main building for Physical Education. There was something wrong with these boys' legs, as they walked crooked. Of course, you were not allowed to talk to them during work hours. You could look and send kisses with your fingers when the nurse was not looking; she learned that from the older girls, the ones who were allowed to go to the Bobby Shop in M to get their hair done.

One day the girls lined up and walked with the attendant over to Cottage L to pick up the dirty laundry of the old women patients. They passed Cottage C with its beautiful glassed verandahs, "excep' they falling down," said Effie; it was where the sickly ones with tuberculosis were put out to get some sun.

Ella was conscious of her ugly wraparound, her ugly shoes that were too big for her, and her ugly, shorn hair as her work line passed the lines of boys who giggled and jiggled their fingers in a V; Ella knew, from the boys on Sumach Street back home, what that meant. "Here wear this!" The nurse's attendant, Deirdre, had said that morning as she had stood in her shift.

The boys were on their way to the Coal Pile or to the swamps, she learned from Effie, who had a boyfriend called Bennie in C whom she was to marry one day. She kept his ring "someplace secret what the nurse won't find." You were not allowed to go up to boys or touch them or talk to them, but they turned and grinned and made signs again with their lips and fingers behind the attendant's back as the girls passed. Now fall was coming, and they were off berry-picking that day, along with the attendants, carrying baskets. She wanted to go with them. She watched their heavy figures in heavy work clothes disappear sadly over the hill.

She began to watch for them across the grounds or out of the window of the Day Room after tea, through the thin rain. Some went out early in the morning in dungarees and rough shirts and funny caps to the farm, said the nurse when she asked. "What you want to know that for, Miss Nosey Parker?" The Dunn Farm was over the road somewhere. There was a barn out there, and a farm house where a group of older boys lived with an attendant, somewhere near the graves. You never saw them, and they did not see you. The boys helped with the milking of cows and feeding of pigs, as well as the hoeing, sowing, and the weeding of crops. Sometimes the boys who went over to help out with the pigs (had Robbie done that?) waved at her at the window, and the attendants did not rebuke them. They were young fellows and earned their wages for the institution. How old were they? In their twenties, perhaps. That meant nothing to Ella, but wages did.

Below was the terrace in full bloom where boys bent in the hot sun weeding. "Chrysanthemums!" cried Miss Nurse Bigelow suddenly.

Ella Hewitt and Effie were assigned to take the dirty towels and other small clothing soiled by the old women in L over to Laundry, a short walk. "Here, Effie Lumsden, take this load over to Group 10 in Laundry, and take Ella with you," Nurse Bigelow had said, flustered. They were short of nursing attendants in Cottage L again.

There was a long, covered glass passage linking the buildings to the Occupational Workshop. Laundry was at the end somewhere; she did not know where, so she followed Effie. Soon they were in a vast room with huge rolling machines that were deafening. Older girls sorted and folded clothing and linens for the various Wards and Cottages. Older boys were at the other end separated from the girls with an attendant, Mr. Anderson. Their job was to lift out the heavy wet sheets from the machines and toss them into the dryers, work too heavy for females. They also pressed the nurses' sheets and uniforms with heavy steaming irons on long tables, in a row, men's work.

Effie handed over the bags of laundry. "From Cottage L, Ma'am, says Nurse Big'low."

"Drat! Another machine down today. Shove it over there, Effie. New girl?"

Ella's slow-growing hair sticking out still was a giveaway.

"She in O. Ella 'Ewitt from Tronno, Ma'am."

A big sturdy boy grinned as he hurled a mound of wet sheets and pyjamas into the dryer. He had short, cropped sandy hair and brown eyes. He winked at Ella. She wanted to kiss him. He lifted his thumb and jerked it backwards. This meant she was to sneak to the back of the room behind the dryers (like behind the outhouse with Ronnie Phelps and Henrietta that time).

"You can't," whispered Effie. "Get locked up in Punishment."

"I wan go wi him," said Ella stubbornly. She felt sudden anger at the nurses and the attendants. He was lifting more heavy sheets into the huge air dryers. She edged closer, pretending to bring towels.

"I'm Jimmy," he called loudly over the din, grinning. "Jimmy Coggs." He was missing some teeth, but no matter.

"Ella."

"Ella? Tha's nice then."

He carried the pile of towels behind the dryers, winking. She followed him quickly, not looking left or right. He grasped her behind lines of sheets and nurses' uniforms hanging to air at the back of the room, before being pressed. There was a utility cupboard. "Give us a kiss, then."

He pulled her close to his chest. He smelled of manure and soap flakes and sweat, but she let him kiss her on the mouth. His big, thick lips tasted of onions. His hands quickly groped her breasts through her overalls. She gasped.

"Nice big ones. You be my girl now. You in Cottage O or M?"

Ella shook her head and thought. "O."

"You come to the dance on Saturday, Social, Ella. I look for you."

Thousands of rompers and towels were hurtling through the machines. "Dryer Four ready. What's happening there, Coggs! Get along."

Ella scrubbed and scrubbed the kitchen floor of Ward 3, Cottage O, to get extra points to go to the Social. She had a pail of water and a scrubber and a bar of soap. She wanted to finish the whole floor, all the tiles gleaming clean to please Nurse Bigelow (who might tell Nurse Marsden, who was "in charge").

The kitchen was behind the dining hall on the second floor that served O-2 and O-3. The first floor, O-1, had its own dining hall, for the little ones. You went down the back stairs with the attendant and the other girls who were assigned to Kitchen Ward Work ("Domestic Science," said Nurse Bigelow). There were large pipes carrying steam around the kitchen. "Watch them, they're hot," warned Mr. Henry, the cook. You had to stay out of his way. There was a vast stove and ovens and a canteen where the trays were laid out in readiness for dinner later.

It did not occur to Ella, as she put on her canvas apron and rolled up her sleeves, and got down on her hands and knees, that she should be going to school in the Administration Building; that she was entitled to put on the navy tunic and white blouse and Oxfords and line up with other girls for Lower Academic School after breakfast. Those girls set out with a monitor to go down to the tramway that led to the main building (in sunny warm weather they walked outside, two by two, slowly). But when they came back to the dorm after morning classes, they changed into work clothes and did Ward Work like herself.

Ella was in Ward School because she was an imbecile, said Effie. She was not allowed to go to the Saturday evening Socials, which were for Academic girls, unless she earned special points and proved trustworthy. There were points for this, points for that.

She dusted the dining hall and washed down the Day Room, cleaned the staircases of all three floors with two other girls from O-3, and, washed out the sinks and the lavatory bowls brown with bilge, along with other backward girls. One sat in a puddle of bilge and would not do any more. The nurse's attendant gave her a good slap, but nothing would budge her. "That's what happens when you get too many idiots," said the nurse's attendant. There was a large canvas bag for soiled linens and menstrual rags from girls' courses in the lavatory area. The bloody rags were to be soaked first in a Javex solution in buckets behind the sinks. "Here," said the nurse's aide. "Four teaspoons." Ella poured in generously. "Lordy, that's enough to asphyxiate us all." Did she have enough points yet? Who would say?

She thought about Effie's lipstick, hidden under her mattress (but which bed? Would she get the same bed tonight?). Back in the scullery she was to help now with the trays, which was part of her domestic servant training for when she would be put out to service one day. The kitchen and scullery was packed with other anxious and confused girls, trying to keep out of the cook's way. One was slopping stew onto dinner plates, and Ella was to transfer the plates to trays to convey to the servery. What was a servery? She felt a deep pain against her legs as she stepped back against the pipes she had been warned about. The tray crashed to the floor and stew splattered and whizzed across the tiles as she fell backwards.

Betty Gillivray screamed. "Drat that girl!"

"It 'urt, miss."

"Fucking 'ell!" The nurse's aide slapped Ella over the head. "Idiot!"

"She'll have to go over to the Infirmary."

"Olwen Richards, you, girl, clean up Hewitt's mess here. These imbeciles we get now are more trouble than they're worth," grumbled the aide.

ACCIDENT AND INJURY REPORT
Name of Patient: Ella Hewitt
Date of Report: June 30/38
Ward: Cottage O
Age: 14

Report of Ward Supervisor
This child has a burn on each leg caused by coming in contact with a hot steam pipe in the scullery. Vaseline dressings applied.
M. Marsden

Report of Superintendent of Nurses
Nurse gave attention to injured area.
B. Stoddart

Report of Physician's Investigation
Small first degree on each leg above ankle. Caused as above. Accidental.
J. R. Stroud, M.D.

46.

Report to Dr. Horne for Minute Book.
April 3, 1935 — March 31, 1936

Location of Patients Employed:
Patients at Industrial Work — 86
Housekeeping — 138
Voc. Classes — 10
Voc. Classes (Mrs. Clarke) — 211
Academic School Classes — 92
Special Occupation (Residences) — 6
Ward Work —107
Patients Unfit for Work by reason of old age or physical disability — up patients — 70
Unfit for work — mental disability — in bed — 41
Unfit for work — mental disability — up patients — 133
Total — 906
Phyllis A. Stubbley, R.N.
Superintendent of Nurses

DR. HORNE NOTED in his Annual Report for 1936 that the institution had been renamed "Ontario Hospital School," with the stress on "School." The epithet had been added to remind the public that Orillia did offer more than custodial care.

The institution had had several names since its inception, most notably the "Orillia Asylum for Idiots and Feeble-Minded" in Dr. Beaton's time. Dr. Beaton had changed the name in 1907 after protests from parents who had objected to the stigma in the word "Asylum" and "Idiots."

He had personally wanted "The Ontario Institution for the Care and Training of the Feeble-Minded" but had finally agreed to "Hospital for Idiots" later changed to "Hospital for the Feeble-Minded," which was later shortened again to "Ontario Hospital" under Mr. Downey. The new title disguised the idea of a custodial asylum altogether.

Dr. Horne continued with the activities and events of the institution:

> May 30, 1936.
> Probations. Increased number of girls probated. I would like to thank The Haven, Toronto, in establishing a second Colony House which has been a great assistance to us in placing trained girls in domestic service. I thank Miss Mann and Miss Charleson for their excellent work in supervising these girls after their arrival at Oxley House and Lorimer Lodge.
>
> No. of girls eloped from Colony House in Toronto — 4
> No. of girls taken shopping — 6
> No. of probationers eloped (discharged) — 2
>
> Hoggery — Trouble with anaemia in our small pigs....
>
> Cottage M — Weekly social evenings and dances in the Recreation Hall. School parties once monthly for school children on the honour roll. Social evenings for senior boys and girls whose work warranted their names being on the honour roll.
>
> Urgent — We cannot add one more bed without endangering the health and lives of the children. Cottage K — Provision needed for increased number of applications we have received for infants. Children's Dorm – one section for care of infants.
> S. J. W. Horne.

Not surprisingly, Dr. Sharpe, government inspector that January in 1937, had expressed concern about the foul odours everywhere. His report had run to over twenty-two pages, noted Dr. Horne.

As most visitors from Queen's Park, Dr. Sharpe had been overwhelmed at times by the stench, for instance in Cottage A, where he had noted fecal odour, and unsorted, soiled laundry piled high a very pronounced odour emanating from it. "Need laundry bags," he had recommended to Dr. Horne. Then he had continued:

> First floor — Dormitory and Ward [S]chool.
> 254 low-grade younger patients total.
> One large dorm — 40 beds which holds 25.
> Mention was made in a previous report of unprotected radiators.
> Accident Reports for 1937 show there were 36 [a]ccidents from burns, 27 of these occurring in the months of Nov. to March.

Again, Dr. Sharpe noted that in Cottage B the floors were wooden and soaked with urine and when scrubbed frequently produced odours. Terrazzo floors would be the answer.

> There is no staff toilet for the use of the staff and the attendants....
> Such toilets are, of course, of the penitentiary type and not enclosed.
>
> The dining rooms in the Infirmary are not supervised by a maid which means that a nurse must take over the task. This is hardly the duty for a graduate nurse who has trained for three years and who is needed to carry out nursing on the ward. Serving of the meal done by patients. Stew, pudding, bread and butter. A patient serving stew had some plates all meat, others no meat at all and no vegetables.

Dr. Sharpe had found cause to object to odours emanating again from soiled laundry. Admittedly, patients and hired help did on average 26,000 pieces of laundry per week with only four washing machines working.

> INFIRMARY
> Odours in the Infirmary due to poor ventilation (try to use suction fans). An objectionable feature was the presence of soiled laundry in the bathrooms — the soiled must be washed, of course, and this must be taken care of in a small slop sink in the bathroom, then placed in bags and left outside the front doors of the infirmaries until picked up.
>
> COTTAGE C
> 227 patients, older high-grade [patients] working on the farm or in industries.
> 10 Attendants + superior, 2 night staff and day – one is employed in the corridors and doing clinic duty.

Basement — sitting room, has toilets for the boys from Dunn Farm. Benches are used and drab.
19 patients on first floor of the better type — i.e., have additional privileges.
5 cases of scabies on 2nd and 3rd floors.

COTTAGE M
227 patients, 26 on first floor, 98 on second, 103 on third.
The single rooms where the disturbed patients and those in punishment are often placed, have been quite badly defaced, and even the outer screens broken almost beyond repair. A few of these rooms should be set aside for this purpose and supplied with suitable guards.

MORGUE — COTTAGE M
The morgue is situated in the basement of Cottage M. Most unsatisfactory especially in summer where it becomes very hot to hold a body for any length of time, and in respect to the fact of its situation, i.e., a morgue below a female ward.

COTTAGE O
Newest on the grounds. Play space limited.
146 patients. Young girls of school age.
Need recreational activity — bundles of energy.
6 nurses in day + supervisor, 1 at night.
Meal — bologna, turnips, pie, bread and butter, milk.
Some of the youngsters on the ward were reading "funny" papers and books which according to the supervisor are plentiful.

Laundry — Taxed to capacity.
It is remarkable there is not more sickness as the result of the working conditions here.

Dr. Horne's reply to Dr. Sharpe and Dr. McGhie, Deputy Minister of Health, was, of course, swift and to the point as a result of Dr. Sharpe's inspection: Dr. Horne stressed the shortage of staff at Orillia, the dilapidated condition of buildings (that were inadequately constructed in the first place, though he did not write that), and the shortage of equipment, due, he added pointedly, to government policies of economy. Battleship linoleum would be requisitioned to retop the tables after April 1, 1937, he assured Dr. McGhie, along with the installation of new Sewage Disposal Plant. (At last.)

Of course, Ella, Effie, Jimmy, and certainly not Hortense in her cage-cot, had little idea that cold April day of the undercurrents of contention simmering between their superintendent and visiting inspectors from Toronto, of whose existence they were not even aware. Though Nurse Marsden over in Cottage O knew, of course she did, as did the various nurses and attendants throughout the Cottages who had been forewarned to get the clothing cupboards tidied up, the files and records in order, the linoleum wiped down, the dorms rectified as far as humanly possible, for Dr. Sharpe's inspection. Though what, indeed, queried Nurse Marsden, were they expected to do about the dead bodies in the basement of Cottage M?

47.

"I DON'T SEE WHY she shouldn't go, Maud." Nurse Beatrice had written in Ella's Ward Progress Report: "Good ward worker. Obedient. B. Mossom."

"She's given no trouble," Nurse Beatrice persisted.

The Hewitt girl had been in Cottage O nearly a year. Nurse Marsden was cautious. There was that red flag on Hewitt's file: "Attracted to fire." This sort could send the whole place up in flames. The Recreation Hall had already been mysteriously set on fire a few years back. "It might encourage others at their Ward Work, something to aim for. After all, she doesn't *look* an imbecile," Beatrice adds.

Ella was to go at last. The dance or Social was to be that Saturday evening in the gym, called the "Ballroom" for the event. Young ladies and lads from Cottages C and M and O Bwho had made the honours list that week would be allowed to attend. Ella at once ran and looked at herself in the cracked mirror over the lavatory. Her short, thick brown hair, and its regulation pudding-basin cut, pressed around her full face. Nothing could be done about it.

There was great excitement in the west wing of Cottage O-3 after dinner amongst those attending, much pulling out of clothes from the cupboard at the end of the long dormitory. Some girls had "good" clothes from home that still fit them, brought by relatives at their admission, marked with their names. Others had to take whatever was handed out by Nurse Bigelow and Nurse Marsden from the pile: corsets, stockings, petticoats, dresses, and indoor shoes.

Nurse Bigelow frowned as she scrutinized each girl hopelessly. There was always a tussle for clothes. The nicer, cleaner dresses used for special occasions were rolled in piles and kept in the dusty cupboard. She pulled out one old, red dress, quite lovely.

Ella at once wanted it. "My, my!" She pushed Jessie Pritchard and Olwen Richards out of the way for that dress. Oh! She wanted it. *Red.* The colour of blood, of rage, of passion, of Mama. It was too small for her, of course; she had big breasts for her age pushing out, but no matter, a red dress to wear in the Ballroom, despite clumpy black shoes and a pair of worn stockings. "Mine!"

"Nah!" snarled Jessie. "Is mine!"

Ella kicked her and slapped her face. She pushed Jessie against the rad.

"Me! Me! Mi-i-ne!"

"You gobbler! Whore!"

Enraged, Jessie pulled out a dinner knife. Hortense shrieked and raged inside her cage-cot in excitement, shrilling with laughter, rattling the bars. She pushed out her arm through the bars and grabbed the dress out of Ella's hand pulling it into the cot.

"A-a-gh!" Enraged, Ella pushed her face against the bars, and tugged at the skirt.

She jerked it back and Hortense pounced.

"She bit me arm!"

There were deep teeth marks in her flesh.

There was the quick tread of rubber soles.

"Enough! No one shall have it!" Nurse Marsden shut the dress decisively into a cupboard and turned the key.

Ella wept at the long shapeless dress she ended up with: cotton with patch pockets.

An attendant was winding the old Victrola gramophone near the stage. It played swing time songs from the musicals: "*The bells are ringing, for me and my gal.*" There was a table down along the side of the room with sandwiches, chips, and pop. Chairs were lined along the walls. Girls sat down stiffly in lines waiting to be asked to dance. A boy had to come up to you and say nicely, "Would you like to dance?" as the social worker Miss Newsome had taught in Social Manners and Etiquette. No holding too tightly out on the floor, either.

"Danshe?"

He was up to her face; she was taller, and, thus, tall for her age. But he was a boy, though not Jimmy, the one from the Laundry (where was he?). She felt surprise at her new height; she had not known she was tall. She stumbled around the floor holding onto his hands, in her ugly dress and cropped hair, but nevertheless beautiful to him. "You got bit?" he said eventually.

Ella shook her head, though the bite mark was now dark blue against her white skin. He breathed heavily in a thick muffled voice, and looked up at her with shining eyes. She smelled his male smell and his hair cream and something else that reminded her of something she had forgotten.

"You be my girl."

He had rough hair. His mouth and cheeks were not like a girl's, but had stubble and cuts from a razor. His teeth were broken and yellowish. He liked Orillia, he said, been there since he was a little boy. Nurse Marsdon had been his mother in the Children's Dorm and loved him, and the attendants were good to him, and some of them were not. He squeezed a hand on her breast, quickly. No one saw, or did they? The attendants stood, amused, along the walls; some went outside for a smoke.

He had played basketball and gone skating with Mr. Atherton, he went on. And, he went on a sleigh ride last winter through the trees, and had chocolate ice cream and cake at the picnic. Orillia was a lot of fun, he breathed.

"Kiss ya," he mumbled, excited. He bought her a pop, an Orangeade, because he had money.

She bent her mouth down to his when the nurses and attendants down the side were not looking. Many were bemused at these couplings out on the floor, tolerant for this night so heavily chaperoned. Why shouldn't the kids have a little fun?

The nurses were still talking excitedly about the abdication of King Edward VIII last year, for the woman he loved, Wallis Simpson (twice a divorcée). Some of the nurses and aides had wept. Now war was coming, in the world beyond Orillia. Hitler was marching into a country called Czechoslovakia ... far from Orillia where the lake lay smooth that night like a pool of ink.

The lights were flickered off, then on again. "Oh-h-h," went everyone, the patients turning towards the attendants. "The evening is over. Get in line please. Girls to the right, boys to the left." The boys went down their back stairs to the tramways below, along the tunnels leading to their Cottages; the girls then went to their tunnels, led by the nursing attendants, who knew the way, and who could read the signposts at each intersection (it was like a town underground, a vast interconnecting tramway of roads and signs).

The girls followed blindly. Ella was overexcited. She had drunk Orangeade, eaten two ham sandwiches and a slice of chocolate cake, and kissed a boy's mouth. His lips had been thick and soft like rubber.

There was much tossing in the dorm all that night after the girls had peed and changed into their night shifts. It was always the same after a dance. Too much excitement, frowned Nurse Marsden. Ella lay hot and disturbed in the dark in her iron cot, locked in, she thought now resentfully. Why couldn't she be with Alfred. That had been his name. Alfred. And Jimmy. Oh Jimmy, the boy in the Laundry. They had stood that time behind the dryers, kissing. She understood, at last, that she was locked away from them — from Alfred, from Jimmy — from boys.

School, Orillia

October 8, 1938
Mr. Henry Hewitt,
71 Berkeley Street,
Toronto

Re: Ella Hewitt
Dear Sir,

We are in receipt of a parcel containing candies, one bracelet, chocolate bars and cookies for Ella Hewitt. Ella is enjoying her treat and was pleased to receive her parcel.

Yours truly,
Mr. Walker
(For S. J. W. Horne, Medical Superintendent)

Typical of people like the Hewitts to send a silly little bracelet and chocolate bars to Ella when what was sorely needed was a set of practical new clothes, tutted Nurse Marsden. Ella had grown taller and her adolescent puppy fat was pushing out of her daydress. Indeed, her bloomers were threadbare. The few clothes she had brought in with her at admission had long since been discarded. Nurse Marsden, had, of course, kept the lists current. The one dress Ella had arrived in that August day in 1937 had been marked on her Clothing Card as "discarded," December 1937. One pair of stockings likewise tossed out in

March 1938. A pair of pants, a vest and one slip had all been replaced by institutional clothes.

She forthwith sent out a pointed requisition list to Mr. Hewitt in Toronto (Form 5M), informing him that his daughter required "articles of clothing mentioned hereunder." It was about time Mr. Hewitt assumed some financial responsibility for this patient:

3 Dresses
Hip size 32" — Sleeve 18½ — Length 41" — Bust 26" — Waist 25"
3 Slips
3 pairs Bloomers
3 Nightgowns
1 pair. Shoes size 5
1 pair. Bedroom Slippers size 5
Playsuit
2 pairs Hose and Ankle Socks.

Did Mrs. Hewitt down on Shuter Street ever forward these items, she who had never had a bedroom let alone bedroom slippers? What did "playsuit" mean? Later, on Ella's Discharge papers, her clothing was listed as "Institutional."

Nevertheless, Ella Hewitt was given a chocolate bar during her break after Ward Work, the rest, Nurse Marsden decided, would be shared Sunday afternoon during tea. That way other patients would not be aware of the source. No word was said in front of patients concerning any gift from home, as it only disturbed them, creating unnecessary trouble.

"Here is a bracelet from your parents, Ella. You may wear it on Sundays," she informed Ella privately, calling her into the Nursing Station. Her "parents"? Ella could not recall the word; it was a far-away word, one she might have heard at the Clinic in Toronto. "From your *father*," stressed Nurse Marsden, trying to keep in mind Ella Hewitt's I.Q. of 45, cited by the Orillia psychologist on admission. This girl was quite dim.

Mama and Dada. Far away. And now here was a tin bangle with precious stones that glittered brightly. Nurse Marsden allowed her to put it shyly round her wrist the following Sunday. She would wear it perhaps for Jimmy at the next Social. But for now, only until bedtime. She flashed it around the Ward.

Hortense shrieked in her cot-cage. She pushed out a hand through the rails for it, but no one took notice. It was just Hortense acting up, which, of course, was why she was locked in there in the first place.

"Oh, is nice. Give us a try!" cried Effie. "You c'n 'ave my pudding."

"Hair clip," insisted Ella.

Effie hesitated. "Okay. You wear clip, I wear bracelet just for a bit."

Ella still had her lipstick under the mattress, now squished, and a sanitary pad. Ella took Effie's clip with the metal flower on it, and snapped it into her hair for the afternoon knowing it was important, what the pretty older girls wore at the Socials.

Effie slipped on the bracelet, a tinny bangle with fake gems and a cheap, brittle clasp from a Five and Dime Store, she guessed. But she could pretend. She could pretend that her mama had sent it to her, care of the Matron, Nurse Marsden, in Ward O, at Orillia. Ella had a mother and father who thought of her, had bought her a bracelet and gone to a post office in Toronto to get stamps and then sent it to Orillia. Effie's mother, Violet, was too poor, poorer even than Florrie Hewitt; she had forgotten her daughter up in Orillia, Effie knew that now. She felt a darkness, a silent despair. But soon she would be transferred into Cottage M, when she turned sixteen and was no longer a ward of Children's Aid Society of Toronto. It would be her big chance, her way out of the institution. She knew this from observing the other big girls, she had confided to Nurse Marsden, who was instrumental in getting any girl into M. You went out on probation to a place called Lorimer Lodge, a halfway house in Toronto, and then you would be freed after six months if you showed good responsible behaviour. The halfway house in Orillia, The Colony out on West Street had burned down in 1932, no one knew how. Effie had seen it once when she was eleven and stayed over at Nurse Marsden's house on the weekends; she had wheeled the old lady Mrs. Marsden, Nurse Marsden's mother, past the big house and envied the young women inside, who were put out as domestics in town. They got half their pay put into a bank account. How wonderful to buy your own scent and lipstick, and tickets to the Orillia Opera House to watch real talking pictures, and listen to the band in Couchiching Park, and meet young men.

But what Effie really longed for was to go back to Ma and Dad in Toronto. There were thousands of people in a city, and factory jobs for such girls as herself. She would marry a nice dependable fellow and — this was the best part — she would have little babies. She already had their names picked, she had confided shyly to Nurse Marsden: Emma, Agnes, Harold, Ernest, and Arthur.

In her Nursing Station, Nurse Marsden pursed her lips. She knew Effie Lumsden was up for probation soon, would likely be transferred to the first floor, for Probation Trainees, in Cottage M, under Nurse Biggs. But she had come to rely on Effie as a useful aide for her mother, Mrs. Marsden, on occasional weekends at her house in town, providing herself with some respite. Effie was smart, she could even catheter the old lady now, and give her enemas when needed, as well as do some mending and stitching in the evenings. In return, she got to sleep in the spare room, with its lovely satin bed covers and matching flowered curtains — a real feather bed of her own.

ACCIDENT AND INJURY REPORT
Name of patient: Ella Hewitt
Date of Report: October 1939
Ward: Cott. O Case #6021
Age: 15
Date of Accident: Oct. 20/39.
Hour: 6:30 p.m. approx.

Report of Ward Supervisor
Bitten on right arm by Hortense D'Arcy, #6598. Skin unbroken.
M. Marsden

Report of Superintendent of Nurses
Contusion only.
M. Stoddart.

Report of Physician's Investigation –
Bite on right forearm. Skin unbroken. Bitten by Hortense D'Arcy.
G. Stroud, M.D.
Relatives or Friends or Committee notified: None.

Ella stood with an arm of soiled bedsheets inside the second floor ward of Cottage L, the old women's dorm. It was full of senile, low-grade patients, said Nurse's Aide Pepper. Some of them were lunatics who should not be there. Beds were crammed everywhere, even down the centre aisle. The noise of the old women was like a low dull hum. A group of them sat on the floor outside in the corridor, something they preferred and that the nursing attendants had no energy left to stop. Ella had been sent to assist Nurse Enright with Laundry as they were short of staff again. There were over 226 elderly patients, grumbled Nurse Enright, with only six nurses on duty and one at night.

Sunlight fell through the grimy windows over equally grimy beds in which rows of old women were propped up, some muffed against self-abuse. In the open bathroom area a woman, old Mrs. Forbes, was struggling naked with a male attendant, Mr. Toby, sent over to help with the violent ones who had to be held down for their baths. Mrs. Forbes floundered and lunged, "Take your 'ands off! Off!"

Ella watched as a line of women were led out by the nursing aide, shuffling slowly in their shapeless shifts. The low-grade imbeciles were being taken to occupational therapy in the Occupational Room in the basement of the Administration Building for tatting and sorting tin foils. They passed by Ella, tall and young with big breasts and thick, short hair. They were loudly gesticulating in protest, whining with their sunken eyes and trembling jaws that they wanted to stay in their warm moist beds. They had a crab-like way of holding their shoulders, she noticed, staring at them in their wraparound housedresses that were stained. Eventually they bowed their heads obediently, a ragged, noisy, disorderly line nevertheless. Old women without men, and women without babies at their breasts, thought Ella. Without protection.

"Come along, Mrs. Mayberry, none of that."

Once outside a few raised their faces to the sun. Mrs. Mayberry began to pull at her tied housedress, to take it off, to tear it to strips. Once, she had run naked, her old breasts flapping, down the Terrace and past Mr. Zarfas, the Steward's office, before getting caught and put in a cold wet pack to get her under control.

There was a stench of human feces and dried sweat and old buildings. Cottage L was the oldest, but how old? "Since the beginning," said Nurse Enright, covering her nose with a pad. Ella had meant, how long had these women been there in Cottage L, which was where you went to, where all females ended up, if you were here long enough. You simply transferred from Cottage to Cottage. And how long had she been in Orillia now? How many months, how many years had she been in O? It did not occur to her, not yet, that you could spend a lifetime in this place.

48.

Inspector's Report of Ontario Hospital School, Orillia
by S. R. Montgomery, M.D.

To: Director of Hospitals, Department of Health, Toronto
March 28, 29, 30, and April 19, 20. 1938.

8 cottages: 4 male, A, B, C, D; and 2 farm homes, F and G;
and 4 female: K, L, M, O + Infirmary.
Took up with the Superintendent the following re: Wards:

COTTAGE A:
248 patients, 70 on the third floor.

...children in restraints. These children were up and around, but their arms were restrained to their bodies. This is a practice which, in my opinion, if once begun increases rapidly. Wooden floors — hold odours of feces and blood. Should be Terrazzo. Shower room — no ceiling except the scantling, there being no plaster or lath. Supervisor's office on second floor. Here are kept the treatment sheets, weight records, clothing cards on each patient. Report Books and physicians' Order Books available.

HERE, AND THROUGHOUT THE HOSPITAL, one is impressed by the multiplicity of files in which records are kept; e.g., There is a file for treatment sheets, another for clothing cards, another filing cabinet for weight records, and so on. I would suggest that there should be an active file for each patient, such file to be contained in a folder in a filing cabinet, and all records pertaining to the individual patient be kept in that file. In addition, the supervisor of the Cottage would be expected to write a bi-monthly note, at least, on every patient. These notes, of course, are not to replace the physician's notes.

COTTAGE B
Low-grade adults. Patients take exercise walking about the Day Room, do not go out, except occasionally in fine weather.

COTTAGE L (low-grade elderly)
Low-grade patients locked up without care.
Patients are allowed to congregate in corridor sitting on floors and there was considerable confusion & much noise even though there is a large sitting room ... large dormitory also very crowded — some beds been placed in centre aisle between the beds. In one of the single rooms, dried feces on the ceiling.

The screens in the single rooms off the dormitories (for violent or punishment) are fastened by screws to the frames. The patients push dirt, paper, etc. between the guard and the window, and of course the window cannot be cleaned unless the guard is removed. Accumulation of dirt ... with the number of incontinent patients and the amount of scrubbing needed....

Recommendation: Some of the windows could be guarded with expanded metal screens.

COTTAGE M (high-grade females)
226 patients. First floor for Probation trainees ... receiving training in occupations with a view to eventual probation; have sitting-room and a radio....
Sitting room (Day Room) only has benches against the wall.
Very crowded.
Does not allow for segregation of patients from the institutional workers. Therefore, not a good rapport between patients and staff.

NURSE'S OFFICE — 1st floor.
Menstrual charts, Clothing charts, in order.
35 sleeping in unheated verandahs.
Roofs of verandahs leaking badly ... in winter the floors are covered with ice.
This roof has been tarred ... with no results.
A false roof is the only solution. Showers not in working order.

DINING ROOM

All girls have to stand and wait until Grace be said with meals getting cold until last girl is served, then they sit down. Perhaps this be stopped and Thanks said at the end.
Meal — March 30: corn beef, potatoes, parsnips, beets, date pie,
bread and butter, and tea.
Tables covered with battleship linoleum, drab and stained.

COTTAGE O

Many young girls not capable of academic training.
194 patients, 50 more than intended — capacity of 144, 50 extra beds. However, there are wide corridors.
Ward class in the Cottage for those who do not attend school.

Treatment sheets, menstrual charts, clothing cards, report books and physicians' order books all in order.
Shower room second floor — plaster chalking off the ceiling.
West dormitory, third floor (O3): plaster off ceiling,
dampness coming through — no paint.

Dining rooms on first floor separated by the scullery.
Food service cafeteria system.
Dinner meal — beets, parsnips, potatoes, date pie, bread and butter, tea.

COTTAGE K

Half the ceiling of the dining room is without plaster, it having fallen down some months ago. It was indeed most fortunate that the incident occurred other than when the patients were in the dining room or serious injuries might have occurred.

INFIRMARY

"G" 70 female patients – 3 were infants.
Accumulated soiled laundry in bathrooms....
Using soap and soda washing dishes.
Sheets on beds unclean — grey slatey colour — may be due to dragging sheets over the floors.
A few patients on boys' side without nightgowns.
Ceilings of Infirmary are low and ventilation very poor.

Heavy odour as if from linen soiled with urine, blood and feces throughout the entire infirmary.

Recommendations —suction fan at end of wards might help.

WARD SCHOOL GROUPS:
Instruction of manual type under an attendant.

Classification	1937	1938
Idiot:	598	646
Imbecile:	710	777
Moron:	461	414
Dull Normal:	60	71
Total:	1,829	1,909

Interesting to note the classification of patients. The Idiot population has increased by 48. Imbecile by 68. Moron decreased by 47.

Another of these irascible inspections, from no other than Dr. Montgomery, Director of Hospitals. Respectful though Dr. Horne knew he must be, he felt it imperative once again to inform Dr. McGhie, the Deputy Minister, the truth about Cottage A.

He took up his pen in protest on July 5, 1939, sitting at the superintendent's desk in the old office where Dr. McGhie himself had sat before him, part of a long line of superintendents going back to feisty old Beaton. At his back, the long window overlooked the terrace and the sloping lawns leading down to the water. He could hear the shouts of children, happy youngsters, he prided himself, at play in the water in the successfully segregated and secluded beaches, their voices mixing with the whirring cicadas in the summer air. Ah, Orillia!

In the immediate background came the more monotonous thud of iron against earth from the low-grade boys' garden group, busy tackling the sod.

He returned to the issue of Cottage A that had certainly caused them "considerable concern," he wrote. The patient population of the Cottage was 253, of whom 140 were of such low grade that they could not be taken to the dining room. Soilers and wetters were attended to at least four to five times a day (60 percent of them were incontinent).

What was needed, he urged, was more staff.

Concerning "odours," he was anticipating the installation of a ventilating fan in a pocket where the odour was most difficult to eliminate. However, smells still remained.

Three new fire doors were needed in A, he informed Dr. McGhie. Renovation to the verandah roofs in Cottages M and C was required. Rewiring of defective circuits in all Cottages was also necessary.

In Cottage K provision was needed to be made by the government for the accommodation of children under six years of age "owing to the increased number of applications" for infants.

> Christmas Concert this year was Little Red Riding Hood.
> An enjoyable evening for patients and staff.
> Annual Picnic: clowns, bands, floats in the parade. Patients and staff had their suppers on the Picnic grounds.
>
> ...We have the usual magnitude of Physical Instruction and Recreation
> 37 baseball teams, football, volleyball, track and field, skating, snowshoeing in winter, calisthenics, Danish exercises, tumbling work, moving pictures, band concerts, amateur plays.
>
> Lovely fall weather, beautiful cut flowers in the dining rooms enjoyed by all patients.

It was winter, but which winter? How many winters had come and gone? Effie said two since Ella had come to Cottage O. Ice lay on the verandah of Cottage M where Effie had now been transferred, to her joy. There was the Bobby Shop downstairs, she told Ella on Sunday afternoons when Ella was allowed over to visit from Day Room. She showed her the two big sitting rooms. They had passes into town. These girls were older, young women really, who were allowed to grow their hair longer and get prettied up in the Bobby Shop in M. They could buy bright red lipstick and sweet personal body powder and stockings with their pin money. Some of the trusted girls were allowed as a treat to sleep out on the verandah even in winter (more space in the dorms for others). They huddled delightfully together under the extra blankets for warmth. They did not notice or care about the cold sharp morning air as they tumbled off their mattresses, or the ice on the floor of the verandah. They were just happy to be out there, away from the eyes of the attendants and senior nurse.

Snow whitened the lawns as Ella stood with Effie that Sunday afternoon; snow matted the grilles and blotted the view of the landscape beyond. Some of the girls were pregnant. Then one day they were not. Ella knew what that meant: blood blobs in a bucket like Mama long ago, when it came out. Nurse Brigham had looked severe, getting out the patient cards and menstrual charts from the nurses' filing cabinet. "Can't watch them every minute."

The bracelet was tight on her wrist. She was bigger, fatter, and taller again, up to five foot nine, said Dr. Stroud at her check-up in the Infirmary. She was more resentful. She no longer scrubbed so hard on the ward floors even as she covered her mouth from the fumes of urine. She was tired and bored with scrubbing the same floors and terrazzo tiles, tired of the same stench and bilge in the toilet areas, of the long hours mopping, of carrying sheets and blankets; tired of turning mattresses over dank with urine, of the dusty smears at the windows overlooking Memorial Avenue to the rear, and those that opened onto the hospital grounds in the front. She looked sadly then rebelliously at the faces of boys pressed sometimes to the windows of Cottage D next door. She wanted to run over to D and C and go up to the boys' dorms, but she understood, at last, that that could never be. Instead, she was to stand on a piece of turf outside with the other girls on her team — always girls — and hit a round, hard, hurtful ball over a high green net. "Make a *fist*, Hewitt! Up and over!" called Mr. Dawson.

"That was jolly fun!" the nursing aides agreed. "Wasn't it? Good to get them outside."

The fire door was locked and the nurse had the keys. The girls of Ward O-3 were taken to listen to the Orillia Band in the concerts from time to time in the Recreation Hall. They watched *Snow White and the Seven Dwarfs* this Christmas, with their own short patients playing the parts on stage. Or had it been it *Little Red Riding Hood?* All Ella remembered was that the audience had been divided — boys on one side, girls on the other. And they had been watched over by lines of nursing attendants on both sides. There had been people in from town, someone called the Mayor and everyone had clapped; he had said what a wonderful event the Christmas Show was in the Hospital and how the townsfolk looked forward to it each year (the standard of acting and elocution put normal children to shame). They clapped and cheered when Dr. Horne stepped up on stage to thank the Mayor and the participants and everyone for coming.

Ella saw women dressed in beautiful furs and cloche hats and long slinky coats and dainty high-heeled boots. There was the scent of perfumes from these lovely ladies, their arms linked through their husbands' arms. Some had brought their children, children different to themselves inside the hospital somehow, but how? They nestled in with their mothers and fathers, and went "Ohh!" and "Aah!" when the Wolf in Granny's glasses and shawl opened his mouth to bite Little Red Riding Hood, who was from Cottage M.

"Cottage O, in line!"

The beautiful men and women and their children departed to their homes in town. She had craned her head to see the rows of boys lining up on their side of the hall. She recognized Jimmy from Laundry. When was that? It seemed so long ago. His hair was parted in the centre, greased and waved on each side. He was dressed in a nice felt suit someone had bought him — and who might that be? She raised her hand and waved. Then he was gone, back to G.

He had seen her. She had waved at him across the rows of patients, a sparkling bracelet on her wrist; he had noted that. One day it would be a ring on her engagement finger, a diamond he had seen in Woolworth's in town one weekend out on his parole pass. He was saving his work wages and the odd quarters he got at times from Mr. Danson at the farm for doing extra jobs for him. Jimmy had also helped Mr. Graham, the head landscape gardener, with his new plan for the cemetery plots a few years earlier. The stone markers were lifted and the ground graded and top-dressed by the boys; it was heavy work but Jimmy was a big, strong, reliable youngster, "a good lad," Mr. Graham had said.

But now Jimmy no longer wanted to live at the Dunn Farm, with twenty men. He did not like what went on at night, but there was no one to stop it. He wanted to move back to Cottage C where the farm boys came for their meals twice a day. Mr. Sanders gave them a quick breakfast of cereal and porridge, bread, butter and ham, in winter, in the old rundown kitchen of Cottage F, but they had lunch and dinner in the dining room in C. In Cottage C he would be able to see Ella more often; there was every chance she would come by Laundry again on some excuse. He was sure to be put in Laundry again, no doubt, as he was strong and able to lift the heavy wet sheets. Or, perhaps he would be back in Carpentry with Mr. Dewdney; he liked working with wood, because it had a nice, sweet smell, not like cow shit. He liked Mr. Dewdney too; the boys all loved him, as he was kind to them, one of the best. A few of the trades instructors were like that, wanting to help Jimmy and other boys like himself "get on."

He put on a clean but not fresh shirt from the pile of clothing that the clothing Matron had set aside for the farm boys to change into from their reeking dungarees. There was an odour of manure. He smoothed his hair with Vaseline, wiped his mouth, and stood out on the upper verandah hoping to see Ella walk by in her funny wraparound dress with her group after Ward School. But she did not come.

Disappointed, he prepared for the twenty-minute walk back to the farm. He was being put to work in the hoggery that week, unaware of how valuable a worker he was. There were 96 head of cattle, he knew, with a daily milk production of 2,500 pounds; 131 swine plus 13 adult sows; and, 1,000 chicks (with 90 percent survival). Like other farm boys in Cottage G, Jimmy also helped with the sowing, furrowing, and picking of the crops. He also assisted with the milking of cows. He was shaken out of bed at two-thirty a.m. for milking at three a.m., making his way wearily in the dark to the sheds without breakfast — that came at eight a.m. He listened to Mr. Graham and the overseer discuss how well the crops were doing. The year before, in 1935, they had harvested 550 bushels of oats. At 35 cents a bushel, that had brought in $192.50. They had brought in 3,000 bushels of mangels (at ten cents a bushel), bringing in $300 for the farm. This year they had got a hundred bushels of oats, making over $140.

Jimmy understood this was a lot of money; he did not think he deserved a part of what Mr. Graham called "the profit," if any. If he had the luck of being rented out to a local farmer, he would get half the earnings with Orillia getting the other half. But now he wanted to be in the Hospital grounds near the girls (Ella with her big ones; he recalled the feel of them through her apron). Instead, he was being promoted to hogs, an honour, smiled Mr. Danson, patting him on the back, "Good lad." He would start with cleaning out the pens; for hoggery was a complex task requiring intelligence. Pigs were very intelligent animals.

Re: Hoggery
From: The Department of Health, Parliament Buildings, Toronto, Dec. 7, 1937

TO: Dr. S. J. W. Horne, Superintendent, Ontario Hospital, Orillia

...11 sows from Ontario Hospital, Woodstock, 9 at Dunn Farm.
Two of the sows now in your hoggery be placed to service the boar purchased last week. Each of the sows and the boar should receive injection of haemorrhagic septicaemia bacterin (Bison Strain).

Diet. In addition to usual diet add — one sack of Glauber's salt be purchased and one ounce of Glauber's salt for each hog be added to feed once or twice weekly. After the animals are unpregnated, a small amount of sodium iodide approximately grains one or two for each hog. As soon as the hogs in your hoggery can be fitted for slaughter ... be disposed of as quickly as possible and hog pen receive a thorough cleansing and spray with white-wash solution containing phenol, creolin, or one of the highly germicidal coal tar products.

Medical Inspection by Dr. J. Sharpe. Department of Health
Jan. 18-21, 1937:

Dunn Farm, or Cottage F:
Farm colony house, ½ mile from the hospital. Quiet older parole type of patient, 23 males reside there, have meals in Cottage C. Supervised day and night by an attendant. House in poor condition — floors bad — some of the windows are out, verandah falling down. In the attic you can see daylight through the walls. Toilet poor in a shed, therefore impractical to use in winter. Lease expires June 30, 1937.

Was the Hewitt girl "egotistical?" Nurse Marsden ticked "No" in the column. She sighed somewhat wearily. On top of night duty that week, as Ward Supervisor she had to fill in over eighty Progress Sheets for the girls of O-2 and O-3 for the Clinical Records (to be checked over by Chief Nurse Doris Stoddart). The government medical inspector from Toronto in his annual inspections of the hospital also had access to them at any given time. Luckily the Progress Sheet on Social Reactions involved mainly Yes and No answers to fourteen questions.

She quickly went down Ella Hewitt's character traits. She tried to recall Ella Hewitt, Case #6021, a tall, chubby-faced, stolid girl who looked older than her age. Was she quarrelsome, quick-tempered, stubborn, reclusive, impulsive? She ticked off "No," "No," "No."

Was she affectionate? Self-confident? Nurse Marsden hesitated. Ella had once been seen to lift her arms up to Nurse Beatrice and try to kiss her (discouraged, of course).

Was she dependable? Timid? Nurse Marsden, bored and unsure whether to tick "Yes" or "No," wrote: "Average," the most useful word in the English dictionary. Insolent? "Average." Profane? "Average." She noted that Ella was not Selfish: "Absent" (another useful little word).

"Obedient," wrote Nurse Marsden, the highest praise accorded to a patient. Finally, she had reached Number 13: Patient's Habits. Had Nurse Marsden observed any of the following in Ella Hewitt? Enuresis? Diuresis? Sciling? Fainting Attacks?: "No," "No," "No," and "No."

Masturbation? Nurse Marsden wrote cautiously: "Has not been observed."

Has patient shown any tendency to elope? "No."

Has patient taken any epileptic seizures since admission? "No."

49.

IT HAD TO DO WITH HER MAINTENANCE FEES, of course. And her age, now that she was nearly sixteen, she was no longer a ward of the Children's Aid Society of Toronto. Dr. Horne had seen that at once. Mr. Hewitt had defaulted in paying the $2 monthly fee for his daughter's upkeep. Mr. Zarfas had rightly informed the Public Trustee at Osgoode Hall in Toronto, whereupon Mr. Hewitt had actually gone to the Pensions Board to plead poverty and put in a complaint against Dr. Horne himself.

The Trust Office of the Public Trustee were now actually requesting an explanation from himself, and a diagnosis of the said patient, Ella Hewitt. It seemed that Mr. H. S. Sparks of the Canadian Pension Commission had telephoned Osgoode Hall claiming that Mr. Hewitt was but a poor pensioner living on a mere $51.95 allowance from the Department of Pensions and National Health (DPNH).

Mr. Hewitt had been to the Christie Street Hospital to complain about $2.00 being demanded for his daughter's upkeep when he had just applied for her probation and discharge (an obvious ploy to avoid payment — the nerve of the man!).

It was the next sentence that incensed:

> *The Public Trustee would certainly like some assistance from you to answer this man's complaint.*

The devil!

Osgoode Hall,
Toronto 2
The Public Trustee

Dr. S. J. W. Horne,
Medical Superintendent,
Ontario Hospital, Orillia

February 3, 1939.

Re: Ella Hewitt — Patient
Dear Sir:

The Canadian Pension Commission ordered the sum of $2.00 to be paid to The Public Trustee during the stay of the child in your hospital. Would you please prepare a statement in duplicate as of this date giving diagnosis, etc. in order that a report may be made to the Commission. Your co-operation will be much appreciated.

This is the second case of this kind today. Is it possible that the parents who are Pensioners remove the children from hospital when they learn there is to be a deduction for the care of such children. Any comment on this would be appreciated in a separate letter which will be regarded confidentially.

Yours very truly,
N. Puley,
Assistant Accountant.

Dr. Horne lost no time setting the Public Trustee to rights:

Ontario Hospital School,
Orillia

October 30, 1939.
The Public Trustee

Re: Ella Hewitt — Patient
To Whom It May Concern:

The above-mentioned was admitted to this Hospital School August 5, 1936. Chronological Age — 13.4. Mental Age — 5.4 yrs. Intelligence Quotient — 40. Diagnosis — High Grade Imbecile. This patient's progress was not good in the Academic School owing to her low mentality and she was transferred to the Ward School Programme.

> On October 10, the father visited the Hospital School demanding her release which was granted and she has been shown to be on probation since that date.
> S. J. W. Horne, MD
> Medical Superintendent
>
> Special remarks: Family on Government Relief
> O. Zarfas.

There had been nothing for it but to discharge the patient, held over in bond to her father, Henry Hewitt, a cunning man. There had been a scene in the Superintendent's office. Mr. Hewitt in a typical, loud, overbearing voice had demanded his daughter's release citing he and his wife "never wanted 'er in fer life." And, "The 'orspital wasn' all it cracked up ter be." Of course, it was no surprise that nothing further had been heard since from Mr. Hewitt, as had been the case with the boys. The family was gone; disappeared into the warrens of Cabbagetown where no doubt Mr. Hewitt would put his daughter out to work in one of the wartime factories, or worse, and make a pretty penny off her. Dr. Horne had been following reports on the radio anxiously as Germany invaded Poland on September 1. On September 3, Britain and France had declared war on Germany. On September 10 , His Majesty King George VI had called upon the Dominion of Canada under Prime Minister Mackenzie King to fight. It had passed unanimously in the Legislature (with the exception of that socialist crank Mr. J. S. Woodsworth who had stood alone voting against war: "I'll be with the children," he had said). Attendants at the hospital were already joining up, sighed Dr. Horne. As an Arch Mason he knew the powers of Lucifer were now being unleashed on the world.

Miss Dorkins frowned. Of course she had not really expected the Lumsden girl to show much improvement; she was after all a designated Imbecile (higher grade). Yet as Ella was discharged, and Miss Dorkins wrote her off in her file, she noted the girl's I.Q. was still at 40, according to Orillia, though of course there had been a time that Ella's intelligence had been deemed higher, much higher, a fact somehow lost now in time, passed over.

She knew only too well how Mr. Hewitt would object. "Ow come she aint learnt 'er letters up there?" Yet had not Ella likely absorbed an extensive new vocabulary from being around the Cottages and Wards of Orillia, and through her relationships with patients and staff, Miss Dorkins was sure; words like "scrubber," "mangle," "dormitory," "dining-room," "bed-pan," "gurney," "restraints," "straight-jacket," "cold pack," "cot-cage," and "Mongoloid."

Too, she would now know words from all the prayers and hymns from Sunday service, and the songs she had heard sung in the Children's Dorm. And then there were all the words she had heard long before Orillia. Here Miss Dorkins had to acknowledge something, insidious, for had she not seen the small child Ella, at only four and a half, bring bandages for her mother's womb, correctly handing over the strips of cloth.

Of course, a slum child like Ella knew words quite beyond the average, nice, little girl in upper Toronto; words like: "spunks," "hookers," "labour pains," "quickening," "afterbirth," "abortion," "pennyroyal," as well as more unsavoury terms that would never be found in any I.Q. test, and, at some level, Miss Dorkins sensed, was that not the point? Ella had also menstruated, as Miss Dorkins knew; she had learned to defend herself, to cope day-to-day, to survive injury and attacks from other patients as well as attendants, surely developing brain skills of sorts?

But she would never again be assessed. Ella Hewitt left as she had arrived: a high grade Imbecile. She was to be a high-grade imbecile with an I.Q. stuck at 40 and a mental age of five years for the remainder of her life, whether she could efficiently help tie up an old woman in restraints or not. Miss Dorkins closed her file.

Ella had known nothing of this, and never would. Dada had come, as she had always known he would. She had no doubt her true life was now to begin. She would rent a room; she would get factory work; she would go to taverns and she would go dancing; she would have pretty dresses and plenty of lipstick and she would meet swell fellers and date them; unaware as yet she would marry Effie Lumsden's brother, Ernest, from Seaton Street, Cabbagetown, and have three children of her own.

All of Orillia fell away, already in the past: the grounds, the workshops and wards, the Laundry, Cottages O and L, the toothless old women fighting in their nighties. All of it already just a dream.

She stood in her worn winter coat outside the Superintendent's office, "clean and free of vermin" as Nurse Marsden had attested. Her father had turned up red-faced, dressed in worn pants, a threadbare waistcoat and collarless shirt, muffler and soft cap, for Ella's release. War had broken out in the old country, he had seen it all over the front pages of the *Star* and the *Globe and Empire,* he informed Dr. Horne. The leader of Germany, called Adolph Hitler — "them Huns again" — had marched into Poland, which had fallen in three weeks. Henry Hewitt knew what that meant. Ella would be a help to them now. At nearly sixteen, he could rent Ella out to do scrubbing or laundry. Or she could do war work. He understood that paid well. No doubt she had learned a thing or two in the hospital.

Ella had waited. There had been words, loud voices in the office. She had had a sense that Dada was on her side. He had emerged, red-faced and fists clenched. She clutched the small canvas bag she had brought with her on her admission two years before, kept in storage by Nurse Marsden. It now contained, counted out by the attendant, one beret, blue; two Institution dresses; two Institution night dresses; two Institution vests; one petticoat.

"Articles of Clothing Belonging to Patient on Discharge or Death," Nurse Marsden had dutifully noted, signing the last form forever for patient Ella Hewitt. Ella had turned down her bed, and packed her few belongings — *quick, quick* — while the eighty other girls of West Ward, Cottage O-3, were downstairs at breakfast. It was essential to be dressed and gone before the girls who were left behind — many forever — would be aware of her absence. There was trouble whenever a patient "disappeared," as Nurse Marsden well knew.

So Ella had stumbled, confused but expectant, through the doorway marked Exit for the last time, and down the back stairs with the nurse's aide, past the crowded dining halls, unseen and unmissed.

But the idiot Hortense had known. She had screeched and rattled her cage-cot, thrashing heavily against the bars (the steel cot stood on sturdy legs), her long howl echoing down the empty dorm.

Oh, Hortense knew. Of course she did. Everything.

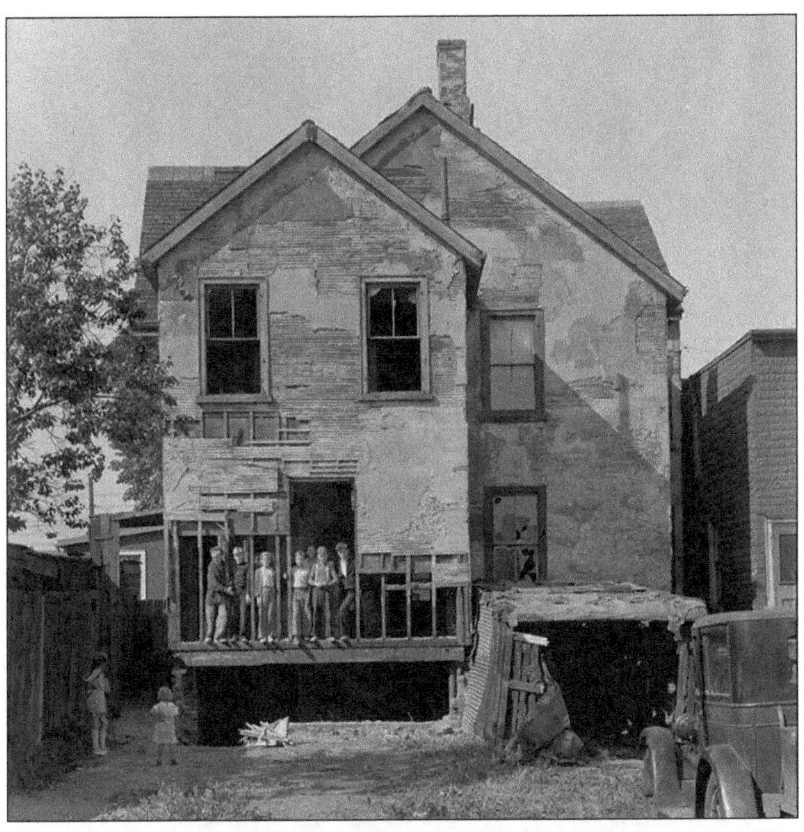

House at Oak Street, between Sumach and River Streets, Toronto, September 22, 1937. Courtesy City of Toronto Archives, Housing Department.

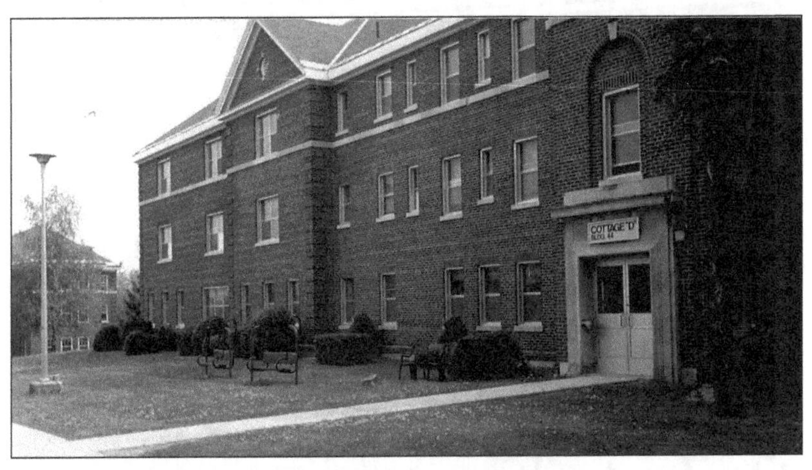

Cottage D today, Huronia Regional Centre, Orillia. Photo: Thelma Wheatley.

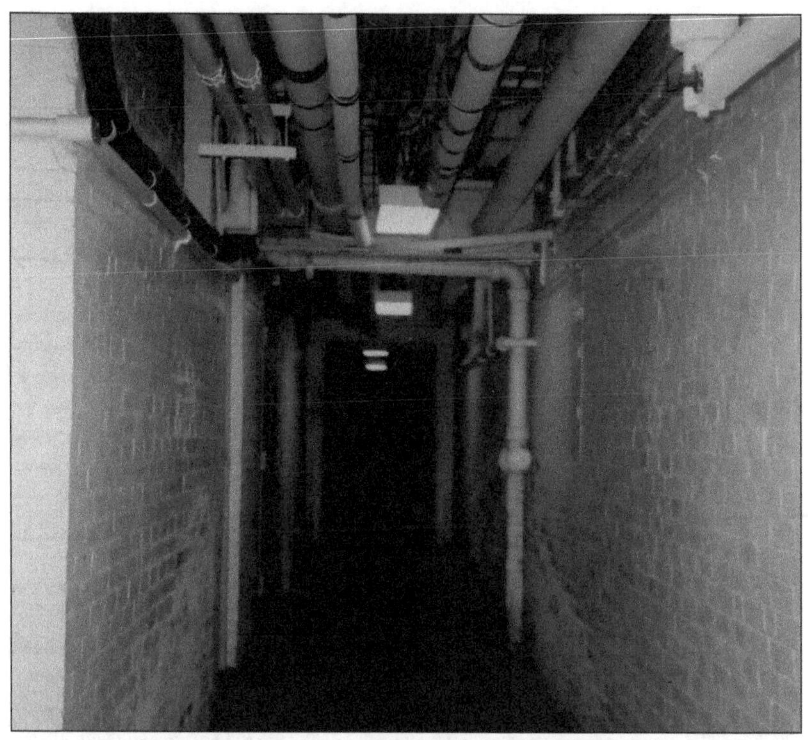

Underground tunnel or tramway Ontario Hospital School, Orillia.
Courtesy Huronia Archives. Photo: Don Heald.

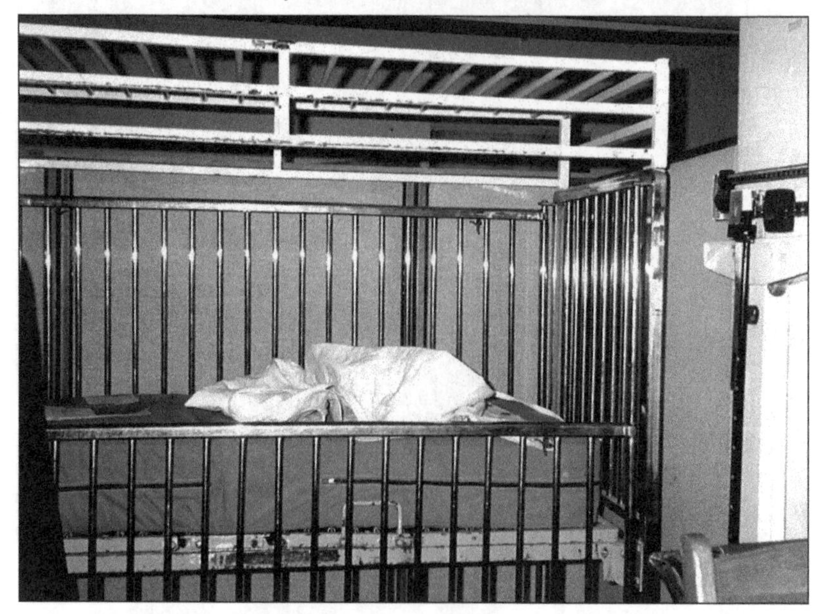

Cage-cot. Ontario Hospital School, Orillia. Courtesy Huronia Archives. Photo: Don Heald.

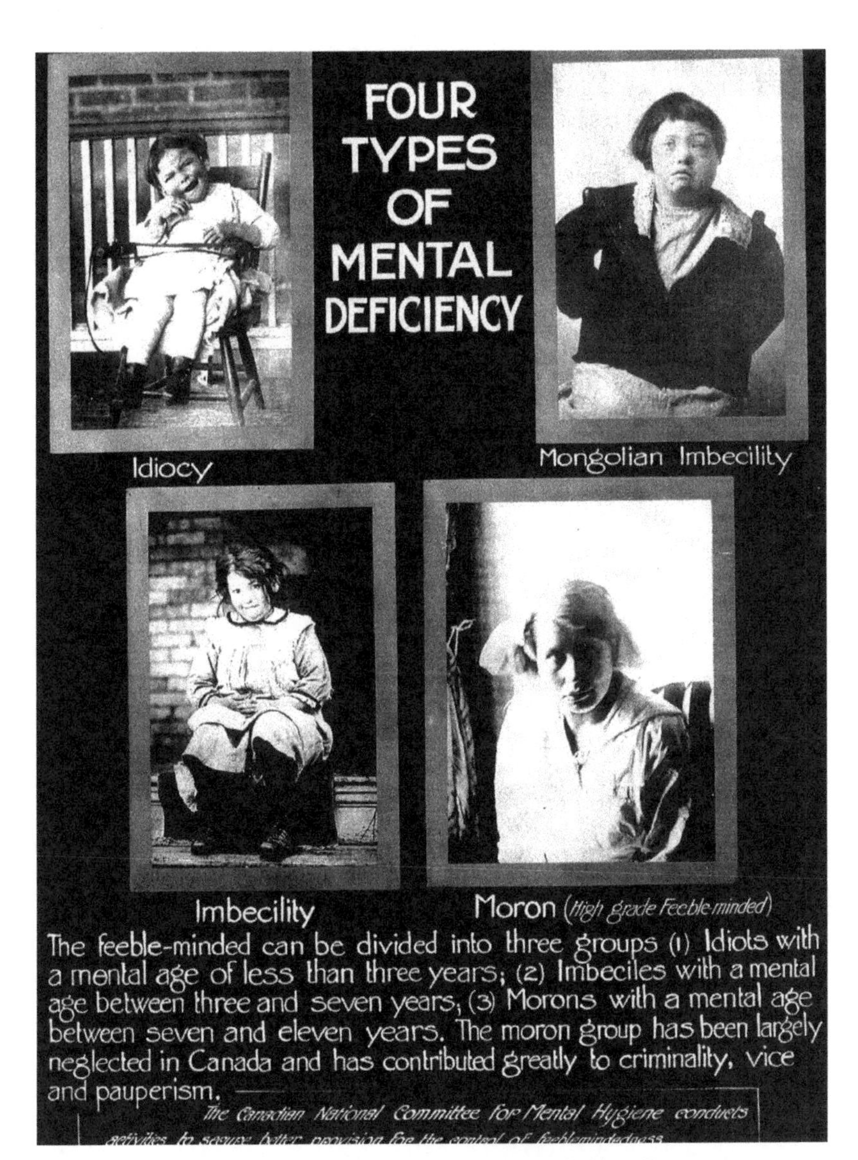

CNCMH eugenic poster, c.1924. Courtesy CAMH Archives, Toronto.

EPILOGUE

DAISY HAD WANTED HER MOTHER'S RECORDS, wanted the truth, and now she had it. It was a somber moment, not least because Daisy had come to realize that "truth" can sometimes unexpectedly change history. For reading the records was not, of course, the end.

More than half a century has gone by since the era of the Ontario Hospital School in Orillia. Ella Lumsden passed away during the writing of this book. She was eighty-two. Joe Potts, Daisy's husband, died suddenly on Palm Sunday, 2013. They did not live to see the closure of the Huronia Regional Centre, as the institution is now called, along with the two other big institutions in Ontario shut down by the government in March 2009, an event that would have given them great satisfaction. In July 2010, the Ontario Superior Court of Justice certified a one-billion-dollar class action lawsuit on behalf of former patients against the government of Ontario, which had operated the facility, for failure to provide proper care and protection for those living within its walls. The claim further charges that the province did little to protect residents after being made aware of such abuses, which included the use of nausea-inducing drugs as punishment and forced labour.

Daisy's history was, in a sense, a microcosm of the greater macrocosm of the phenomenon called "institutionalization," which spanned a whole era, from the eugenicists in the early 1900s to "de-institutionalization" in the 1980s. At that time nearly three thousand patients, many of whom had lived "on the inside," as it were, of Orillia for over thirty years, many longer, were transferred to communities "on the outside" to live new lives of freedom. Daisy has lived to see the closure of Orillia in 2009, and to be part of that one-billion dollar class action lawsuit against the province of Ontario and Huronia Regional Centre.

The class action, initiated by a social worker, Maralyn Dolmage, claims compensation for abuses suffered by former patients at the Orillia institution, formerly the Ontario Hospital School. Maralyn Dolmage had worked at Orillia for a few years, from 1969-72, and had spoken out against abuses at that time. Now, over thirty years later, she assisted two former patients, Marie Slark and Patricia Seth, whom she had known well "on the inside" in the 1960s, to instigate the current lawsuit against the government of Ontario on behalf of all former patients. Maralyn and her husband Jim Dolmage were appointed Guardians of the two litigants.

The lawsuit was certified in July 2010, by the Ontario Superior Court of Justice against the province of Ontario, which had operated the facility. The province and Huronia Regional Centre are named as the defendants in the action while former patients Marie Slark and Patricia Seth are the plaintiffs. Koskie Minsky, LLP, the Toronto law firm representing the ex-patients are highly regarded in class-actions. The trial is scheduled to take place on September 30, 2013, and to last six weeks.

The lawsuit created a stir in the community. The courtroom was packed at Osgoode Hall, Toronto, for the initial hearings in fall, 2006, many present being former patients, now in middle age. There was excitement over the idea of "one billion dollars" which patients understood to be a large sum of money of which they and their parents were to be beneficiaries, including Daisy and her mother, should the class action be won. Money is good, Daisy observed, but it did not compensate for the loss of family and your childhood, she added slowly.

The press took up the case. The *Globe* and the *Toronto Star* were ablaze with head-lines: "Invisible No More" — a popular catch-phrase — "A Troubled History," "A chance for Huronia's 'invisible' to be seen and heard," "The long journey out of HRC."

The class action cites alleged abuses that include failure to provide proper care and protection for patients, physical, sexual, and psychological abuse, and "spiritual harm." The claim further charges that the province did little to protect residents after being made aware of such abuses amounting to "*breach of fiduciary duty.*"

This last claim concerning fiduciary trust is perhaps the most disturbing in relation to parents. This is a sensitive issue, given the circumstances. For many parents are aware that they themselves had not always "protected" their children as they would have wished, even after being made **cognisant** of abuses in the institution. Many parents knowingly placed their children in harm's way, fully aware that Orillia was a dangerous, overcrowded, abusive, unsafe environment, a virtual "fire hazard." Parents continued the process up to the 1980s, grateful for the "option" of institutionalizing when they could no longer cope. Others simply put their children away not caring what became of them, never to return.

These are painful complex realities underlying the class action, sensitive and complicated to address. Since putting one's child away was always voluntary in Canada, parents held a certain implicit power they might not have been fully aware of. Their consent was necessary to the process, a symbiotic relationship with government authorities and medical professionals. If we look closely at Daisy's story, we see that gaining control over parents was essential to institutionalization. As Dr. MacMurchy noted, parents needed to be "taken firmly in hand." Parents thus had to be coerced into accepting two basic concepts: that putting put their "mentally defective" child away was for the child's " own good" — a phrase constantly reiterated throughout the century — with the state assuming all rights of wardship; and the notion that trained staff in an institution could provide far superior care to home care. It was the parent's *duty* to acquiesce. Parents put up little opposition in the first half of the twentieth century. In fact, it never really occurred to them to resist, to form, for instance, a parents' association. Being primarily poor and uneducated, they were no match for the well-educated, affluent lobby groups that regularly put pressure on the government; such organizations as the Young Men's Christian Associations, the Moral and Social Reform Council, the University Women's Club, and the Provincial Association for the Care of the Feeble-Minded, in which there was not one parent representative. It was these upper middle-class professionals and activists in Toronto, not the parents, who decided on the issues at stake and confronted the government, even about improving the conditions in the Orillia Asylum.

And so when Daisy's grandparents, Florrie and Henry, stepped ashore their new country of Canada in 1913, mere children at the time, they could not have known they were part of a vast callous emigration scheme to provide cheap labour for the dominion.

Florrie and Henry, children of the English Poor Laws, numbered among eighty thousand British boys and girls shipped off to the Dominion from England and Scotland, along with 125,000 children from Wales, between 1868 and 1925, at the behest of the powerful hated Guardians of the Poor Laws. The 'Home' children — an ironical epithet if ever there was one — had had little knowledge of the role organizations had played throughout the transactions, philanthropic groups such as the well-meaning Salvation Army, the Waifs and Strays of the Church of England, nor that the Canadian government had encouraged the scheme through subsidised transatlantic fares, free railway transport, and per capita payment to the recruiting agencies. They were the "gutter" children, part of the "dangerous classes." And what of their parents? Few knew their children had been transported without their knowledge or consent. By 1908, six per cent of boys and eight per cent of girls from the "Barnardo Homes for Children," a philanthropic organization, had been shipped to Canada illegally from Britain. But what did the concept of "illegal" mean to a parent of the workhouse labouring under the harsh Union Poor Laws?

Some Home children were grateful to Canadians who had treated them well but many were neglected and abused with no recourse to law. Most boys left the farms once their indenture was up, turning to mining, logging, railroad construction, telegraphy, or like Henry Hewitt, to work in factories for wages. Most girls left domestic service and became factory workers or salesgirls, and got married in their twenties.

A registry is now available online for about four million descendants of the Home children, long lost to their parents and families. Over 9,000 links are now available online for the United Kingdom and Ireland, and a British Home Children site for 100,000 children sent from England and Wales with an official genealogy website of the English and Welsh census information for 1901. It has given Daisy a sense of identity, a truth to her grandparents' history she had never suspected.

Daisy took a long look at the faded archival photograph of the Home girls arriving in New Brunswick on the landing stage, dressed in long sturdy coats and funny little hats, and sturdy white shoes, as if dressed for church, clutching their portmanteaux no doubt handed out for the journey. Any one of them might have been her grandmother Florrie; the rows of little girls not knowing what lay in store for them on that cold hard shore. There is a sense of a lowering grey Canadian sky, the water is steel grey edging the wharfs, a gleam of sun breaks through over the scene, so long ago.

The era of "the eugenicists" was a powerful, tempestuous time in Canada, particularly in Toronto. Intense articles and pseudo-scientific papers on the topic of the "feeble-minded" flowed from the pens of medical doctors, clergymen, psychiatrists, social workers, even the superintendent of the girls' reformatory out on Kingston Road, Miss Lucy Brooking. "The Menace of the Feeble-Minded," "Sterilize the Unfit!" "The Problem of Wayward Girls and Delinquent Women," "Sterilization of Imbecility," "The Defective and Insane Immigrant," and "Feeble-Mindedness in Canada: A Serious National Problem" – "We Pay!" were just a few of the titles, not to mention the vituperations of leading psychiatrists.

Of course, one must not to be too quick to judge and condemn another era from the modern vantage point of one's own, replete with a social network, public education for all, and the Canadian Charter of Rights and Freedoms. Theirs were legitimate concerns, for Toronto and Canada had been inundated with over three million poor immigrants during the nineteenth and early twentieth century, overwhelming Toronto in particular, which had increased its population by more than a quarter million. There were recurring cholera, diphtheria, and scarlet fever epidemics, raging bouts of syphilis against which there was no effective modern medicine, contaminated milk giving rise to the dreaded "summer diarrhea," a high rate of infant and maternal mortality, thousands of wretched hovels "below College" with thirty thousand outdoor privies overflowing with bilge, and a starving restless population suffering from the recurring economic slumps, as well as a Great Depression that lasted through the 1930s. The fear that a new under class would overwhelm and outbreed the upper classes, known as the "fertility differential" — hotly debated — was all the more ominous. Basically, it meant the poor were having far more children than the rich and would eventually outnumber them. It had to be stopped, but how? The obvious solution was birth control for the poor. But here we see the paradox of class distinctions of the time, for whereas the middle and upper class had availability to birth control, being educated, the poor were virtually denied owing to poor education. As Dr. Farrar, director of the Toronto Psychiatric hospital, noted, the poor were too stupid to be relied on to follow the directions correctly, sterilization having to be the preferred alternative. (Marie Stopes, who founded the first birth control clinic for poor women in London, found that working class women were ignorant of their anatomy, not even knowing the location of the vagina or cervix, and were loath to undress.) But also doctors themselves found it "repugnant," according to Dr. MacMurchy and failed to provide information. The only answer seemed to be institutionalizing the degenerates, and ultimate sterilization.

As arguments raged, women like Florrie submitted to endless childbirth.

While the authoritative Dr. MacMurchy claimed to have a certain compassion for the poor — "the rich baby lives, the poor baby dies" — she and her colleagues did not seem to connect the dire poverty all around them to the low wages worker had to survive on, dictated by "the market." Dr. Clarke, always concerned about procuring high income for medical men, offered Dr. Ernest Jones a starting salary of $600 per annum to work in the feeble-minded Clinic with extra hours in pathology and neurology at the Asylum, not a great sum considering that Joseph Atkinson, editor of the *Star*, earned $5,000 per annum, but still considerably more than common labourers who had to manage on $6 a week, and some working girls on $2 per week sewing knickerbockers (and having to supply their own thread), in the clothing trades' sweat-shops. Clarke railed against the government for granting Mother's Allowance to the poor and felt that $2 to $5 a week was more than adequate for factory girls sticking labels on bottles in a bottling factory. "They are well paid for what they do."

Low wages and unemployment were the root cause for unrest and rebellion among the workers. But to alleviate suffering by raising their wages meant cutting profits. The only recourse of the workers was the "strike," a new phenomenon smacking of Bolshevism to the eugenicists. There were twenty-five strikes alone in Toronto, in 1919. The Winnipeg General Strike of 1919 with its "bloody Saturday," struck terror into the upper class, many of whom, like Dr. MacMurchy and Dr. Clarke, lived in the new elite neighbourhood of "Rosedale," on the north side of Bloor Street, and feared the degenerates rising up in their hovels south of College. The General Strike brought to mind the recent Russian Revolution in 1917, that saw the Czar murdered along with his wife and children, and the aristocracy laid low, as the workers seized power — all followed avidly in the Toronto newspapers by those who could read.

If the weapon of the labouring classes was the strike, the most powerful tool acquired by the medical profession was the "I.Q. TEST." This became the lynch pin of control over parents, the hinge on which institutionalization revolved. The powerful "Stanford-Binet I.Q. test," with its "50" I.Q. dividing line, so arbitrarily chosen by Dr. Helen MacMurchy back in the early 1900s, and never challenged by parents, intimidated rich and poor alike. For now there was a whole slew of new, indecipherable terms — imbecile, idiot, moron — developed by Lewis Terman at Stanford, who had once written his Ph.D. thesis on "Genius and Stupidity: A Study of the Intellectual Processes of Seven 'Bright' and Seven 'Stupid' Boys".

This complex array of diagnostic terms empowered those who employed them, the psychometrists, psychologists and psychiatrists.

Can we ever know the true potential of people like Daisy's family, caught in endless cycles of poverty and neglect, subjected to the tyranny of "50 I.Q."? Twelve year-old Ella Hewitt, for instance, was acknowledged by the psychologist at Orillia on admission as "a bright appearing child, but undernourished," despite her I.Q. of 40, a significant drop of eleven points from her previous test at the Toronto Psychiatric Hospital, when she had scored 51. No comment on the discrepancy.

Ella's score of 51 deemed her eligible for admission to an auxiliary class. But what happened highlights the fate of a poor girl like Ella. She was sent instead to St. Mary's Catholic School, starting at the late age of seven, and after only two months in Jr. 1, was "excluded," a reprehensible act by today's standards but commonplace.

There could be many reasons why Ella did not attend school, let alone an auxiliary class. The social worker described the Hewitt children as "with barely a shred of clothing to their backs," and Ella as covered in vermin, which would hardly have endeared her to the nuns of St. Mary's. Poor children like the Hewitts regularly ran wild in the streets, easily evading the truancy officers who were hardly going to run after them down filthy back alleys. Was Ella too developmentally delayed or out of control (she never obeyed her parents noted the social worker and threw violent tantrums) to warrant schooling? It is also possible that Henry Hewitt was aware of the possibility his children might end up in the "idiot asylum" in Orillia if they attended Auxiliary Classes in the public school system, as he must have seen happen to many poor children in the neighbourhood. The fact that he later capitulated shows the exigencies of the Hewitt's poverty during the Great Depression and the persuasive authority of medical professionals who easily intimidated the poor. Ella's fate was sealed.

The I.Q. tests gave rise to a more subtle form of intimidation: stigma and shame. Of course the very nature of this shame was rooted in the general medical *view* of a "mentally defective" child as basically ugly, deformed, with nothing to offer his parents or society. Parents could hardly be blamed if they too felt revulsion and horror at the sight of their severely retarded offspring, regarded by medical doctors as "reversions" to a distant ancient past in the human chain, a reprehensible sort of throw-back of Darwin's "descent of man." Dr. Beaton in Orillia had called them "the loathsome ones."

Eugenicists stressed the biological nature of retardation, an "inherited defect" that could be passed down from generation to generation, a "taint in the blood." Parents who produced such children were themselves labelled as "tainted" genetically. The aetiology favoured throughout the records, "*familial,*" was a frightening term to most parents, since it implied something hidden inside one's body, deep within the genes that only a trained doctor could "tell," thus giving the medical profession psychological power over many a parent, whether rich or poor, but especially the uneducated.

Daisy soon guessed that "*familial,*" cropping up constantly in her records —"Etiology: *familial*" — meant that her retardation was "*inherited.*"

This was confirmed by the discovery of a "family tree" on a faded sheet of paper slipped inside her records. It had been drawn up by some nameless psychometrist "interested" in tracing the Hewitts' "retardation" going back to the great grandparent, but without their knowledge or permission. "Mentally defective" family members were indicated by striped boxes or circles next to their name, boxes assigned for the males and circles for females. Daisy, her mother, her two uncles, a paternal aunt (her father's sister Effie Lumsden), her mother's cousin, Aunt Henrietta's son Cuthbert and possibly "others" hinted at by psychiatrists, had been committed to Orillia on the base of these assumptions. Daisy was shocked. She had known that her mother had been in Orillia, but not a whole slew of relatives including, apparently, Lizzie who, she now discovered from one of the records, had been "slated for Orillia" in 1955, if she but knew. This was averted when Lizzie's foster mother had stepped forward and extended her care up to age sixteen, another bitter pill for Daisy to swallow.

Orillia was all about secrecy and shame, for both parents and the children placed there, as Daisy recognized. She was well aware of the stigma of being a patient and for decades had kept her history a secret. "Orillia was nothing to be proud of," she observed. The reading of her records and this book has had a paradoxical effect on her. She was excited, enthused with each section she read. One day she deliberately confided to a neighbour that she had been in the Orillia institution. The neighbour responded, "Oh! I didn't know you were an Institution Girl, one of 'Them'." Daisy was hurt, but challenged her friend, that she should be ashamed and that "being put away could of happen to a lot of people." Something had changed in Daisy. A few days later, according to Daisy, her friend knocked on her door and apologized, "I thought about what you said, Daisy and you're right. It ain't your fault what happen."

And so Daisy at last came to the most sensitive, painful part of the records, her mother's "promiscuity." When she finally read the words: "*admits to one sexual experience with her brother,*" Daisy said she felt "sick to her stomach." Her eleven-year-old mother had had "sex" with her seventeen year old brother Robbie — "Uncle Robbie" to Daisy — all the more terrible since the social worker's words in the "family history" did not sound like rape to Daisy. Why had her mother not screamed and begged for mercy as she herself had, or called out to Grandad (perhaps in the same room, another horror to contemplate), all the more horrific in that it seemed only to confirm once again the family's degeneracy and her mother's waywardness, and hence her own shame. There was an unacknowledged legal aspect to Ella's affair. Here was an unreported crime. For Robbie was seventeen, an adult, and as such should have been removed from the home situation by the social worker to put eleven year-old Ella "out of harm's way." But Robbie had also been deemed an "imbecile," and as such could not be held responsible for his action before the law. The parents favoured Robbie, so Ella took the blame and was removed from the home. She had been betrayed by her parents, blamed for the act, while Uncle Robbie had got off scot-free.

Daisy did not weep. There was no real sorrow or empathy for her mother. That was reserved for Florrie — "Granny" — whom she had loved, for Granny, she recalled, had always had a little "something" for the children when they visited. Daisy had been fond of her. She recalled guiltily that Florrie had been deaf, that "she read lips." Now she realized that Grandad had burst Granny's eardrums in a temporary fit of violence, attributed to something called "shell-shock," another aspect of the tragedy uncommented on by the social workers who were given to dwelling on his "*insanity*" — the fact that he had "put his head in a gas oven" and had actually tried to jump from the roof-tops — obviously "insane," but no treatment ever offered. Daisy simply wept quietly to herself, and put the records aside for a while.

Still Daisy could not forgive her mother, linked as she was to her own sexual betrayal. "No matter what, I was just a kid and she shouldn' have done what she done." For what else had Ella's betrayal of Daisy been decades later on that cold, snowy day at Christmastime in her mother's bleak apartment while her father was at work, if not "incestral," with its murky Freudian undertones. What mother would enjoy the rape of her daughter with an insane man she had picked up outside the mental asylum on Queen Street, reasoned Daisy. For just as her mother had been betrayed and sent to Orillia, so Daisy felt betrayed, identifying the lack of legal action with her forced return to Orillia. Of course, again, there are deeper levels here. For both the CAS and the administration had carelessly put Daisy "in harm's way" by allowing her to go home to parents they knew were unsatisfactory and dangerous. To cover up their own negligence, it is likely that Daisy's rape was passed over as a "story."

This inability of Ella Lumsden to mother her children, as Daisy saw it, was the root of their suffering, for Daisy had dearly loved her father and little sister and brother, and mourned the loss of the loving united family that she had always longed for, with all the eagerness of her loving heart.

It was then that Daisy wept the most bitterly concerning her mother. "Gone," she cried; like so much else.

The closure of Huronia Regional Centre, Orillia, along with the Rideau Regional Centre in Smith's Falls and Southwestern Regional Centre in Blenheim, on March 31, 2009, was a momentous occasion for people with disabilities across Canada, for us all. People with disabilities came from Newfoundland to British Columbia, from sea to sea, to attend the Remembrance Ceremony at Queen's Park, Toronto, where people gathered for a candlelight vigil: "Hold this candle up and say that you have Freedom." We gave thanks and honoured, in particular, the members of the Ontario Legislature who fought to replace the old *Developmental Services Act* with the new *Social Inclusion Act,* which does away with institutions, and all who sought to influence the politicians to change the law. Orville Endicott, Community Living Ontario's legal counsel, spoke, saying it was time for rejoicing, but also for sadness for the thousands of former patients, many of them still young children, who had been needlessly separated from their families, and that we offered our "longing for them to healed of their wounds and restored to loving friendships." People linked arms, singing "Amazing Grace." There were cheers and tears. Church bells rang. The battle had been won. The old Asylum for Idiots and Feeble-Minded, high on the hill overlooking the broad expanse of Lake Simcoe, silent and serene, had received its death-knell.

Daisy and I paid a final visit to Orillia one summer day. The institution was silent, the residents long departed. But Orillia still stands, with its three entrances, A, B, C, and long red-brick buildings behind a row of wrought iron railings, in full view at the curve of Memorial Avenue off highway 400. One and a half hour's drive north of Toronto.

All was eerie, still, the past rising once again with all its joys and sorrows, the scene of so many battles fought, won, and lost amongst parents and officials, now extinguished by time. We wandered about the grounds past wards and cottages boarded up. Sunlight swept over the vast lawns that led down to Lake Simcoe, glittering below. Wild turkeys strutted where children once had played. Our shoes echoed on the paved paths that connect the various cottages and trades buildings and great Administrative Building. Hidden underground was the maze of tunnels, the tramways that had transported food on trolleys to the inmates and where so much had taken place, still undisclosed. Orillia's buildings are dangerous now, many containing asbestos that is lethal to workers who might have to dismantle the place. The old infirmary is also boarded up, too toxic to enter, warned a guard.

We passed a blank stretch of scrub land, dried and stony, where once had stood Cottage M and L and infamous B demolished long since, half a century ago, as if they had never been, left to memory only.

Old Cottage C for Boys, however, was a hive of activity: it now contains the County Court House and Gaming Commission for Ontario. Its old hallways all hustle and bustle, its driveway crammed with SUVs. Cottage O for Girls, where Daisy had resided, is renovated with modern windows and sandblasted brick. It is now used as a residence for police cadets. Many of the buildings still have the old names embedded in the brick: *Nurses' Residence, Building 47, Cottage K* — a place of history little known to most Canadians, a place of the past.

We cross the road by the new OPP building where once the institution farm had stood, coming to the Huronia graveyard, hidden from view. A shadow droops from the maple, a buzzard hovers: the graves of Orillia stretch row on row, nameless slabs in the burning sun identified only by their case numbers, these ones long gone, locked in the past, something lost at the heart of Orillia, of the human soul itself. For who will remember Orillia or its truth, complex and subtle as the whisper of wind through the fading leaves, the thousands of inmates forever silenced, their unspoken lives seemingly lost in time, but for Daisy's courage in allowing her story to be told on their behalf, all the more vital since Daisy's records from the old Toronto Psychiatric Hospital have now been destroyed in accordance with the new policies of the day.

Yet Daisy has survived, she and her family who overcame all odds with that fortitude of old. Henry and Florrie and Ella, deemed illiterate, morons, part of the "unfit" had amazingly won out, gaining the release of their children where so many had failed, showing the power of the human spirit. "Don't pretty them up," Daisy had said of their story, "They was what they was," a part of history that for too long has been swept under the table, yet still a living memory for the few, mourned and cherished. And perhaps we may, at the last, acknowledge our communal responsibility for the suffering of the most vulnerable of our citizens, and come to that place of forgiveness, and mercy, remembering, as William Faulkner once said, "*The past is not dead. It's not even the past.*"

ACKNOWLEDGEMENTS

My special thanks, first, to Don Heald, for his kind and practical support and patience throughout; my daughter Mandy Alexander; Cyril Greenland, an early mentor; voluntary reader Joan Sutcliffe who listened for hours and read early drafts, Jane McCaig for her encouragement, reading the manuscript and for important help with the Cabbagetown section of the book; Gordon Kyle, a valuable reader of the early manuscript; Judith Sandys who also read the early manuscript; Pat Bishop for her love and support; Lorraine Williams who first led me to Inanna Publications; Beth Donaldson who helped with early research; Dell Brown who took me round the pubs of Cabbagetown; Sandy Macpherson who also showed me the back streets of Cabbagetown; Arthur and Bernice Lepper, both residents of Cabbagetown, for sharing reminiscences; Laurie and Muriel Morgan for reminiscences of early Toronto, and Dr. Morgan's help with medical facts; Captain Doris Routly of the Salvation Army, Toronto, former Matron of "The Nest" Girls Home, for her reminiscences; the late Jim Burns, former principal of William Burgess Public School, East York, Toronto, for his memories of the Orillia institution and of the Opportunity Class; Marilyn Hew, teacher at William Burgess for useful information about the Opportunity Class as a child, and her memories of "The Nest" in the 1950s; Ed Swinton, whose late brother was attendant at the Orillia institution, for useful reminiscences of Dr. Horne, Superintendent; Werner Jacobson, former attendant and volunteer archivist at the Orillia institution; Edith Mole, and Irene Hill, administrators at Huronia Regional Centre, Orillia, for kind access to the archives; Jessica Heald who set up my great web-site; John Lofaso; Barbara Werhspan; Bill Belfontaine; the late Eleanor West, teaching colleague at Parkholme School for Developmentally Challenged, Peel

Board of Education, for vital first-hand recollections of the "cot-cages" at the Orillia institution in the 1960s; my mother-in-law, Helen Orchard, former residential counsellor at the Mental Retardation Centre, Surrey Place, Toronto; the late Pierre Berton for early encouragement and information on his visit to Orillia in 1959; Jake Scragg and Options, Mississauga, for invaluable help with digitalizing photographs; David Watson, psychic; Sherry McKechern and Robert Graham for ongoing support over the decades; Maureen Maguire, former librarian at Huronia Regional Centre; Audrey Cole, parent advocate for patients in the institutions; Orville Endicott for legal assistance; Jim O'Donnell; "X," former worker at the institution, for information on patient abuse in the 1980s; Adele Gibbard, parent, and her invaluable assistance in her recollections of Ward O-3, Ontario Hospital School, in the 1960s and of staff abuse of patients; her son Brian Gibbard, former patient, for his courageous recollections of life as a patient.

I am grateful to Philip Melville, retired psychiatrist and Head of Women's Dorm at the Toronto Psychiatric Hospital for his lively recollections of the hospital in the 1960s. Also I am indebted to Ron Ward, Coordinator of the Freedom of Information and Protection of Privacy Act at the Ontario Archives, for advice and to research assistants at Ontario Archives; and to Jim Dolmage for reading the manuscript and his wife Maralyn Dolmage both for their tenacity as Guardians for the Litigants and initiating the class-action law-suit on behalf of citizens who were former patients in Ontario institutions; Susan Leventhal, msw, for her insights into legal aspects of wardship; John Court, Archivist, for invaluable help in research and archival photographs at the camh Archives, Queen Street, Toronto. I also wish to acknowledge Carolyn Strange's book, *Toronto's Girl Problem: The Perils and Pleasures of The City*, and Mariana Valverde's book, *The Age of Light, Soap and Water: Moral Reform in English Canada*, which provided excellent resources for the social background of the early 1900s; also Harvey Simmons' book, *From Asylum to Welfare*, for useful material on Orillia and the "feeble-minded."

I am deeply grateful to the courageous former patients of Orillia for their testimony: Desi Harnum for providing access to his patient records and for many recollections of patient abuse and life in the institution, Brian Gibbard, Mike D., Barry Thachuk, Michael Callahan, Robert, Marie

Slark, Julia Hadley and many more who wish to remain anonymous; also Joe Clayton, former patient of Rideau Regional Centre, Smith's Falls.

Last but not least, I would like to specially honour "Daisy Lumsden," and her mother, the late "Ella Lumsden" (née Hewitt), for sharing their experiences and for Daisy, in particular, for her courage in coming forward with her story.

Finally, most of all, my editor at Inanna Publications, Luciana Ricciutelli, for her ongoing faith in this book.

Endnotes

PROLOGUE

Orillia: The institution was generally called 'Orillia' by professionals and parents after the town of Orillia, Ontario, where the institution was built in 1876. It changed names many times: The Asylum for Idiots and Feebleminded, 1876; Orillia Hospital for Idiots and Feebleminded, 1907; Hospital for the Feeble-Minded up to 1920; Ontario Hospital, Orillia, to 1936; Ontario Hospital School, 1936-1974; Huronia Regional Centre, 1974 to 2009. However, names often continued to overlap in usage. Thus, the 'Idiot Asylum' and 'Hospital for the Feeble-Minded' continued in use for many years.
Daisy's records: Daisy Lumsden's records and files, that include records from the Children's Aid Society of Metropolitan Toronto and the Salvation Army Girls' Home, called 'The Nest,' Toronto, are contained in Daisy's file in the Salvation Army Archives, Toronto. The records of her years as patient in Ontario Hospital School, Orillia, are accessed from Daisy Lumsden's Patient File, Case No. 65043, Ontario Hospital School Orillia, Records Office, Huronia Regional Centre, Orillia, obtained in 1999. The file also contains her patient records from Toronto Psychiatric Hospital. Hereafter referred to as: Daisy Lumsden's Patient Records.

PART ONE

Chapter One
All references to letters are from Daisy's Lumsden's Patient File.
Ernest Lumsden ... Isabella: There were three separate branches of Children's Aid Societies: the Children's Aid Society of Toronto, the Infant's Homes and the Protestant Children's Home; 33 Charles Street East was used by CAS as a Children's Shelter in 1928. In 1932, 32 Isabella Street was bought for Administrative Offices. On May 31, 1951, the two agencies amalgamated and became the Children's Aid and Infants' Homes of Toronto. See John McCullagh, A *Legacy of Caring: A History of the Children's Aid Society of Toronto* (Toronto: The Dundurn Group, 2002: 39, 57). Hereafter: McCullagh.
The Nest: The Nest was a Girls' Home in Toronto on Broadview Ave., run by the Salvation Army. Daisy's records also include full reports from the CAS, 1952-1959, up to and including the date of her admission to Orillia, August, 1959,

which are contained in her records from the Salvation Army.
Effie Lumsden's records: Lost in transit to date, but referred to in Daisy's patient records as Effie Lumsden Case #5721 in the Clinical Abstract and Family History forms, Ontario Hospital School, Orillia, Sept., 24, 1959.

Chapter Two
Miss Prewse, Infants Home, Shelter: On May 31, 1951, the two agencies, Children's Aid and Infants Homes of Toronto amalgamated becoming the largest child welfare organizations in North America. They worked out of the CAS offices at 32 Isabella Street and at the Charles Street shelter, the Huntley Street Receiving Centre and the Infants Homes old offices at 34 Grosvenor Street (McCullagh 110). The CAS address on Daisy's records was cited as: Children's Aid Society, 33 Charles Street East, Toronto.

Chapter Three
"J. J. Kelso himself ... had stressed that if a family 'failed'": It was acknowledged by Kelso that "parents are the natural guardians of the children" *Annual Report CAS, 1894* (cited in McCullagh, 39, 57).

Chapter 4
The Nest, Captain Rawlings, Lady Eaton: In January 15, 1941, Lady Eaton opened The Nest for girls from age four to fourteen who came from broken homes. The girls were to stay at The Nest until their own homes were re-established (The Salvation Army Archives, Scarborough, Ontario).
"Salvation Army does not serve the mentally retarded": The care, responsibility and planning for mentally handicapped children was a contentious issue between the CAS and the provincial government. The society's approach was that handicapped children should not be their responsibility because of the difficulty of finding foster homes (particularly for children with Down's Syndrome).
"Finances had been settled": Under the *Children's Protection Act*, municipalities were required to contribute a 'reasonable sum' — not less than $1 a week — for each child from its jurisdiction who was in the care of the CAS. This eventually became an annual grant. The government made it clear that their mandate was not to be fully engaged in providing community services to the mentally retarded people; only had limited responsibility. See Harvey G. Simmons, *From Asylum To Welfare* (Downsview: National Institute on Mental Retardation, 1982: 171-172, n.33). Hereafter: Simmons.
"To Dear Mother and father": Daisy's letter to 'her mother and father,' no date. Unposted. Daisy Lumsden's Patient file.

Chapter 5
"The agency went ahead with plans for placement in Orillia": Daisy Lumsden's Patient File, Clinical Abstract, September 24, 1959, Ontario Hospital School, Orillia. Application for her admission (to Orillia) was made by the CAS on September 25, 1956, and again on May 7, 1959: "Girl was admitted on August 21, 1959, certified as mentally defective."
Opportunity Class, William Burgess Public School: An Opportunity Class for slower learners, integrated into William Burgess Public School, one of the few offered at the time by the East York Board of Education in the 1950s ("The

Opportunity Class," Mimeograph, Toronto: Ontario Department of Education, Auxiliary Branch, 1950 and 1964, cited in Gerald Hackett, *The History of Public Education for Mentally retarded Children in the Province of Ontario 1867-1964*, D.Ed. thesis, University of Toronto, 1969: 246). Hereafter: Hackett). Daisy's report cards in the Opportunity Class found in Daisy Lumsden's Patient Records.
"The issue of Mrs. Lumsden's operation": Daisy Lumsden's Patient File, Conference Notes, January 1956, The Nest. It was noted that Mrs. Lumsden "underwent a hysterectomy operation" and that "consequently she is anxious to have her family reunited." Further, the CAS felt "under pressure" from Mr. and Mrs. Lumsden "with regard to having their children" and that "they may have to consider granting their request."
"The Nest was an open secret": Maralyn Hew, teacher and former pupil at William Burgess Public School, remembers the Opportunity Class and the teacher Miss Webb, when she was herself a pupil in the school in the 1950s. Protocol and a sense of honour prevented children from referring to The Nest as a girls' home (personal interview with Maralyn Hew at William Burgess Public School, June 28, 2005).
"The day at William Burgess": William Burgess Public School Archives.
"The greatest iceberg": Quoted from 'Habits' by Alonzo Newton Benn, *The Young Soldier*, June 24, 1950, Salvation Army Archives. His cry, "Around me were wretchedness, misery," was said in 1910 at the Commemoration Stone laid at Mile End Waste, England. Booth's third son, Commandant Herbert Booth, was the Canadian Territorial Commander from 1893 to 1897. Booth's poem "While children suffer" was first expressed in the early years of his ministry, in the formation of the "East London Revival Society" which became The Christian Mission. Booth's visit to the Holy Land where he hoisted the Army Flag on Mount Calvary, cited in "His Hold On God," Salvation Army pamphlet, "The Salvation Army Highlights from the Life of General William Booth" (The Salvation Army Archives).
"Enclosed is a form ... transfers to Orillia": Letter from Lieutenant Lovering to Miss Tickles, Children's Aid Society, June 10, 1959. Daisy Lumsden's Patient File.

Chapter 6
"Two Physician's Certificates of Incompetence": Every child admitted to Orillia had to have two certificates of incompetence signed by physicians. Since Daisy was a ward of CAS, her parents did not have to sign.
Toronto Social Service Index: Morton Teicher, in 1948, as chief social worker at the in and out-patient departments at the Toronto Psychiatric Hospital, tried to change "the social service exchange" whereby information about a child was passed between agencies without the client's knowledge or permission. Teicher felt that this was unethical (Morton Teicher, "Let's Abolish the Social Service Exchange," *Social Work Journal* 33.1 (January 1952): 28-31, cited in Shorter 243).
"First admission under the guardianship of the Toronto Children's Aid Society": Daisy was under the guardianship of CAS until she turned sixteen, even though she was held inside an institution. This age was extended to age eighteen.

Chapter 7
"Some were Mongoloids": This term was used for children with Down's syndrome until into the 1980s (for definition and usage see David Wright, *DOWNS:*

The History of a Disability, New York: Oxford University Press, 2011: 191). Hereafter: Wright.
"The aides threw pieces of food": This incident was related to me by Adele Gibbard, mother of a child in the Orillia institution. Adele set up a group of mothers in Mississauga, Ontario, who visited Orillia twice a month. She related that if one complained, visiting privileges could be suspended or stopped by the superintendent (personal interview with Adele Gibbard, summer 1999; 2005).
"A certain number of normal girls on the wards": Adele Gibbard was aware of girls of normal intelligence in the institution (personal interview with Adele Gibbard, summer 1999, 2005).

Chapter 8
"Dr. Snedden, the Inspector from the Department of Health, always checked": Inspection Report by Dr. F. W. Snedden, Nov. 29 and 30, and Dec. 3 and 4, 1956, hereafter: Inspection Reports. The School of Nursing at Orillia opened in 1928 and closed down in 1945."
"Children's Dorm, big-headed babies": Orillia provided space for a number of children suffering from terminal hydro-cephalus. Dr. Snedden noted that the Children's Dorm accommodated 146 patients from age two to eight years. It provided cot accommodation along with one section for infants.
"*You shouldn' have to dress like that, Daisy. We workers complained to Dr. Snedden*": Dr. Snedden did report complaints from staff about the type, pattern and outmoded style of girls' clothing, under 'Patients Clothing.'
"*A considerable proportion are of low-grade intelligence*": Dr. Snedden's report throughout, like other inspectors' reports, shows how aware the inspectors were of physical, sexual, and psychological abuse taking place in the institution, and their descriptions deliberately draw attention to inhumane conditions.
Dr. Lionel Penrose: Director of Psychiatric Research for the Province of Ontario, circa 1940. Medical Inspection of Ontario Hospital School, Orillia, June 18-21, 1940, including section on "Medical Research Investigations at Orillia Ontario Hospital, Government Reports Ontario, 1939-1945 (CAMH Archives).

Chapter 9
"*What's Wrong at Orillia*": see Pierre Berton, "What's Wrong at Orillia: Out of Sight, Out of Mind," *Toronto Daily Star,* January 6, 1960. Hereafter: Berton.
"*Orillia Packet & Times* glowing account": see *Daily Packet & Times*, January 7, 1960: 1.
"Donald MacDonald buildings for human storage ... Ontario Legislature": See Janet Shea, *A Short History of the Ontario Hospital School, Orillia, 1875-1970* (Toronto: Monograph typescript, n.d., c.1980: 188, n.7). Hereafter: Shea.
"*Morton Schulman & "Cot-Cages"*: see newspaper articles, "Staff Shortage Hits Retarded Children" (*Toronto Daily Star* April 6, 1971:1); "Crib Cage Problem to Get Top Priority" (*Toronto Daily Star* April 7, 1971: 1). Parents' reaction to the "cage cot" controversy, 1971: One father with a twenty-three-year-old son in Orillia praised the institution and accepted the necessity for staff to use a cage-cot for his son. "My son was in a bed with sides but no top for some time. He was frustrated and had to be protected from hurting himself" (*Orillia Packet & Times* April 7, 1971:1).
"*Cedar Springs*": The government had wanted to build another huge institution,

similar in size to Orillia and Smith's Falls, at Cedar Springs. It was planned to have 2,400 beds. Parents objected and opposed the plan, and it was reduced to 1,000 beds in 1961. See Betty Anglin and June Braaten, *Twenty-Five Years of Growing Together: A History of the Ontario Association for the Mentally Retarded* (Toronto: Canadian Association for the Mentally Retarded, 1978). Hereafter: Anglin and Braaten.
Dr. Don Zarfas: Psychiatrist highly esteemed by the Association for Mentally Retarded Children in Ontario (Anglin and Braaten).
One On Every Street: Government-sponsored propaganda movie showing life, education and treatment for patients at Ontario Hospital School (Fletcher's Film Productions, narrator Allan McPhee, 1960. RG 29-24-2-4, AO).

Chapter 11
"You ain't a ward no more": Children's Aid Society wardship ended at age sixteen.
"The stuff Eddie told them!": Eddie and Steve's stories are based on true events of sexual abuse, related to the author in interviews with former patients (see author interviews).

Chapter 12
"Straight jackets": A straight jacket made by former patients at Ontario Hospital School Orillia is on display in the Huronia Regional Centre Archives, Orillia.
"The Pavilion": Named for Dr. Bernard McGhie, superintendent of Ontario Hospital, Orillia, 1927-1930, who brought about important changes in the institution. All references to Daisy's behaviours are cited from Daisy Lumsden's Patient File.
"Mellaril 100mg. Daily for homosexual tendencies": Daisy Lumsden Patient File. March 19, 1965. "Medication: Mellaril 100mg. p.m. for homosexual tendencies."

Chapter 13
Duty Book: Dr. Binnington, Dr. Bartley, Dr. James, entries in Duty Book, September 5, 1963, October 10, 1964. Dec. 5, 1964. Daisy Lumsden's Patient File.
"Habeas corpus": Since both Ernest and Ella Lumsden were illiterate and Ella of limited intelligence, it is obvious that their lawyer, Charles Farquar Q.C, advised them concerning a writ of *habeas corpus*. A writ of habeas corpus ("You have the body") is a judicial mandate usually to a prison official ordering that an inmate be brought to the court so it can be determined whether or not that person is imprisoned lawfully and whether he/she should be released
"Mrs Lumsden had already complained to CAS and the Juvenile and Family Court.... She nevertheless could be dangerous": Letter from Charles Farquar, Q.C., to Dr. MacLean Houze, Dec. 10, 1964. It is significant that Mr. and Mrs. Lumsden appealed to the Children's Aid Society and the Juvenile Court.
Donald MacDonald: Donald MacDonald was head of the provincial Co-operative Commonwealth Federation (CCF) in 1953. He was a Toronto MPP from 1955 to 1982.
"Without any good and sufficient reason ... boy-crazy": Mr. Farquar, the lawyer, is challenging Dr. Houze's right to claim responsibility for Daisy in a court of law, implying the institution has no real legal basis for detaining her.
"Dr. Houze added one final, surely telling comment ... We have over 500 children on our waiting list": Daisy Lumsden Patient File, Letter from Dr. M. Houze to Charles Farquar, Q.C., Dec. 14, 1964.

Chapter 14
"Daisy eloped": Daisy Lumsden Patient File,Treatment Record, Dec. 24, 1965. No details are given of punishment or ill-treatment of Daisy by staff, simply that she "eloped" and "returned a half hour later."

Chapter 15
"Victoria Glover": Letter from Victoria Glover to the editor of the *Toronto Daily Star*, September 29, 1949.
"Parents ... started up school ... grass-roots movement": see Anglin and Braaten (6-10).
John Brown, Director of Warrendale: see John Brown, "Warrendale to Browndale," *Experience and Experiment*, Ed. Jalal Shamsie (Toronto: Leonard Crainford 1977: 97-115). Hereafter: Brown, J.

Chapter 16
Toronto Psychiatric Hospital & Clarke Institute of Psychiatry: In June 1966 the old TPH moved to a new building on College Street, Toronto, as the 'Clarke Institute of Psychiatry', in honour of Dr. Charles Kirk Clarke, first Professor of Psychiatry at University of Toronto, 1908.
"TPH famous for lobotomies (leucotomy)": see Edward Shorter, ed., *TPH: History and Memories of the Toronto Psychiatric Hospital, 1925-1966* (Dayton, OH: Wall & Emerson, Inc., 1996: 130-135, 177, 189, 190). Hereafter: Shorter.
Milieu Therapy: The 'milieu' approach moved the philosophy of care on the female ward from a hierarchical system based on medical and professional authority to a more equal sharing of power (author phone and e-mail interview with retired psychiatrist Dr. Philip Melville, Wednesday, January 30, Thursday, January 31, 2008; see, also, Shorter 210-212).

Chapter 17
"Clinical Record ... rape": All references to Daisy's treatment and interviews are from Daisy Lumsden's Patient File.
"Objections from Dr. Crawford Jones": Daisy Lumsden Patient File, Conference notes regarding Daisy Lumsden, Ontario Hospital School, Nov. 5, 1965. The Psychological Report at that time stated: "Daisy's parents have been a continual source of concern to us on account of their repeated interference, threats, and verbal and written abuse and phone calls."

PART TWO

Chapter 19
Charles Kirk Clarke: Charles Kirk Clarke, M.B., M.D., LL.D., born in Elora, Ontario, Feb 16, 1857, son of Hon. Lieut.-Col. Charles Clarke and Emma Clarke. Clinical Assistant Toronto Hospital for Insane, 1874-1878; Assistant Physician at same Institution, 1878-1880; Assistant Superintendent Hamilton Hospital for Insane, 1880-1881; Assistant Superintendent Rockwood Hospital for Insane, Kingston, 1881-1885; Superintendent of same Hospital, 1885-1905; Superintendent, Toronto Hospital for Insane, 1905-1911; Medical Superintendent, Toronto General Hospital, 1911 and 1917-1918. Royal; Commissioner to investigate and report on methods of treatment of the Insane in Europe, 1907.

Professor of Psychiatry, University of Toronto, 1908, Dean of Medical Faculty, 1908, Medical Director, Canadian National Committee for Mental Hygiene (CNCMH). Co-Editor, *American Journal of Insanity*, 1904. See Cyril Greenland, *Charles Kirk Clarke: A Pioneer of Canadian Psychiatry* (Toronto: The Clarke Institute of Psychiatry, 1966: 4, 24). Hereafter: Greenland.
"Girls ... dressed in latest fashions, cheap frills ... and furbelows": see Carolyn Strange, *Toronto's Girl Problem: The Perils and Pleasures of the City, 1880-1930* (Toronto: University of Toronto Press, 1995: 116). Hereafter: Strange. See also Mariana Valverde, *The Age of Light, Soap, and Water: Moral Reform in English Canada, 1885-1925* (Toronto: McClelland & Stewart Inc., 1991: 169-88). Hereafter: Valverde.
"Pleasures of the city ...cheap vaudeville shows": Strange (122, 145); "girlie" shows (116-119); public dances halls (117, 243, n.4); see also Christopher St. George Clark, *Of Toronto the Good: A Social Study: The Queen City of Canada As it is* (Montreal: Toronto Pub. Co. 1898). Hereafter: Clark.
"Thousands at loose...": see Strange (51); statistics of domestic servants (126, 233, n. 68); see, also, Genevieve Leslie, "Domestic Service in Canada, 1880-1920," *Women At Work: Ontario, 1880-1930*, Eds. Janice Acton et al. (Toronto: Canadian Women's Educational Press, 1974: 71-127). Hereafter: Leslie.
Salvation Army: 1903-1914 brought over 15,000 women in as domestic servants. See Barber, Marilyn, "The Women Ontario Welcomed: Immigrant Domestics for Ontario Homes, 1870-1930," *Ontario History* 72.3 (September 1980):148-72, and "Sunny Ontario for British Girls, 1900-30," *Looking Into My Sister's Eyes: An Exploration in Women's History*, Ed. Jean Burnet (Toronto: The Multicultural History Society of Ontario, 1986: 55-69). Hereafter: Barber.
"Uncertified lodgings south of College": see Strange (177); room registry, different types of lodgings reflecting class and status (127, 175-9, 180-183).
Mrs. Willoughby Cummings: see Strange (229).
Toronto Local Council of Women (National Council of Women of Canada): see Paul Adolphus Bator, *"Saving Lives On The Wholesale Plan": Public Health Reform In The City Of Toronto, 1900-1930* (Abstract for Ph.D., May 24, 1979: 220, 235 n.7, 239). Hereafter: Adolphus Bator; *Report on the Care of the Feeble-Minded, 1913* at the Twentieth Meeting held in Montreal, QC, May 1-9, 1913; see also Veronica Strong-Boag, *The Parliament of Women: The Nations Council of Women of Canada, 1893-1929* (Ottawa: National Musuems of Canada, 1976). Hereafter Strong-Boag.
"Committee on Feeble-Minded Women, 1912": At the Annual Meeting of NCW Toronto, the Committeee on Feeble-Minded Women called for the sterilization of women of child-bearing age who were feeble-minded (Valverde 94; NCW Annual Report, 1913: 52).
"Protection of Girls ... White Slavery Committee ... Committee on Feeble-Minded Women": see Strange (49, 104);
"Shoulder to shoulder": see NCWC Handbook (cited in Strange 99, 241, n. 22); see also Valverde (77-103).
"Penalties for White Slavers": National Council of Women and the Moral and Social Reform Council of Canada together lobbied parliament with reform proposals.
Jail farm: Referred to in Dr. Clarence Hincks' article, "Feeble-Mindedness in Canada: A Serious National Problem."
"Nation's germplasm": see Edwin Black, *War Against The Weak* (New York:

Thunder's Mouth Press, 2003: 17). Hereafter: Black.
"Sir Francis Galton ... Hereditary Genius": see Galton's article, "'Eugenics: Its Definition, Scope and Aims' and 'Restrictions in Marriage'" (cited in Black 17, 42, 246n).
Women's Christian Temperance Union (WCTU): see Valverde (58-59, 61); Strange (91, 95). WCTU members wore a knot of white ribbon on their dress to symbolize purity.
"Hotbed of vice": Dr. Margaret Patterson, quoted at March 19, 1913 meeting of TLCW (see Strange 105).
"Lady Falconer ... Mrs Florence Huestis": Lady Falconer, wife of Sir Robert Falconer, President of University of Toronto (Valverde 61-62, 125). See also Angus McLaren, *Our Own Master Race: Eugenics in Canada, 1885-1945* (Toronto: Oxford University Press, 1990: 94, n.77, 35, 37, 83, 108, 110). Hereafter: McLaren.
"Alarming drop in domestics": National Council of Women, 1900 (cited in Strange 32-33); discusses the issue of the day: why did girls prefer factory work to domestic work (Strange 38-39); the "domestics' crisis" among upper class women (Strange 42-43); Dr. Clarke's views (Strange 233, n.68); drop in domestics, quote the Telegram, see Michael Piva, *The Condition of the Working Class in Toronto, 1900-1921*(Ottawa: University of Ottawa Press, 1979: 23). Hereafter: Piva.
"Royal Commission on the Relations of Labour and Capital, 1898": see Strange (28-33); *Report of Royal Commission* (minority report), see Strange (29, 33-37); second (majority) report (29, 30, 33-37); Piva (142-43, 144-45, 168-169).
Ontario Bureau of Industry: A government agency 1887 investigated why women workers were rejecting domestic work as servants and turning to factory, manufacturing and retail work. See Alice Klein and Wayne Roberts, "Beseiged Innocence: The 'Problem' and the Problems of Working Women – Toronto, 1896-1914," *Women At Work: Ontario, 1880-1930*, Eds. Janice Acton et al. (Toronto: Canadian Women's Educational Press, 1974: 211-59). Hereafter: Klein and Roberts.
"Mr Meeks ... Knights of Labour ... Miss Burnett": see Strange (231, n.27, 32, 36); Miss Burnett testified to the Commission (Strange 36).
"Elizabeth Neufeld ... Central Neighbourhood House": see Strange (244, n. 13). Central Neighbourhood House, Headworker's Report, April 1913, City of Toronto Archives (cited in Strange 120-122, 104-5, 124-5, 143, 152).
"Rev. Mackenzie ... low wages": cited in *Toronto World*, March 31, 1915; Piva (28-29, 76-77).
"Lower-class women ... supplementing their wages": see Strange (110-111). *Report of the Social Survey Commission, Toronto, Presented to City Council, October Fourth, 1915*: cited in Strange (242, n.44).
"Insufficient wages": see Strange (110-111). See also Lori Rotenberg, "The Wayward Worker: Toronto's Prostitute at the Turn of the Century," *Women At Work: Ontario, 1880-1930*, Eds. Janice Acton et al. (Toronto: Canadian Women's Educational Press, 1974: 33-69). Hereafter: Rotenberg and Acton.
"One boy of sixteen": cited in Clark (104).
Carrie Davies: the Carrie Davies trial was described in David Frank,"Sex and Violence in Toronto,"*Evening Telegram*, February 9-27, 1915; see, also, *Daily News* February 26, 1915: 84. Donations to Davies via the *Telegram* office, cited in the *Telegram*, 22 February, 1915; Strange (83-85).

"Ward Clinic": see Greenland (*Charles Kirk Clarke,* 15-16). Includes a photograph of the Ward Clinic.
"Clarke's dream ... psychiatric clinic": see Cyril Greenland, "The Origins of the Toronto Psychiatric Clinic," *TPH: History and Memories of the Toronto Psychiatric Hospital, 1925-1966,* Ed. Edward Shorter (Dayton, OH: Wall & Emerson, Inc., 1996: 19-59); Shorter (19-36).
"Elaine O": see Geoffrey Reaume, *Remembrance of Patients Past, Patient Life at the Toronto Hospital for the Insane, 1870-1940* (Don Mills, ON: Oxford University Press, 2000: 82-83, 282 n.81). Hereafter: Reaume.
"New science of psychiatry ... old alienists": See Court useful discussion of this issue and the animosity and competition between the old "alienists" who worked in insane asylums and the "new" modern psychiatrist who wanted to give treatment in modern hospital settings.
"Clarke once said: 'I love psychiatry, but hate politics'": *American Journal of Insanity* (cited in Greenland, *Charles Kirk Clarke,* 10).
"Dr. Ernest Jones": Dr Clarke's letter to Hon. W. J. Hanna, dated October 23, 1908 (Greenland, *Charles Kirk Clarke,* 18-19).
"Dr. Helen MacMurchy ... Immigration Act": see MacMurchy, *Fifth Report on Feeble-Minded* (1910: 32) ; *Eighth Report on the Feeble-Minded* (1914: 17-18).
"Demise ... Ernest Jones ... little evidence": see Philip Kuhn, "Romancing with a Wealth of Detail: Narratives of Ernest Jones's 1906 Trial for Indecent Assault," Studies in Gender and Sexuality 3.4 (2002): 344-378. Hereafter: Kuhn.

Chapter 20

"80,000 Home children": Between 1868 and 1924, 80,000 British boys and girls were sent from the poor urban areas of Britain, especially London, Manchester and Glasgow to Canada to work as indentured labourers, many without the knowledgeable consent of their parents. See Joy Parr, *Labouring Children: British Immigrant Apprentices to Canada* (Toronto: University of Toronto Press, 1980: 1, 11). Hereafter: Parr.
"Passenger warrant system": Agents were often paid $5 per head. The British Women's Emigration Association, established in 1884 sent 16,000 females to Canada as domestic servants (Barber "The Women Ontario Welcomed" and "Sunny Ontario").
Advertisements ... "Canada Wants Domestic Servants": Before the First World War, the government of Canada circulated thousands of pamphlets. In 1910, 100,000 copies of "Canada Wants Domestic Servants" were distributed in Britain. See Ellen Scheinberg,"Bringing 'Domestics' to Canada: A Study of Immigration Propaganda," *Framing Our Past: Canadian Women's History in the Twentieth Century,* Ed. Sharon Anne Cook, Lorna R. McLean and Kate O'Rourke (Montréal: McGill-Queen's University Press, 2001: 336-342).
"Children of the Poor Laws": Many children, unaccompanied by their parents, came from Britain's work houses. The *Poor Law Amendment Act* of 1834 established boards of Guardians to administer and oversee the workhouses and poorhouses where conditions were harsh for relief of the poor and paupers. See David Thomson, *The Problem of Mental Deficiency, Eugenics, Democracy and Social Policy in Britain, 1870-1959* (Oxford: Clarendon Press, 1998: 68-73).
Poor Law Guardians: Poor Law Guardians supported emigration of destitute parish children to relieve overcrowding in the workhouses and relieve unem-

ployment in England (Parr 30).
"*Master wanted his way*": Sexual exploitation of domestic servants was a concern and government officials were aware of it (Clark 104). *Royal Commission into Relations of Capital and Labour, 1898*, included reports of adolescent boys sexually exploiting servant girls (see Strange 28-33).
"*Lie on her back and keep still*": Based on a true anecdote provided by the late Cyril Greenland, Professor of Social Work, McMaster University, who had known a servant girl who had been instructed to do this very thing to avoid pregnancy (personal interview with Cyril Greenland).

Chapter 21
Imperial Order Daughters of the Empire: Philanthropic nationalist women's group linked to National Council of Women and Women's Christian Temperance Union.
"*Welcome Hostel*" : Established by National Council of Women to help immigrant girls and women (Barber, "Immigrant Domestic Servants" 8; "Sunny Ontario" 60).
"*Songs and jokes at burlesque*": "I'm not too young ... Ta-ra-rah-BOOMPS-de-yah": Credited to Henry J.Sayers, manager of the George Thatcher Minstrels, 1891.

Chapter 22
Dr. Helen MacMurchy: No biography was ever written of this remarkable woman. Yet the newspapers of the day, the *Toronto Daily Star*, the *Globe,* the *Telegram* and *Mail and Empire,* regularly followed her career and much biographical information is provided by them. Born 1862. Taught for twenty years at Jarvis (Toronto) Grammar School, later Jarvis Collegiate, under her father, head-master Archibald MacMurchy from Scotland. Canadian official to the British Royal Commission, 1905, Inspector of the Feeble-Minded for Ontario, 1906-1919, "double inspectorate" of Inspector of Feeble-Minded and Assistant Inspector of Hospitals and Charities; Inspector of Auxiliary Classes, 1914; Head of Federal Department of Health, Child Welfare Division, 1920. Commander of Order of the British Empire (CBE) 1934. See William Brown, *Making Representation: Dr Helen MacMurchy and the "Feeble-Minded" in Ontario, 1906-1919* (Ph.D. dissertation, University of Toronto, 2005). Hereafter: Brown, W.
"*Trusty old bike*": *Toronto Daily Star,* June 7, 1923.
Rev. John Shearer: Head of the Presbyterian Church's moral and social reform department, 1907-1915. Feared a 'wide-open Sunday' might cause Toronto to become a sinful city (Valverde 54-57; Strange, 98, 99-101).
"*The Ward*": St John's Ward, slum at foot of City Hall (today Nathan Philipps Square) (Piva 120, 126, 128, 129). *Mail and Empire*, 1897, referred to the Ward as a "disgrace to this city." Biographical details given of Dr. MacMurchy in the *Toronto Daily Star*, June 7, 1923, cite that MacMurchy "spent much of her labour in the Ward."
"*Jews ... rag-pickers*": The Ward was the poorest Jewish area in the city and rag picking was the main occupation, also, for women, garment making in the sweat shops of Eatons nearby or on Spadina Avenue. See James Lemon, *Toronto Since 1918: An Illustrated History* (Toronto: James Lorimer & Company, 1985: 51).
"*Unemployed march on City Hall 1909*": see Piva (74).
"*Contaminated milk*": MacMurchy's efforts, with the support Dr. Charles Hasting's, Medical Officer of Health, resulted in the *Milk Act*, 1911 (see MacMurchy "Infant Mortality").

"The rich baby lives...": Full quote: "The destruction of the poor is their poverty. The rich baby lives, the poor baby dies" (see MacMurchy "Infant Mortality" 5).
British Royal Commission on the Care and Control of the Feeble-Minded, 1904-8: see Simmons (54-61; 67-90). See, also, Kathleen Jones, *A History of the Mental Health Services* (London: Routledge and Kegan Paul, 1972: 191). Hereafter: Jones.
"No child, even the most severely retarded...": *Annual Report,* 1889: 99 (cited in Shea 58).
"The ideal ... train inmates ... self-sufficient ... Dr. Langmuir": *Annual Report of the Inspector of Asylums, Prisons and Public Charities*, 1871-2: 17.
"Inspector Reilly ... girls of puberty": *Annual Reports of the Inspector of Asylums, Prisons and Public Charities*, 1883: 170.
"Feeble-minded girls ... pauperism. Board of Guardians": Mr Baldwin Fleming, General Inspector to the Local Government Board (see Jones 191, 196).
"*Beaton ... family of seventeen idiots*": Dr. Beaton's *Annual Report to the Inspector of Prisons, Asylums and Public Charities*, March 9, 1889.
"*We must not permit the feeble-minded ... mothers*": see MacMurchy, *Annual Report on the Care of the Feeble-Minded in Ontario,* 1915: 13.
Marie Stopes: The story of the love affair between Helen MacMurchy and Marie Stopes, plus excerpts from MacMurchy's love letters dated 1909, cited in Hal*l (Passionate Crusa*der, 78-80), form the basis for this episode. MacMurchy destroyed her letters from Stopes, but MacMurchy's letters to Stopes are in the British LibrarY, Bl-s.
"Mary Dendy": The first test for feeble-mindedness, she asserted, was women who came into the workhouse with an illegitimate child, which would prove "evidence of weakness of mind" and a "lack of moral fibre'," cited in the *Royal Commission on the Care and Control of the Feeble-Minded*, Vol. 1, London 1908: 44, 51.
*"Beaton ... idiots in workhous*es": see Ontario Sessional Papers, 1892, Vol. 24, Pt.1, No.7, p. 24 (cited in Simmons 41*)*.
"Dendy's visit to Toronto": see Simmons (73); Hackett (77).
"*Jews less number of children with defects"*: see Simmons (73, 91).
"*Germany ... auxiliary classes*": Germany had, at this time, the most humane treatment and education of feeble-minded children in Europe. Germany was the first country to set a standard for the education and specialized treatment of the feeble-minded in the nineteenth century (Hackett 123). See also, Leo Kanner, *A History of the Care And Study of the Mentally Retarded* (Springfield, IL: Charles C. Thomas Publisher, 1964: 41-42, 67, 112-113). Hereafter: Kanner.
"Commissioner Star": cited in *Toronto Daily Star,* 22 January 1913: 2.
"*For no skill, no knowledge, no training*": see MacMurchy, *Annual Report on the Care of the Feeble-Minded in Ontario,* 1908: 13.
Journal of Psycho-Asthetics: Founded in 1896 by the Association of Medical Officers of American Institution for Idiotic and Feeble-Minded Persons. See Martin Barr, *Mental Defectives: Their History, Treatment and Training* (New York: Arno Press, 1904: 90). Hereafter: Barr.
"*Clarke ... thirteen defective ... murderers*" and "*fierce passions*": see MacMurchy, *Annual Report on the Care of the Feeble-Minded,* 1912: 23.
Marriage Act: Ontario Statutes, 1911. Added a prison sentence of not more than twelve months to $500 penalty first imposed by the 1896 *Marriage Act* on those issuing licenses to the idiotic or insane (Simmons 278, n.106).

British Mental Deficiency Act, 1913: The *Mental Deficiency Act* was an act of Parliament of the United Kingdom. It repealed the *Idiots Act,* 1886, and established a Board of Control for Lunacy and Mental Deficiency. One MP voted against it, Josiah Wedgwood, who said it was the "Spirit of the Horrible Eugenic Society" which wanted to "breed up the working class as though they were cattle." See Anne Digby, "Contexts and Perspectives," *From Idiocy to Mental Deficiency: Historical Perspectives of People With Learning Disabilities*, Ed. David Wright and Anne Digby (London: Routledge, 1996: 1-21). Hereafter: Digby.

Chapter 23

"*Esme Derrick ... childbirth*": MacMurchy wrote advice for home birthing in the *Supplement* to the *Canadian Mother's Book.* See Dianne Dodd, "Helen MacMurchy: Popular Midwifery and Maternity Services for Canadian Pioneer Women," *Caring and Curing: Historical Perspectives on Women and Healing in Canada,* Eds. Dianne Dodd and Deborah Gorham (Ottawa: University of Ottawa Press, 1994: 135-161). Hereafter: Dodd.

"*The Slump*": In 1913, the economy entered a severe depression period, resulting in the appointment of a Commission on Unemployment. By January 1914, about 15,000 people out of work, by October, 20,000 (Piva 76-77).

"*Houses of Refuge: Houses of Refuge Act,* 1913. By 1914 there were 71 houses of refuge with a total of 7,986 inmates. Conditions in the houses of refuge were worse than at Orillia (Simmons 106).

"*Vaudeville songs, burlesque, etc.*": Joan Morris and William Bolcorn, *Vaudeville Songs of the Great Ladies of the Musical Stage,* Elektra/Asylum/ Nonesuch Records, 1976.

Chapter 24

"*A good example*": cited in MacMurchy, *Annual Report on the Care of the Feeble-Minded,* 1917.

"*Henry's attestation papers*": These were received from the Federal Department of War, war records, via the Internet, and are now in Daisy Lumsden's records.

"*Women's dispensary, Dovercourt*": There were a few medical clinics for poor women in Cabbagetown and west end of Toronto. The Women's Dispensary was on Parliament and Queen Street in 1903, and then at 18 Seaton Street in 1910. There was also the Evangelina Settlement clinic at Queen and River Streets, northeast corner, in 1914. See Colleen Kelly, *Cabbagetown in Pictures* (Toronto: Toronto Public Library Board, 1984). Hereafter: Kelly.

Chapter 25

"*Justice Starr*": see Starr, J. Edward, "Charities and Corrections," *The Public Health Journal* 4.10 (October 1913): 567-70.

"*Aments ... amentia*": see MacMurchy, *Annual Report on the Care of the Feeble-Minded*, 1907, noted the inconsistencies in the usage of the term 'feeble-minded'. She referred to the generic term used by Dr. Tredgold of Britain, "ament," meaning "one whose mind from birth has been defective" (also cited in Brown, W. 129).

"*Dr. Clarence Hincks ... Dr. Withrow*": see Charles G. Roland, *Clarence Meredith Hincks, M.D., 1885-1964: A Biography* (Toronto: Hannah Institute & Dundurn Press, 1990). Hereafter: Roland.

"*Alfred Binet*": see Black (76).
Dr. Henry Goddard: Psychologist appointed Head of the laboratory at Vineland School for Feeble-Minded Boys and Girls in New Jersey. Goddard recognized the potential in the new Binet tests. He introduced Binet-Simon test into his work in 1908 at the school. Often referred to in her reports by MacMurchy.
"*Galton*" and "*Binet*": Galton introduced the term "eugenics" in 1883 (see Galton).
"*Stigmata ... size of cranium*": Dr. Alfred Tredgold was the most influential British psychologist of his day, and Dr. MacMurchy regularly consulted his book, *Mental Deficiency (Amentia)*. Tredgold believed "the whole body of mental defect was implicated in the pathology. The whole body is marred by defects of anatomical development and physical function" (Alfred Frank Tredgold, *Mental Deficiency (Amentia),* London: Balliere Tyndsall & Cox, 1914: 78). Hereafter: Tredgold.
"*Binet and the "educationalists and Dr. MacMurchy*": Binet questioned the validity of only physical examination by a doctor for diagnosis of mental deficiency, beginning a schism between the medical and educational/psychology professions concerning who was to be responsible for identification and diagnosis for special education (see Hacket 101). See, also, Alfred Binet and Theodore Simon. *Mentally Defective Children,*Trans. W. B. Drummond (New York: Longmans, Green & Co., 1914: 88).
William Stern: William Stern, with his equation, had set in motion the first intelligence test. See Ken Richardson, *The Making of Intelligence* (New York: Columbia University Press, 2000: 36). Hereafter: Richardson.
"*Dr. Hincks and the supra-normals*": see Hincks ("The Scope and Aims" 22; Hackett 103-104). Though Hincks did not put his views concerning this formally into writing until 1919, he had formulated these views from his collegial work with Dr. Clarke by 1916, the date of this chapter of events.
"*Goddard and the new borderline group of morons*": Goddard noticed a higher-functioning group who looked 'normal' and scored higher on the tests, but were still feeble-minded. He called this group 'morons'. The morons were the most dangerous as they looked 'normal', could therefore pass in society and reproduce more defective offspring (Black 78).
"*The new classification system*": This was L. M. Terman's classification finalized in 1916 (cited in Hackett, Table 1, p. 14).
"*Dr. Martin Barr and 'moral imbecile*'": 1860-1938. Chief physician at the Pennsylvania Training School for Feeble-Minded Children at Elwyn.
"*Sexual pervert, etc.*": see Barr (131); Brown, W. (205).
"*The girls coming through the Clinic*": All names and history of patients examined by Clarke and his colleagues coming through the Psychiatric Clinic from Juvenile Court are taken verbatim from Clarke's articles about his work at the Clinic (see Clarke, "The Story of..."; "A Study of 5,600 Cases"; "Occupational Wanderers").
"*Syphylitic babies ... Hutchinson's teeth*": A sign of congenital syphilis. Named after Sir Jonathan Hutchinson, an English surgeon and pathologist who first noted them (Tredgold 242).
Dr. Withrow: see Clarke ("The Story..." 32).
"*Miss Jane Grant ... Eliminate the feeble-minded*": see Clarke ("The Story..." 31, 33). See, also, Robert Pos, "History of Psychiatry at Toronto General Hospital 'til 1975"(The History of Canadian Psychiatry Research in Progress Seminar,

Toronto, Friday, May 1, 1992: 42,46). Hereafter: Pos.
“Rev. S. W. Dean ... the sty makes the pig”: Rev. S. W. Dean of the Fred Victor Mission in Toronto. “The Church and the Slum,” Social Service Council of Canada Congress, Ottawa 1914: 127 (cited in Valverde 134).
Emma de Veber Clarke: Clarke married Margaret de Veber in 1880. They had five children. Clarke’s eldest daughter, Emma de Veber fulfilled her father’s aspirations and worked at the clinic as head social service nurse. Dr. Hastings, Medical Officer of Health later made her in charge of the mental hygiene work of the Department, while her brother Eric Kent Clarke became a respected child psychiatrist. She devoted herself to the field of mental health, and never married, remaining loyal to her father.
Miss Grant ... slums”: Clarke was ambivalent about the role of social workers and seemed to divide them into two groups: those who believed in the influence of heredity as cause of the problems of the poor, whom he labelled ‘radicals’, and those who agreed with himself, favouring heredity (Clarke, “Occupational Wanderers”; Pos 42).
“Deaconesses ... Training School”: see Valverde regarding the middle-class Methodist philanthropic woman in the church involved in the Methodist and Presbyterian Moral and Social Reform movement in Toronto (157).
Alice Chown: Alice Chown operated in Kingston. She favoured wearing loose Grecian tunics and walking barefoot (Valverde 155).
“Living pictures of awfulness of sin” : United Church Archives, pamphlet, “These Twenty Years (1886-1906)” (cited in Valverde 143).
“Dr. Douglas ... Dr. Hastings”: Dr. Douglas’ night-time raids, *Bulletin,* 1913 (cited in Valverde 137). Dr. Hastings’ “external appearances, etc.” documented in his Report on conditions in the slums, 1911 (cited in Valverde 195, n.35).
Emmeline Jarvis: Emmeline Baumont Jarvis wrote a book of poetry, ‘Leaves from Rosedale,’ published in 1905, in praise of Rosedale. Both Jarvis Street and Jarvis Collegiate were named after Samuel Jarvis (Mrs. Morrison, *Christian Guardian*, November 29, 1911: 25 cited in Valverde 157).
“National Welfare Exhibit, 1916”: see MacMurchy, *Annual Report on the Care of the Feeble-Minded in Ontario,* 1916: 62-64.
“The Jukes”: see Dugdale, a study of the descendants of five Juke sisters (R. L. Dugdale, *The Jukes: A Study in Crime, Pauperism, Disease and Heredity*. 4th ed. New York: Putnam, 1888). See, also, L. M. Terman, *The Measurement of Intelligence* (Cambridge, MA: Houghton Mifflin, 1916: 10-11).
“Toronto is roused at last!”: Clarke quoting Dr. Hincks (“The Story of ...” 33).
“MacMurchy and Clarke’s attack on Premier Hearst and Mr. Rowell”: see C. K. Clarke to N. W. Rowell, April 27, 1916 (cited in Simmons 81-85).
“Mr. Downey and Marion Harvey”: Miss Harvie’s quote regarding girls of “normal intelligence” (Shea 115). See, also, Simmons (104).
“Government lacks grasp, vision, etc. and the survival of the unfittest”: see Bator, (230-231, n.53). In the 1920s, before the Stock Market Crash, the government introduced old age pensions and Mother’s Allowance to help the very poor, but this was not a general program for all.
House of Refuge Act: Reformers wanted the municipalities to establish local institutions to house socially defective people, paupers, unemployed. In 1903, the province passed an act compelling the erection of houses of refuge; 1913, again insisted on houses of refuge (Simmons 100, 106).

"*It is necessary to control the sex lives of these classes*": see Hincks ("The Scope and Aims" 28).
"*Dr. Clarence Hincks and the* CNCMH": see Roland (40-41).
"*Dr. Clarke's violent diatribe against immigrants*": see Clarke ("The Defective and Insane" 462-65).
"*Lucy Brookings*": see Lucy Brookings, "We Pay," *Public Health Journal* 5 (April 1914): 212-218.
"*CNCMH agenda and surveys*": The surveys done in the provinces proved the correlation between immigration and insanity, criminality, feeble-mindedness and unemployment. The surveys helped to influence Alberta's decision to pass the *Eugenical Sterilization Act* in 1928 (Simmons 59; Roland 78).
"*Why haven't we got results? ... blowing up parliament!*": see Roland (60-61).
"*Mr. Downey ... Among The Children*": All references are from Mr. Downey's article, which gives useful, revealing information of the lives of the children and how Downey and the government viewed them. Mr. Downey succeeded Mr. Beaton as superintendent in 1910 and stayed until his sudden death in 1928.
"*Miss Marion Harvie*": Teacher and principal, 1922-1926, Ontario Hospital, also known as the Hospital for the Feeble-Minded. Miss Hale became principal of the academic school at the Ontario Hospital Orillia in 1928 (personal interview with G. Hackett, July, 1958; see also Hackett 429).
"*Beaton ... filthy and repulsive*": *Annual Reports of Inspectors, 1880*, pg. 370, (cited in Hackett 48).
"*Miss M. V. Nash*": Principal of the little school at Orillia under Dr. Beaton, 1905 (Hackett 63).

Chapter 26

"*What 'ad ter go from red ter brown...*": Poor women, like Florrie, had to rely on the practical experience of neighbours to help with birthing. Canadian women isolated forced to have babies without the aid of a doctor or midwife was a concern of Dr. Helen MacMurchy. She wrote a Supplement to her popular book, *The Canadian Mother's Book*. The helper was to take off her dress, scrub her hands and arms in soap and hot water, then change the mother's pads and check the colour of her 'discharge' which could change 'from red to brown to green in colour' (Dodd, "Helen MacMurchy: Popular Midwifery" 140).
"*Biggest Anglo-Saxon slum in North America*": see Hugh Garner, *Cabbagetown*, (Toronto: Mc-Graw-Hill Ryerson Limited, 1950), author's Preface to the 1968 edition. Hereafter: Garner.
"*There are no poor in Canada*": see J. A. Hobson (Minister of Labour), *Canada To-day* (London: Unwin, 1906: 3-4); *Report of the Department of Labour, 1912* (Ottawa, 1913).
"*Strikes ... Winnipeg General Strike*": see Piva (169).
"*Observation ward ... Toronto General Hospital*": see Pos (53).
"*Shellshock ... Committee of Enquiry*": see Clarke and Farrar.
"*Dr. Barnardo's agency*": see G. Wagner, *Children of the Empire* (London: Weidenfeld and Nicolson, 1982: 230-231).
Emma Clarke: In September, 1919, the City Council of Toronto appointed Dr Clarke's daughter, Miss Emma De V. Clarke, to take charge of the mental hygiene work of the Department (Roland 37; Pos 42).
"*Winnipeg Strike ... Port Rouge*": see Kenneth A. McNaught, *Prophet in Pol-*

itics, A Biography of J. S. Woodsworth (Toronto: University of Toronto Press, 1959: 105-7).
"Calomile ... V.D, Clinic": see Jay Cassel, *The Secret Plague: Venereal Disease in Canada, 1838-1939* (Toronto: University of Toronto Press, 1987): 131-132, 181-182).
"CNCMH traveling exhibit": The Canadian National Committee for Mental Hygiene, CNCMH, (today the Canadian Mental Health Association, CMHA) launched a full-scale public relations campaign in the 1920s to educate the public in the principles of mental hygiene. The posters in the travelling exhibits, 1924, were to help people identify mentally defective people in their midst. The exhibition travelled across Canada stopping off at major cities, Montreal, Toronto, Vancouver. CNCMH advocated the segregation and sterilization of the mentally defective and mentally ill citizens. The labels of people identified in the poster legitimized forced segregation and sterilization (see page 365 in this volume).

Chapter 27
"Penn'royal an' carbolic ... Norforms Zonite": Pennyroyal was a well-known herb that reputedly brought on a miscarriage or abortion, as was the use of carbolic acid. The cost of a private abortion would have been far beyond the means of a destitute woman like Florrie (see McLaren 43).
St. Vincent de Paul Catholic Children's Aid Society of Toronto: In 1893, the Catholic Children's Aid was established. The Children's Aid Society of St. Vincent de Paul was a shelter for young women lawbreakers provided by the Sisters of the Good Shepherd in Toronto.
"New York stock market crash!": Government forced people to work for food vouchers but no vouchers for soap or medicines. See Max Braithwaite, *The Hungry Thirties, 1930-1940* (Toronto: Natural Science of Canada, 1977: 11-12). Hereafter: Braithwaite.

Chapter 28
"A wart on the landscape": see Shorter (45).
"Five thousand club": Pamphlet 1921, Canadian National Committee for Mental Hygiene (CNCMH).

Chapter 29
"Reading Married Love*"*: see Marie Stopes, *Married Love: A New Contribution to the Solution of Sex Difficulties*. 9th ed rev. (London: G. P. Putnam and Sons, Ltd., 1920 [1918]).
"Objectionable books": see Angus McLaren and Arlene Tigar McLaren, *The Bedroom and the State: The Changing Practices and Politics of Contraception and Abortion in Canada, 1880-1980* (Toronto: McClelland & Stewart, 1986: 157, n.1). Hereafter: McLaren and McLaren.,
"Miss Stopes" and *"the fertility differential between the classes ... Galton"*: McLaren and McLaren (55, 56, 79, 82, 84-85). In 1892, the Criminal Code in Canada made it an indictable offense to provide information or advertise contraceptives and abortifacients. Until 1969, the provision of contraceptives was illegal. At the same time, contraceptives were sold undercover by agents and advertised under code names (see Mclaren and McLaren 9, 19, 23, 24, 28).
"Unsanitary, dirty hands": see Mclaren and McLaren (107).

"Dr. Ogino and Dr. Knaus": see Mclaren and McLaren (20).
"Dr. Withrow ... birth control clinic ... Ruth Dembner": see Mclaren and McLaren (82-88); Strange (169-173).
"Miss Stopes' Mother England": based on thousands of letters Stopes had received over the years from desperate, working poor mothers.
"Queen Mary and Stopes": Marie Stopes's correspondence is in the British Library (BL-S). Cited in Ruth Hall, *Passionate Crusader: The Life of Marie Stopes* (New York: Harcourt Brace Jovanovich, 1977: 168). Hereafter: Hall.
"Withrow and Stopes": MacMurchy was correct in intuiting a link between Dr. Withrow's birth control clinics in Toronto and the influence of Marie Stopes, whom he admired. After he was released from prison and regained his medical license in 1933, he resumed correspondence with Stopes (McLaren 83).
"She knew what she had to do": see Hall (92).

Chapter 30
"Hewitts latest check-up": Robbie Hewitt Patient File, Case Book No. 1115, Abstract of Clinical History from Division of Family Welfare Social History, examined at Outpatient Department, Toronto Psychiatric Hospital, November 1932. RG 29-25-2, Resident Files, 1876-1971, Provincial Archives of Ontario.
"Delivery boy, Ronnie Phelps": Henrietta subsequently gave birth, out of wedlock, to a son, Cuthbert Hewitt, in early 1933. Henrietta did not marry Ronnie Phelps, and nothing more was heard of him or any relatives he may have had. Henrietta subsequently married a different tradesman, Percy Wilkins. Cuthbert was subsequently placed, as a ward of the Children's Aid Society, in Orillia at age fourteen (Cuthbert Hewitt Patient File, Case Book No. 8227, Abstract of Clinical History, Ontario Hospital School Orillia, May 1946. RG 29-25-2, Resident Files, 1876-1971, Archives of Ontario).
"Rainhill mental asylum": The Rainhill County Lunatic Asylum opened January 1, 1851, a stone building housing 1,000 patients. In December 1911, there were 975 men and 1,015 women, a total of 1,900 patients..
"Applications and Certificates of Incompetence": There were two ways for parents to commit their 'mentally defective' or 'feeble-minded' child into the Orillia institution: 1) The most common was through the Lieutenant-Governor's warrant. The child then became a ward of the province. 2) A formal medical certificate, the "Certificate of Incompetence,"signed by two physicians after examining the child and confirming idiocy. With the warrant method, the government covered the costs of the medical exam and transportation to the asylum. Method 2, the costs were covered by the parents. See Park, Deborah. "Changing Shadows: The Huronia Regional Centre 1876-1934" (M.A. Thesis, York University, 1990).
"Henrietta ... the Haven": Examining physicians could transfer 'fallen' women from houses of refuge such as the Haven in Toronto, run by the Salvation Army, and place them in an institution such as Orillia and Cobourg, according to the 1919 *Houses of Refuge Act* (Simmons 132).
"The baby was to be handed over ... Henrietta been told": Unwed mothers who kept their babies were not eligible for Mother's Allowance (McCullagh 61).

Chapter 31
"EVICTED": Evictions were common in the 1920s and 1930s in the slums of Toronto (Cotter 108).

PART THREE

Chapter 32
"*Wooden station hospital grounds*": The institution had its own CNR station stop named 'Orillia Institute, a.k.a. Orillia Asylum'. Up to 1909 it was called Orillia Asylum Platform (Shea 29).
"*Hewitt, Robbie, 62 inches ... Dr. Tredgold feeble-minded ears*": Robbie Hewitt Ward Admission Record, Patient File No. 4952, Resident Files, 1876-1971, RG 29-25-2, Archives of Ontario.

Chapter 34
"*Upper and Lower Academic ... sang songs*": During the superintendency of Dr B. McGhie, 1928-1930, McGhie re-organized the school curriculum calling on the resources of the psychology department, University of Toronto. Upper and Lower academic schools were established as well as 'ward work' for those unable to participate in school, and probation work for those who were high-functioning with high or normal I.Qs. (Academic Instruction Programme, 1928-1930, RG 29-24-1-1, AO).
"*Clinical Record*": All excerpts from the Clinical Record of Robbie Hewitt are in Robbie Hewitt's Patient File.

Chapter 35
"*Letter from Dr. E.P. Lewis, Director of OPC, Toronto Psychiatric Hospital, to Dr. S. J.W. Horne*": Robbie Hewitt's Patient File.

Chapter 36
"*Freight trains ... hobos*": "riding the rails" was a serious offense punishable with a night in "clink." CNR and CPR officials employed "bulls" to guard the freight trains from thousands of men and women trying to cross the country in search of a job (Braithwaite 12). Men took to riding the rails from city to city in search of work. St Lawrence Hall, Toronto was converted into a flop house with steel bunks (Cotter 105).
"*The Horne boys ... Mr. Zarfas's sons*": Donald Zarfas, son of Mr J. A. Zarfas, the bursar, grew up in the institution with his brother. Don Zarfas eventually became a famous child psychiatrist and became Director of CPRI, devoting himself to improved treatment for intellectually handicapped children. Mr J. A. Zarfas remained bursar until the mid 1950s. All anecdotes about Dr. Horne as a Captain in the Great War, and as an Arch-Mason Recollections of Ed Swinton. Author Interview, July 16, 2007.
"*Letter from Henry Hewitt to Dr. Horne*" (dated only Dec. 7th but likely in 1932) and "*Letter from N. L. Walker for Dr. Horne, to Henry Hewitt, December 19, 1932*": Robbie Hewitt's Patient File.

Chapter 37
"*They were properly clad*": Dr. Fletcher's Medical Inspector's Report, Ontario Hospital Orillia, February 10, and February 11, 1931. All excerpts from Dr. Fletcher's report in Chapter 6 are from Dr. Fletcher's Inspection Report, Inspection Reports, 1931-1961, RG 29-24-1-7, AO.
"*Dr. McGhie ... four continuous baths*": Hydrotherapy was a principal treatment

for calming excited mental patients in asylums and was carried on in Orillia. Dr. McGhie had petitioned the government for continuous baths for hydrotherapeutic treatment (letter to Dr. Edward Ryan, Director of Medical Services, Parliament Buildings, Toronto from Dr. B. T. McGhie, June 30, 1928).
"*During the past year a complete survey of our Mongolian patients*": Dr. Horne's Superintendent's Report for 1932 to the Department of Health, Parliament Buildings, Toronto (Annual Reports, Correspondence, 1827-1948, RG 29-24-1-3, AO).

Chapter 39
"*Dr. Horne's Minute Book*": Twice a day, after early morning roll-call and bedtime roll call at 9:00 pm, attendants were to report to the superintendent who recorded the information in a Minute Book. See superintendent's Minute Book on display in the local Orillia Museum, Orillia, dated 1895, 1905, 1910.
"*Robbie lay, his feet shackled*": Shackling inmates' feet and hands was a common punishment in reformatories and asylums (Brown, W. 118).
"*Report of Elopement*": Register of Elopements, 1917-1967. RG 29-25-6, AO.

Chapter 40
Superintendent's Annual Report, Nov. 19, 1934: Annual Reports, Correspondence, 1827-1948, RG 29-24-1-3, AO.
Dr. B.T. McGhie's Inspection Report of Ontario Hospital, Orillia, July 31, 1933: Inspection Reports, 1931-1961, RG 29-24-1-7, AO.
Dr. Horne's Annual Report 1933 to Dr. B.T. McGhie: Annual Reports, Correspondence, 1827-1948, RG 29-24-1-3, AO.
"*Patients placed on probation ... Lorimer Lodge*": Dr Horne's Annual Report 1933. Colony House, a residence for mildly retarded women in the town pf Orillia was established by Katherine Day, the chief Social Worker at Orillia. It was opened by Dr. Horne on July 20, 1931. The number of girls in residence averaged 12 to 15. They were placed in homes in the area to do housework and half their wages went to the institution. Local women complained that the girls of Colony House were taking jobs from them and in June 1932 the house was destroyed by fire. After the fire, Orillia continued to send girls on probation to the Haven in Toronto. The Haven was originally established in 1867 as a half-way house for women discharged from prison but taken over for mentally retarded girls from Orillia and Cobourg after 1925. In 1965, the Metropolitan Toronto Association for Retarded Children took over the Haven, later called Lorimer Lodge. Lorimer Lodge agreed to take in girls from Colony House on probation after the 1932 fire (Simmons 127, 128).
"*Pest house ... absolutely dangerous creatures*": Dr Alexander Beaton, Medical Superintendent of the Asylum for Idiots and Feeble-Minded, Annual Report, 1883 (cited in Shea 68). Dr. Beaton became disenchanted with visitors to the asylum from the town whom he felt displayed a morbid interest in the inmates, expecting to see "repulsive" objects. An article in the *Orillia Expositor* reported in 1876 on the first "batch" of idiots arriving at the asylum, noting that a large crowd of townspeople had gathered to watch the "parade of idiots" to the asylum (Hackett 69).

Chapter 41
Letter to Dr. Horne from A. W. Laver, Commissioner, Department of Public Welfare,

(no date but likely 1935, see date on next letter): Robbie Hewitt's Patient File.
Letter to A.W. Laver from N. L. Walker for Dr. Horne, July 19, 1935: Robbie Hewitt's Patient File.
"*Demission lists in 1934*": Dr. Horne's Annual Report for 1934 (Annual Reports, Correspondence, 1827-1948, RG 29-24-1-3, AO).
"*Survey of girls on probation*": In 1933, Marion E. Haugh, a Social Service Internee at Orillia, did a survey of the girls' on probation at Orillia, basing her findings on the case records of 53 girls who had gone out on probation between 1929-1933. Haugh found that the average I.Q. of the girls was 65 and the lowest was 43. Some of the girls had come to Orillia because they had nowhere else to go or because they were in trouble with the law. Out of fifteen girls in one group, there were three orphans, four illegitimate children and eight whose homes had been deemed 'unfit'. All had been sent by the Children's Aid Society. The second group of thirty-eight girls had been admitted by warrant or sent by the Juvenile Court. Sixteen were unmarried mothers, eleven having one child, four with two children, and one having seven illegitimate children. Eight had been admitted for 'abnormal sexual tendencies', three charged with promiscuity, four with 'moral weakness' and one with nymphomaniacy (Simmons 128, n.42).

Chapter 42
Ella Hewitt: All psychological references to Ella Hewitt are found in Ella Hewitt, Patient File, Clinic No.1106, Outpatient Department (OPD) 1936, Toronto Psychiatric Hospital, in Patient File, Ontario Hospital Orillia, Case Number 5734. Resident Files, 1876-1971, RG 29-25-2, AO.
"*Not eligible for an Auxiliary Class*": The feeble-minded with 50 and below I.Q. belonged in the Orillia asylum.
"*Eugenics Society of Canada (ESC)... The Aims and Objectives*": The ESC met for the first time on November 6, 1930. Doctors and physicians formed the single largest group within the ESC. See Dianne Dodd,"The Canadian Birth Control Movement 1929-1939," (M.A. Thesis, Department of Education, University of Toronto, 1982).
"*Dr. Hincks's surveys*": Dr. Hincks' survey of mental hospitals in B.C. and other Canadian provinces, published in 1921, attributed social immorality, the rise in the number of mental defectives and insane in asylums and mental hospitals to low-class mentally defective Eastern European immigrants being allowed in to Canada, justifying the use of eugenic sterilization that helped encourage the passing of the *Sterilization Act* (see Jane Harris-Zsovan, *Eugenics and the Firewall: Canada's Nasty Little Secret*, Winnipeg: J. Gordon Shillingford Publishing Inc., 2010: 18). Dr. Hincks maintained this attitude towards eugenic sterilization of the 'unfit' even after World War I (Hinks, "Sterilize the Unfit" 39-40).
"*Sterilization of people of inferior stock ... birth control techniques*": see C. B. Farrar, "Sterilization and Mental Hygiene," *Canadian Public Health Journal* 22 (January 1931): 92-94; McLaren (118).
"*Miss Vera Moberley ... sterilization*": Executives of both the Infants Home (CAS) and the West End Creche supported eugenic sterilization of the 'unfit'. The Neighbourhood Workers Association called for sterilization of 'low grade families' (McLaren 118).
"*Kaufman ... court case ... trial ... contraceptives*": see McLaren (84, 115, 116).

"*Reeve of Newmarket, Mr. Dale*": In November, 1935, Dr. L.W. Dale called for the sterilization of children in York County shelters (McLaren 121).
"*Mayor of Fort Erie*": ibid.
"*Pope Pius XI ... Papal Bull of 1930*": Pope Pius XI condemned sterilization of the mentally retarded, in his encyclical on marriage, "Casti Connubi," December 31, 1930, which was read aloud and distributed throughout Catholic churches (Simmons 114-115).

Chapter 43
"*Editor of the Star ... COMMON SENSE*": *Toronto Daily Star*, May 10, 1933.
"*Road Hog Sterilization*": Letter To the Editor, *The Mail and Empire*, June 19, 1933.
"*Sterilization of the Unfit*": Letter to *The Mail and Empire*, Toronto, May 16, 1933, signed by "A MOTHER."
"*End the 'consent' clause in the* Sexual Sterilization Act *of 1928*": Consent could now be given by the spouse or by the parents or guardian. Alberta ultimately removed the need for consent to sterilize mental defectives in 1942.
"*Agnes MacPhail ... United Farm Women ... seed-bearers*": United Farm Women of Alberta supported sterilization of the 'unfit' (*Toronto Star*, 4 December, 1935); The President of the United Farm Women, Mrs Gunn, once said that "democracy was never intended for degenerates" (McLaren 97).
"*It is unnatural, it is repugnant*": see MacMurchy (*Sterilization? Birth Control?* 5).
"Dr. Macmurchy Would Halt "Propagation of the Unfit": MacMurchy's book on Sterilization of the unfit was denounced by a Montreal Jesuit priest (*Toronto Star*, June 27, 1934).
"*University Women's Club ... honour*": see "University Women Honour Dr MacMurchy,' *Mail & Empire*, December 5, 1933.
"*Spirited letter ...Toronto Housing Report*": *Mail and Empire*, May 14, 1933;
"*The premier feared the loss of Catholic votes in Ontario*": see Simmons (114, 124-125).
"*Delegation to Queen's Park ... Eisendrath*": Premier Mitchell Hepburn, General Correspondence, 1935, Box 335, Public Archives of Ontario, cited in Simmons (120).
"*Dr. Hutton knew ... castrations in Poor Law Hospital*": In Februrary 1930, a twenty-two year old man was castrated by Dr. Lionel Westrope at High Teams Institution in Gateshead, London, for excessive masturbation (Eric Donaldson, "*Operations on Mentally Deficient Patients in the Poor Law Hospital*, cited in Black 231).
"*Opposition from ... Dr. McGhie ... statistics*": see McLaren (106-109, 157).
"*Walter Lippmann, influential...*": see Walter Lippmann, "The Mental Age of Americans," *New Republic* 32.415 (October 25, 1922): 213-215. See, also, Michael D'Antonio, *The State Boys Rebellion: The Inspiring True Story of American Eugenics and the Men Who Overcame It* (Riverside, NJ: Simon & Schuster Paperbacks, 2004: 14-15).
"*Success of Nazi sterilization policy*": Lieutenant-Governor Dr. Herbert Bruce's address to the Eugenics Society of Canada in 1935, in which he praised Germany's sterilization of 50,000 "misfits," April 24, 1936 (cited in McLaren 122).
"*Dr. Horne's survey of high grade girls, 1944 ...'improvables' and 'potentials'*": see Simmons (125, 132); Sterilization File, 1933-1944, RG 29-24-1-18, AO.

Chapter 44
"Needlessly saved ... quiet euthanasia American hospitals ... Germany": Dr. Farrar, Dr. Hincks and Dr. Hutton, president of the Eugenics Society of Canada, argued that the problem of the feeble-minded in Canada was compounded by medical science which now saved the lives of mental defectives and the unfit who once would have died. "The struggle for survival," claimed Dr. Hutton, "has been reversed by advances of medicine with the result that the feeble-minded and the unfit who once would have died, now survive" (*Canadian Medical Association Journal* 11 (1921): 23-25 cited in McLaren 90). Under Hitler, policy changed and the Nazi leadership initiated Aktion-4 to euthanize incurables, (*unheilbar kranken*), held in long-term care in German mental hospitals. Between October 1939 and August 1941, it is estimated that the T-4 programme killed between 70,000 and 95, 000 mentally and physically disabled adults as well as 5,000 children.

Chapter 46
"*Report to Dr. Horne by Phyllis Stubley, April 3, 1935-March 31, 1936*": Annual Reports, Correspondence, 1827-1948. RG 29-24-1-3, AO.
"*Dr. Horne's Annual Report, May 30, 1936*": ibid.
"*Dr. J. Sharpe's Inspection Report, January 1937, Cottage 'A' and Cottage 'B'*": Inspection Reports, 1931-1961, RG 29-24-1-7, AO.

Chapter 48
"*Dr. Sharpe's Inspection Report, March 28, 29, 30; April 19, 20, 1938*": Inspection Reports, 1931-1961, RG 29-24-1-7, AO.
"*Christmas Concert this year...*": Dr. Horne's Annual Report, July 5, 1939 (Annual Reports, Correspondence, 1827-1948, RG 29-24-1-3, AO).
"*Some of the girls were pregnant*": Jim Burns, late principal of William Burges-Public School, East York, Ontario, during the 1950s. Jim Burns grew up in Orillia opposite the institution. He recalled that as a young boy of about six or seven, he heard his grandfather, who was a construction engineer working on the site of the institution building two new cottages in the 1930s, coming home one day and declaring: "Some of the girls in Cottage M are pregnant" (personal interview, with Jim Burns, July 2005).
"*Hoggery ... 96 head of cattle ... 550 bushels of oats*": Farm & Garden, 1929-1940, RG 29-24-1-6, AO.

Epilogue

"Eighty thousand British boys and girls": All references to "Home" children are cited in Parr. All articles cited are to in the Bibliography.
"Daisy's records from Toronto Psychiatric Hospital destroyed: The "destruction of patient records" policy initiated by Centre for Addiction and Mental Health (CAMH) in 2011 involves the destruction of patients' records 35 years after last contact, going back to 1976. The policy applies only to files from the old Toronto Psychiatric Hospital and the Clarke Institute of Psychiatry.

Select Bibliography

PRIMARY SOURCES

Archives of Ontario:

Annual Reports of the Inspector of Asylums, Prisons, and Public Charities. Toronto: Province of Ontario, 1868-1909.

Annual Reports of the Inspector of Auxiliary Classes. Toronto: Province of Ontario, 1915-1919.

HURONIA REGIONAL CENTRE SUB-SERIES RG 29-24-1

Archives of Ontario, RG 29-24-1-1. Academic Instruction Programme. 1928-1930.

Archives of Ontario, RG 24-1-3. Annual Reports – Correspondence. 1827-1948.

Archives of Ontario. RG 29-24-1-5. Canadian Conference of Charities & Correction. 1916.

Archives of Ontario. RG 24-1-6. Farm and Garden. 1929-1940.

Archives of Ontario. RG 24-1-16. History – Typescript. 1981.

Archives of Ontario. RG 29-24-1-7. Inspection Reports. 1931-61.

Archives of Ontario. RG 29-24-1-12. Nurses and Attendants Curriculum. 1934-36.

Archives of Ontario. RG 29-24-1-13. Nursing School Course Instruction. 1930-1943.

Archives of Ontario. RG 29-24-1-14. Ontario Hospital School – Correspondence. 1928-1942.

Archives of Ontario. RG 24-1-15. Ontario Hospital School – History – Notes. 1958-1978.

Archives of Ontario. RG 24-1-18. Sterilization. 1933-1944.

HURONIA REGIONAL CENTRE: SUB-SERIES RG 29-25

Archives of Ontario. RG 29-25-1-2. Register of Application for Admission. 1908-1936.

Archives of Ontario. RG 29-25-1-5. Register of Admission. 1934-1960.

Archives of Ontario. RG 29-25-1-6. Register of Elopements. 1917-1967.

SUB-SERIES RG 29-25-2

Archives of Ontario. RG 29-25-2. Resident Files. 1925-1935 only. 1876-1971.

BOOKS, ARTICLES, REPORTS

Barr, Martin. *Mental Defectives: Their History, Treatment and Training*. New York: Arno Press, 1904.

Binet, Alfred and Theodore Simon. *Mentally Defective Children*. Trans. W. B. Drummond. New York: Longmans, Green & Co., 1914.

Brookings, Lucy M. "We Pay." *Public Health Journal* 5 (April 1914): 212-218.

Bruce, H. A. "Sterilization of Imbecility." *Social Welfare* 16 (September 1936): 95-97.

Clarke, Charles Kirk. "Mental Hygiene Survey of the Province of Nova Scotia", *Canadian Journal of Mental Hygiene* 3 (April 1921): 1-45.

Clarke, Charles Kirk. "Occupational Wanderers."*MacLean's Magazine* April 15, 1922.

Clarke, Charles Kirk. "The Defective and Insane Immigrant." *The University (Toronto) Monthly* 8 (June 1908): 273-278.

Clarke, Charles Kirk and C. B. Farrar. *One Thousand Psychiatric Cases From The Canadian Army.* Toronto: The Canadian National Committee For Mental Hygiene, 1920.

Clarke, Charles Kirk. "The Story of the Toronto General Hospital Psychiatric Clinic." *Canadian Journal of Mental Hygiene* 1.1 (April 1919): 30-37.

Clarke, Charles Kirk, with C. M. Hincks and M. Keyes. "A Study of 5,600 Cases Passing Through the Psychiatric Clinic of Toronto General Hospital, Also a Study of 188 Clinic Cases and 767 Cases of Illegitimacy."*Canadian Journal of Mental Hygiene* 3 (July 1921): 11-24.

Clark, Christopher St. George. *Of Toronto the Good: A Social Study: The Queen City of Canada As It Is*. Montreal: Toronto Pub. Co. 1898.

Clarke, Eric. "Survey of the Toronto Public Schools." Toronto: Department of Public Health, 1919-20.

Downey, J. P. "Among The Children." *Bulletin of Ontario Hospitals for the Insane* 11.2 (January 1914): 119-124.

Farrar, C. B. "Sterilization and Mental Hygiene." *Canadian Public Health Journal* 22 (January 1931): 92-94.

Fernald, Walter E. *History of the Treatment of the Feeble-Minded*. Boston: Geo. Ellis Co., 1912.

Fotheringham, John, Mora Skelton and Bernard Hoddinott. *The Retarded Child and His Family.* Toronto: Ontario Institute for Studies in Education, Monograph Series/11, 1971.

Galton, Francis. *Inquiries into Human Faculty and Its Development*. London: Macmillan & Co., 1883.

Goddard, Henry Herbert. *Feeble-Mindedness: Its Causes and Consequences*. New York: The MacMillan Company, 1914.

Hastings, Charles. *Report of the Medical Health Officer Dealing With the Recent Investigation of Slum Conditions in Toronto Embodying Recommendations for the Amelioration of the Same*. 1911. CTA.

Freedom of Information and the Protection of Privacy. Archives of Ontario Handout No. 17, AO.

Haugh, Marion. *A Survey of the Girls' Probation Scheme at the Ontario Hospital, Orillia, in Regard to Success or Failure*. Unpublished ms. Department of Social Sciences, University of Toronto, May 18, 1933.

Hincks, Clarence. *Annual Reports on the Care of the Feeble-Minded in the Province of Ontario,* 1907-1919. Ontario Sessional Papers. AO.

Hincks, Clarence. Biographical File. Academy of Medicine. University of Toronto Archives.

Hincks, Clarence. "Feeble-Mindedness in Canada: A Serious National Problem." *Social Welfare* 1 (November 1918): 29-30.

Hincks, Clarence. "Feeble-Mindedness in Canada: Governments and the Feeble-Minded." *Social Welfare* 1 (February 1919): 103-104.

Hincks, Clarence. "The Scope and Aims of the Mental Hygiene Movement in Canada." *Canadian Journal of Mental Hygiene* (1919): 20-29.

Hincks, Clarence. "Surveys in Canada." Paper presented at the Mental Hygiene Division of the National Conference on Social Work, Atlantic City, May, 1919. Archives CNCMH.

Hincks, Clarence. "Sterilize the Unfit." *Macleans Magazine* February 15, 1946.

"History of Auxiliary Classes in Toronto." Pamphlet, n.d. Records, Archives and Museum, Toronto Board of Education.

Lippmann, Walter. "The Mental Age of Americans." *New Republic* 32.415 (October 25, 1922): 213-215.

MacMurchy, Helen. *Annual Reports on the Care of the Feeble-Minded in the Province of Ontario, 1907-1919.* Ontario Sessional Papers, AO.

MacMurchy, Helen. Biographical File. Academy of Medicine. University of Toronto Archives.

MacMurchy, Helen. *Organization and Management of Auxiliary Classes.* Toronto: L. K. Cameron, 1915.

MacMurchy, Helen. "Letters to Marie Stopes." British Library, London, UK.

MacMurchy, Helen. "Organization and Management of Auxiliary Classes." Toronto, Department of Education, Educational Pamphlets, No. 7, 1915.

MacMurchy, Helen. *Sterilization? Birth Control?A Book for Family Welfare and Safety.* Toronto: Macmillan, 1932.

MacMurchy, Helen. *The Canadian Mother's Book.* Ottawa: F. A. Ackland, 1926.

McGhie, Bernard T. "The Problem of the Subnormal in the Community." *Canadian Public Health Journal* 28 (March 1937): 105-110.

McGhie, Bernard T. and E. D. MacPhee. "Training and Research in a Hospital for Subnormals." Ontario Hospital (Orillia) Publications, Vol. 1. No. 1. Toronto Ontario, February 1929. CAMH Archives.

Miner, Maude E. "The Problem of Wayward Girls and Delinquent Women." *Academy of Political Science Proceedings* 12.4 (1912): 604-612.

Penrose, Lionel S. "The Inheritance of Mental Defect." *The Scientific Monthly* L11 (April 1941): 359-364.

Shuttleworth, G. E. and W. A. Potts. *Mentally Defective Children: Their Treatment and Training.* 5th ed. Philadelphia: Blaikston's Son & Co., 1924 [1913].

Stogdill, Charles. "Special Education Facilities in Public and Secondary Schools Operated by the Toronto Board of Education, including 'Classes for the Mentally Handicapped': A. Junior Opportunity Class." Toronto Board of Education Archives, October 1, 1956.

Stopes, Marie. *Married Love: A New Contribution to the Solution of Sex Difficulties.* 9th ed rev. London: G. P. Putnam and Sons, Ltd., 1920 [1918].

Terman, L. M. *The Measurement of Intelligence.* Cambridge, MA: Houghton Mifflin, 1916.

Tredgold, Alfred Frank. *Mental Deficiency (Amentia)*. London: Balliere Tyndsall & Cox, 1914.

NEWSPAPER ARTICLES

"A Day at the Orillia Hospital for the Mentally Deficient." *Orillia Packet and Times* 11 (October 1928): 12-14
"A Great Lady Passes Away." Editorial. *Toronto Telegram* 10 October 1953: A6.
"Arrival of Idiots." *Orillia Expositor* September 28, 1876: 3.
Berton, Pierre. "What's Wrong at Orillia: Out of Sight, Out of Mind." *Toronto Daily Star* January 6, 1960: 31.
"Dr. Helen MacMurchy Assumes High Office. Distinguished Career. Double Inspectorate." *The Star* June 19, 1913.
"Dr. Helen MacMurchy." Editorial. *Toronto Daily Star* 13 October 1953: 6.
"Dr. MacMurchy Would Halt 'Propagation of the Unfit'." *The Star* June 27, 1934.
Fenton, Faith. "A Day In The Idiot Asylum." Part 1. *Empire* (Toronto) January 3, 1891: 5.
Fenton, Faith. "A Day In The Idiot Asylum." Part II. *Empire* (Toronto) January 10, 1891: 5.
Frank, David. "Sex and Violence in Toronto."*Evening Telegram*, February 9-27, 1915.
"The Idiot Asylum," *Orillia Expositor* October 12, 1876: 3.
"Leading Woman Physician Dr. H. MacMurchy, 91, Dies." *Toronto Daily Star* 9 October 1953: 2.
"Metro Objects to Tax for Retarded Schools." *Toronto Daily Star* May 6, 1964: 22.
Newman, Jean. "Our Retarded Children are Lost in Ontario's Big Institutions." *Toronto Daily Star* May 24, 1963: 7.
"No More Isolated Retarded Hospitals – Dymond." *Toronto Daily Star* February 26, 1964: 67.
"Orillia Charges 'True'." *Toronto Daily Star* January 7, 1961: 1-2.
"Probe May Bring End to Shackling." *The Globe* 6 March 1912.
"The Housing Report." Helen MacMurchy's Letter to the Editor. *The Star* November 29, 1934.
"University Women Honour Dr. MacMurchy." *Mail* December 5, 1922.

SECONDARY SOURCES

Adolphus Bator, Paul. "'Saving Lives on the Wholesale Plan': Public Health Reform in the City of Toronto, 1900-1930." Abstract for Ph.D., May 24, 1979.
Anglin, Betty, and June Braaten. *Twenty-Five Years of Growing Together: A History of the Ontario Association for the Mentally Retarded.* Toronto: Canadian Association for the Mentally Retarded, 1978.
Barber, Marilyn. "Sunny Ontario for British Girls, 1900-30." *Looking Into My Sister's Eyes: an Exploration in Women's History.* Ed. Jean Burnet. Toronto: The Multicultural History Society of Ontario, 1986. 55-69.
Barber, Marilyn. "The Women Ontario Welcomed: Immigrant Domestics for Ontario Homes, 1870-1930." *Ontario History* 72. 3 (September 1980): 148-72.
Bator, Paul Adolphus. "'Saving Lives on the Wholesale Plan': Public Health Reform in the City of Toronto, 1900-1930." Abstract for Ph.D., May 24, 1979.

Beck, Marie, Ruth Parmlee Rawlings and Sophronia Williams. *Mental Health Psychiatric Nursing*. Toronto/St. Louis: The C.V. Mosby Company, 1984.

Black, Edwin. *War Against The Weak*. New York: Thunder's Mouth Press, New York, 2003.

Braithwaite, Max. *The Hungry Thirties, 1930-1940*. Toronto : Natural Science of Canada, 1977.

Brown, John. "Warrendale to Browndale." *Experience and Experiment: A Collection of Essays*. Ed. Jalal Shamsie. Toronto: Leonard Crainford 1977: 97-115.

Cassel, Jay. *The Secret Plague: Venereal Disease in Canada, 1838-1939*. Toronto: University of Toronto Press, 1987.

Court, John. " Historical Synopsis – Establishing the Department of Psychiatry at the University of Toronto." Online publication, Department of Psychiatry, University of Toronto, Dec. 2004, rev. and updated, April 2011.Web. Accessed March 2012.

Cotter, Charis. *Toronto Between The Wars: Life in the City 1919-1939*. Richmond Hill, ON: Firefly Books Ltd., 2004.

D'Antonio, Michael. *The State Boys Rebellion: The Inspiring True Story of American Eugenics and the Men Who Overcame It*. Riverside, NJ: Simon & Schuster Paperbacks, 2004.

Digby, Anne. "Contexts and Perspectives." *From Idiocy to Mental Deficiency: Historical Perspectives of People With Learning Disabilities*. Eds. David Wright and Anne Digby. London: Routledge, 1996. 1-21.

Dodd, Dianne. "Helen MacMurchy: Popular Midwifery and Maternity Services for Canadian Pioneer Women." *Caring and Curing: Historical Perspectives on Women and Healing in Canada*. Eds. Dianne Dodd and Deborah Gorham. Ottawa: University of Ottawa Press, 1994. 135-161.

Dowbiggin, Ian. *The Quest for Mental Health. A Tale of Science, Medicine, Scandal, Sorrow, and Mass Society.* New York: Cambridge University Press, 2011.

Dowbiggin, Ian. *Keeping America Sane: Psychiatry and Eugenics in the United States and Canada 1880-1940*. Ithaca: Cornell University Press, 1997.

Dowbiggin, Ian. "Keeping This Young Country Sane: C.K. Clarke, Immigration Restriction, and Canadian Psychiatry, 1890-1925." *The Canadian Historical Review* 76.4 (December 1995): 589-627.

Dugdale, R. L. *The Jukes: A Study in Crime, Pauperism, Disease and Heredity*. 4th ed. New York: Putnam, 1888.

Fabrega, H. and K. K. Haka. "Parents of Mentally Handicapped Children."*Archives of General Psychiatry* 16 (1967): 202-209.

Frazee, Catherine, Kathryn Church and Melanie Panitch, Curatorial Tteam: *Out from Under: Disability, History, and Things to Remember.* School of Disability Studies, Faculty of Community Services, Ryerson University, and Royal Museum of Ontario, 2008.

Hobson, J. A. *Canada To-day.* London: Unwin, 1906.

Jones, Andres and Leonard Rutman. *In the Children's Aid: J.J. Kelso and Child Welfare in Ontario*. Toronto: University of Toronto Press, 1980.

Garner, Hugh. *Cabbagetown*. Toronto: McGraw-Hill Ryerson, 1968.

Glazebrook, G. P. de T. *The Story of Toronto*. Toronto: University of Toronto Press, 1971.

Gould, Stephen Jay. *The Mismeasure of Man*. New York: W. W. Norton & Co., 1981.

Greenland, Cyril. *Charles Kirk Clarke: A Pioneer of Canadian Psychiatry*. Toronto: The Clarke Institute of Psychiatry, 1966.

Greenland, Cyril. "The Origins of the Toronto Psychiatric Clinic." *TPH: History and Memories of the Toronto Psychiatric Hospital, 1925-1966*. Ed. Edward Shorter. Dayton, OH: Wall & Emerson, Inc., 1996. 19-59.

Hall, Ruth. *Passionate Crusader: The Life of Marie Stopes*. New York: Harcourt Brace Jovanovich, 1977.

Hall, Ruth, ed. *Dear Dr. Stopes: Sex in the 1920s*. Harmondsworth: Penguin, 1981).

Harris-Zsovan, Jane. *Eugenics and the Firewall: Canada's Nasty Little Secret*. Winnipeg: J. Gordon Shillingford Publishing Inc., 2010.

Jones, Kathleen. *A History of the Mental Health Services*. London: Routledge and Kegan Paul, 1972.

Kanner, Leo. *History of the Care and Study of the Mentally Retarded*. Springfield, IL: Charles C. Thomas Publisher, 1964.

Kelly, Colleen. *Cabbagetown in Pictures*. Toronto: Toronto Public Library Board, 1984.

Klein, Alice and Wayne Roberts. "Beseiged Innocence: The 'Problem' and the Problems of Working Women – Toronto, 1896-1914." *Women At Work: Ontario, 1850-1930*. Eds. Janice Acton, Penny Goldsmith and Bonnie Shephard. Toronto: Canadian Women's Educational Press, 1974. 211-259

Kuhn, Philip. "Romancing with a Wealth of Detail: Narratives of Ernest Jones's 1906 Trial for Indecent Assault." *Studies in Gender and Sexuality* 3.4 (2002): 344-378.

Lemon, James. *Toronto Since 1918: An Illustrated History*. Toronto: James Lorimer & Company, 1985.

Leslie, Genevieve. "Domestic Service in Canada, 1880-1920." *Women At Work: Ontario, 1850-1930*. Eds. Janice Acton, Penny Goldsmith and Bonnie Shephard. Toronto: Canadian Women's Educational Press, 1974. 71-127.

Mazumdar, Pauline. "Changes in Policy in the Treatment of the Mentally Retarded in Ontario." Presentation at the Psychiatric Historical Group, Clarke Institute of Psychiatry, Toronto, February 10, 1978. CAMH Archives.

McCullagh, John. *A Legacy of Caring: A History of the Children's Aid Society of Toronto*. Toronto: The Dundurn Group, 2002.

McLaren, Angus. *Our Own Master Race: Eugenics in Canada, 1885-1945*. Toronto: Oxford University Press, 1990.

McLaren, Angus and Arlene Tigar McLaren. *The Bedroom and the State: The Changing Practices and Politics of Contraception and Abortion in Canada, 1880-1980*. Toronto: McClelland & Stewart, 1986.

McNaught, Kenneth A. *Prophet in Politics, A Biography of J. S. Woodsworth*. Toronto: University of Toronto Press, 1959.

Panitch, Melanie. *Disability, Mothers and Organization: Accidental Activists*. New York: Routledge, 2008.

Piva, Michael. *The Condition of the Working Class in Toronto, 1900-1921*. Ottawa: University of Ottawa Press, 1979.

Pos, Robert. "History of Psychiatry at Toronto General Hospital 'til 1975." For discussion at The History of Canadian Psychiatry Research in Progress Seminar, The Archives, Queen Street Mental Health Centre, Toronto, Ontario, May 1, 1992.

Reaume, Geoffrey. *Remembrance of Patients Past: Patient Life at the Toronto*

Hospital for the Insane, 1870-1940. Don Mills, ON: Oxford University Press, 2000.

Richardson, Ken. *The Making of Intelligence.* New York: Columbia University Press, 2000.

Roland, Charles G. *Clarence Meredith Hincks, M.D. 1885-1964: A Biography* Toronto: Hannah Institute & Dundurn Press, 1990.

Rotenberg, Lori. "The Wayward Worker: Toronto's Prostitute at the Turn of the Century." *Women At Work: Ontario, 1850-1930.* Eds. Janice Acton, Penny Goldsmith and Bonnie Shephard. Toronto: Canadian Women's Educational Press, 1974. 33-69.

Scheinberg, Ellen. "Bringing 'Domestics' to Canada: A Study of Immigration Propaganda." *Framing Our Past: Canadian Women's History in the Twentieth Century.* Ed. Sharon Anne Cook, Lorna R. McLean and Kate O'Rourke. Montréal: McGill-Queen's University Press, 2001: 336-342).

Simmons, Harvey G. *From Asylum To Welfare.* Downsview, ON: National Institute on Mental Retardation, 1982.

Skelton, Mora. Personal communication with John Fotheringham, summer 1992, "The Mental Retardation Clinic." *TPH: History and Memories of the Toronto Psychiatric Hospital, 1925-1966.* Ed. Edward Shorter. Dayton, OH: Wall & Emerson, Inc., 1996. 296-303.

Edward Shorter, ed. *TPH: History and Memories of the Toronto Psychiatric Hospital, 1925-1966.* Dayton, OH: Wall & Emerson, Inc., 1996.

Shea, Janet. *A Short History of the Ontario Hospital School, Orillia, 1875-1970.* Toronto: Monograph typescript, n.d., ca.1980. CAMH Archives.

Starr, J. Edward, "Charities and Corrections." *The Public Health Journal* 4.10 (October 1913): 567-70.

Stephen, Jennifer. "The 'Incorrigible', the 'Bad,' and the 'Immoral': Toronto's 'Factory Girls' and the Work of the Toronto Psychiatric Clinic." *Law, Society and the State: Essays In Modern Legal History.* Eds. Louis A. Knafla and Susan W. S. Binnie. Toronto: University of Toronto Press, 1995.

Strange, Carolyn. *Toronto's Girl Problem: The Perils and Pleasures of the City, 1880-1930.* Toronto: University of Toronto Press, 1995

Strong-Boag, Veronica Jane. *The Parliament of Women: The Nations Council of Women of Canada, 1893-1929.* Ottawa: National Musuems of Canada, 1976.

Thomson, David. *England in the Nineteenth Century: 1815-1914.* Harmondsworth, UK: Penguin Books, 1978 [1960].

Thomson, Matthew. *The Problem of Mental Deficiency, Eugenics, Democracy and Social Policy in Britain, 1870-1959.* Oxford: Clarendon Press, 1998.

Valverde, Mariana. *The Age of Light, Soap, and Water: Moral Reform in English Canada, 1885-1925.* Toronto: McClelland & Stewart Inc., 1991.

Wagner, G. *Children of the Empire.* London: Weidenfeld and Nicolson, 1982.

Wheatley, Thelma. "'He'll Never Amount To Anything': A Visit to Huronia Regional Centre, August 1995." *The Beacon* 9.1 (October 1995): 6.

Willard, Joseph W. "Inquiry into the Management and Operation of the Huronia Regional Centre, Orillia: A Report to the Honourable James Taylor, Minister of Community and Social Services." Toronto, Ontario, November 1976.

Williston, Walter. *Present Arrangements for the Care and Supervision of Mentally Retarded Persons in Ontario.* Toronto: Ontario Department of Health, 1971.

Wolfensberger, Wolf. *The Principle of Normalization in Human Services.* Toronto:

National Institute on Mental Retardation, 1972.
Wright, David, *DOWNS: The History of a Disability.* New York: Oxford University Press, 2011.

DOCUMENTARIES: VIDEOS, DVD, RADIO BROADCASTS

Danny and Nicky. Prod. Douglas Jackson. National Film Board of Canada, 1969. (The lives of two boys with Down's syndrome are compared: one growing up in the institution in Orillia and the other at home.)
"Keeping This Young Country Sane." *Ideas.* Canadian Broadcasting Corporation, 1999.
One On Every Street. Video and DVD. Fletcher's Film Productions, narrator Allan McPhee, 1960. RG 29-24-2-4, AO. (Government-sponsored documentary of life inside Ontario Hospital School, Orillia.)
"The Gristle in the Stew: David Gutnick Looks at the Institutionalization of Mentally Disabled Children in the 1960s." *Sunday Edition.* Canadian Broadcasting Corporation, November 24, 2011.

THESES

Park, Deborah. "Changing Shadows: The Huronia Regional Centre 1876-1934." M.A. Thesis, York University, 1990.
Brown, William. *Making Representation: Dr. Helen MacMurchy and the "Feeble-Minded" in Ontario, 1906-1919.* Ph.D. dissertation, University of Toronto, 2005.
Dodd, Dianne. "The Canadian Birth Control Movement 1929-1939." M.A. Thesis, Department of Education, University of Toronto, 1982.
Hackett, Gerald. *The History of Public Education for Mentally Retarded Children in the Province of Ontario 1867-1964.* Ph.D. dissertation, University of Toronto, 1969.
McConnachie, Kathleen. *Science and Ideology: The Mental Hygiene & Eugenics Movements in the Inter-War Years, 1919-1939.* Ph.D. dissertation, University of Toronto, 1987.

INSTITUTIONS VISITED

Huronia Regional Centre, Orillia (aka The Asylum for Idiots and Feeble-Minded, and Ontario Hospital School, Orillia): August, 1995; July, 1999; July 2005; 2009; 2010; 2012.
Huronia Regional Centre Cemetary/Graveyard: July, 1999; 2009;2010.
Rideau Regional Centre, Smith's Falls: July, 2010.
Children's Psychiatric Research Institute (CPRI), London, Ontario, 1995.
Cobourg Institution, Cobourg, Ontario: August 2010.
Local Jail, Cobourg: August 2010.
Thistletown Regional Centre, Etobicoke, Ontario, Summer, 1981.

Other:
Parkholme School for Mentally Retarded, Brampton, Ontario (Peel Board of Education): 1998.

Applewood Acres School for Senior Mentally Retarded Students, Mississauga, Ontario, 1990s-2009.
Mental Retardation Centre, Surrey Place, aka Toronto Psychiatric Hospital (currently Surrey Place Centre), Toronto: 1968.
William Burgess Public School, Toronto: June 28, 2009.
Beverley Street School, Toronto: April 1996.
Lucy McCormick School for Senior Mentally Retarded Students, Toronto: April 1996.

INTERVIEWS

Berton, Pierre, phone interview summer 2002, regarding his recollections of his visit to Orillia December, 1959, and his column "What's Wrong At Orillia," exposing abuses and conditions at Ontario Hospital School Orillia, in the *Toronto Daily Star,* January 6, 1960.
Burns, Jim, Principal of William Burgess P.S., East York, Toronto, in the 1950s. Memories recalled of the "Opportunity Class."Phone interview, July 2005.
Former patients of Ontario Hospital School, Orillia, who offered their recollections and experiences: Michael Callahan, Mike D., Julia Hadley, the late Brian Gibbard, Desi Harnum, Gail Lynam, Marie Slark, Barry Thachuk, and others who wish to remain anonymous. Also Joe Clayton, former resident of Rideau Regional Centre, Smith's Falls, Ontario.
Gibbard, Adele, parent of child placed in Ontario Hospital School in the 1960s and organizer of mother volunteers group at the Orillia institution, Mississauga 1995.
Greenland, Cyril, reminiscences as visiting social work inspector of Ontario Hospital School, Orillia, in the 1960s, summer 2004, 2006.
Hew, Maralyn, former pupil at William Burgess Public School in the 1950s, for her recollections of the "Occupational Class" in the school and The Nest run by the Salvation Army on Broadview Ave., Toronto, June 28, 2005
Jacobson, Werner, former attendant at Ontario Hospital School, and archivist Huronia Regional Centre, Orillia. August, 1995. Lepper, Arthur and Bernice, long-time residents of old Cabbagetown, Toronto. Phone interview, January 21, 2007.
McCaig, Jane, Resident of Cobourg. Reminiscences of her grandmother who hired domestic servants from Cobourg Asylum. Dec. 29. 2006.
Melville, Philip, reminiscences as psychiatrist in charge of the Women's Ward, Toronto Psychiatric Hospital in the 1960s, summer 2009.
O'Donnell, Jim, former resident of Cabbagetown, recollections of his childhood in Catholic Cabbagetown in the 1930s, Wasaga Beach, September, 2012.
Person "X." Phone interview, 2005, former counsellor at Huronia Regional Centre in 1980s. Anonymous.
Swinton, Ed, brother Frank Swinton was an attendant working on the wards in the Cottages in 1950s. Born and raised in Orillia with personal recollections of Dr. S. Horne, Superintendent of Ontario Hospital School in the 1930s. Phone interview, July 16. 2007.

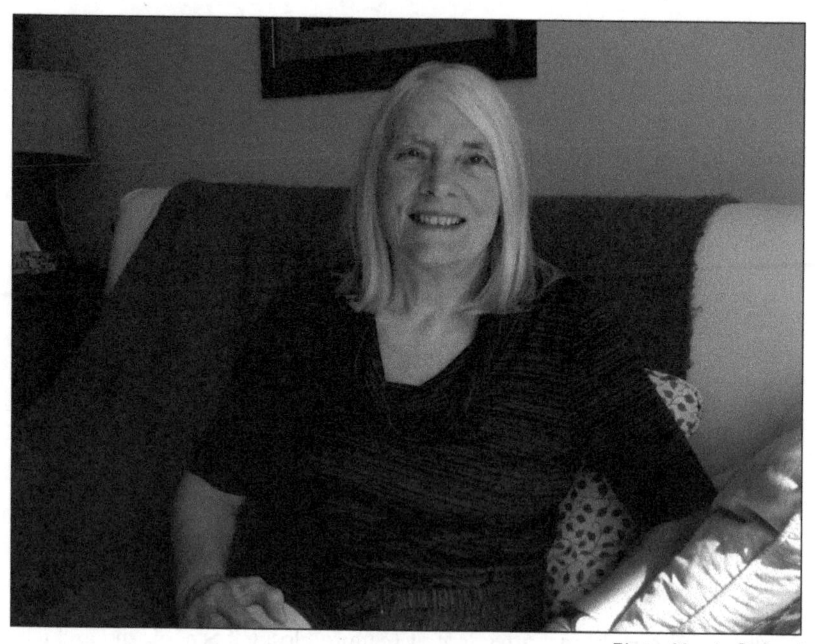

Photo: Mandy Orchard

Thelma Wheatley, grand-daughter of a Welsh coal-miner, is the author of *My Sad Is All Gone: A Family's Triumph Over Violent Autism* (2004), a book about raising her autistic child. Her award-winning short fiction and poetry has been published in a number of literary journals across Canada. She is a committed advocate for develpmentally challenged individuals and is in demand as a speaker on violence, autism and institutionalization. She is on the Board of the Friends of the Archives, CAMH, and is currently co-editor of the *Friends of the Archives Newsletter.* She lives in the greater Toronto area.